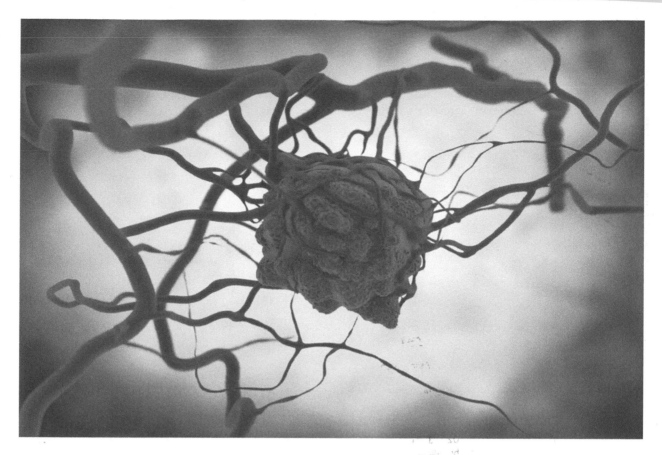

BMJ Clinical Review:

Clinical Oncology

Edited by
Babita Jyoti & Eleftheria Kleidi

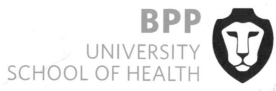

BPP
UNIVERSITY
SCHOOL OF HEALTH

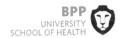

First edition August 2015

ISBN 9781 4727 3932 2
eISBN 9781 4727 4405 0
eISBN 9781 4727 4413 5

British Library Cataloguing-in-Publication Data
A catalogue record for this book is available
from the British Library

Published by
BPP Learning Media Ltd
BPP House, Aldine Place
London W12 8AA

www.bpp.com/health

Printed in the United Kingdom by
Ashford Colour Press Ltd

Unit 600, Fareham Reach,
Fareham Road,
Gosport, Hampshire,
PO13 0FW

Your learning materials, published by BPP Learning
Media Ltd, are printed on paper sourced from
sustainable, managed forests.

The content of this publication contains articles from The
BMJ which have been selected, collated and published
by BPP Learning Media under a licence.

The contents of this book are intended as a guide
and not professional advice. Although every effort
has been made to ensure that the contents of this
book are correct at the time of going to press, BPP
Learning Media, the Editor and the Author make no
warranty that the information in this book is accurate
or complete and accept no liability for any loss or
damage suffered by any person acting or refraining
from acting as a result of the material in this book.

Every effort has been made to contact the copyright
holders of any material reproduced within this
publication. If any have been inadvertently overlooked,
BPP Learning Media will be pleased to make the
appropriate credits in any subsequent reprints or
editions.

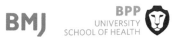

About the publisher

BPP Learning Media is dedicated to supporting aspiring professionals with top quality learning material. BPP Learning Media's commitment to success is shown by our record of quality, innovation and market leadership in paper-based and e-learning materials. BPP Learning Media's study materials are written by professionally-qualified specialists who know from personal experience the importance of top quality materials for success.

About The BMJ

The BMJ (formerly the British Medical Journal) in print has a long history and has been published without interruption since 1840. The BMJ's vision is to be the world's most influential and widely read medical journal. Our mission is to lead the debate on health and to engage, inform, and stimulate doctors, researchers, and other health professionals in ways that will improve outcomes for patients. We aim to help doctors to make better decisions. BMJ, the company, advances healthcare worldwide by sharing knowledge and expertise to improve experiences, outcomes and value.

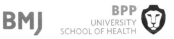

Contents

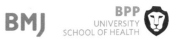

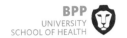

About the editors

Dr Babita Jyoti is a Radiation Oncologist with a special interest in Paediatric Proton Therapy. She graduated in Medicine in India followed by training in UK and obtained MRCP (UK) & FRCR (UK). She trained as a Clinical Oncologist at Clatterbridge Cancer Centre. She is currently working at the University of Florida Health Proton Therapy Institute in Paediatric Proton Therapy. She has been a PBL tutor and an OSCE examiner at Manchester Medical School.

Mrs Eleftheria Kleidi is a Specialty Registrar in Upper Gastrointestinal Surgery at Leighton Hospital, Crewe. She qualified from the Medical School of the University of Crete in 2004. After her foundation years, she started her training in general surgery in Athens and obtained her CCT in 2013. Since then, she has been specialising in UGI surgery and Bariatrics and was awarded the scholarship of the College of Surgeons of Greece for training in the UK. She completed her PhD in Bariatrics at the University of Athens in 2015.

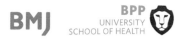

Introduction to Clinical Oncology

The field of clinical oncology is one of the most rapidly developing with new trials resulting in new diagnostic and therapeutic modalities. The BMJ clinical reviews provide a clear, up to date account of the topics. This review includes a broad update of recent developments and their likely clinical applications.

Our attempt was to select and include the clinical reviews that provide a thorough, useful, and clear knowledge on Clinical Oncology. Advances and updated principles are hereby presented including screening, diagnostic and treatment. It should rather be used as an adjunct to the expansion of knowledge on the fields of oncology.

Clinical oncology is a major participant in any multi-disciplinary team deciding on cancer patient management. As such, its updates influence all members of the team. This book is intended as a comprehensive resource for all oncology practitioners in order to assist the management through the illness trajectory. In addition, this book serves as a guide to oncology for primary care practitioners and other health care workers seeking practical information on the diagnosis and management of patients with cancer.

Oncology remains the science in which the continuous advancement of knowledge is the cornerstone for the welfare of cancer patients. We do hope that you will find this book useful towards this direction. Its aim is also to stimulate readers to read further with additional sources of information. Many articles include a part entitled "How patients were involved in the creation of this article" in an attempt to advance patient partnership and contribution to the clinical reviews."

In this book, every effort has been made to contribute to the advancement of knowledge in oncology by carefully selecting clinical reviews from the recent publications in The BMJ. These books are an outcome of international cooperation and we are very grateful to authors for their substantial contribution to this book.

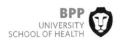

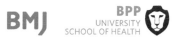

Investigation and management of unintentional weight loss in older adults

Jenna McMinn foundation year 2, medicine[1], Claire Steel specialist trainee year 6 in medicine for the elderly[2], Adam Bowman consultant physician[3]

[1]Queen Elizabeth National Spinal Injuries Unit, Southern General Hospital, Glasgow G51 4TF, UK

[2]Department of Medicine for the Elderly, Monklands Hospital, Airdrie, UK

[3]Department of Medicine for the Elderly, Glasgow Royal Infirmary, Glasgow, UK

Correspondence to: J McMinn, Department of Medicine, Southern General Hospital jennamcminn@gmail.com

Cite this as: BMJ 2011;342: d1732

<DOI> 10.1136/bmj.d1732
http://www.bmj.com/content/342/bmj.d1732

Unintentional weight loss occurs in 15-20% of older adults (those over 65) and is associated with increased morbidity and mortality.[1] Clinical and epidemiological studies have reported even higher prevalence in certain populations, with as many as 27% of community dwelling elderly people and 50-60% of nursing home residents being affected.[1] [2w1]

Weight loss may be the presenting problem or an incidental finding during a consultation for other reasons. There are no published guidelines on how to investigate and manage patients with unintentional weight loss, and responses range from doing nothing (if it is viewed as a normal part of the ageing process) to extensive blind investigation because of the fear that it represents underlying cancer. Observational studies have shown that in as many as 25% of cases no identifiable cause is found, despite extensive investigation.[3] [4] It is not clear how far clinicians should go to investigate older patients with unintentional weight loss in the absence of an obvious medical cause.

We review the available evidence (mainly epidemiological and observational studies) and outline a structured approach to investigation and management of the older patient with unintentional weight loss.

When is unintentional weight loss clinically important?

Age related physiological changes occur in elderly people and contribute to the so called "anorexia of ageing." These include a reduction in lean body mass, bone mass, and basal metabolic rate; reduced sense of taste and smell; and altered gastric signals leading to early satiation.[5] However, observational studies of healthy older adults report this normal age related weight loss to be only 0.1-0.2 kg a year,[6] and most elderly patients maintain weight over a reasonably long period of 5-10 years.[7] Substantial weight loss should not be dismissed as natural age related change and should be investigated.

Although no universally accepted definition of clinically important weight loss exists, most observational studies define it as a 5% or more reduction in body weight over 6-12 months.[3] [4] [8] To take into account the variability of baseline weight, weight loss is best expressed as a percentage rather than an absolute value; a loss of 2-3 kg is less important in a 90 kg patient than in a frail elderly patient who is underweight already.

Reported mortality within 1-2.5 years of clinically important weight loss ranges from 9% to 38%,[1w2] and those particularly at risk include frail elderly people,[w1] those with low baseline body weight,[w3] and elderly patients recently admitted to hospital.[1] [7]

Substantial weight loss has been shown to be associated with an increased risk of in-hospital and disease related complications,[9] increased disability and dependency,[7] higher rates of admission to residential home or nursing home,[w1] and poorer quality of life.[w4] At the extreme, cachexia (the disproportional loss of skeletal muscle rather than body fat, which leads to skeletal and cardiac muscle wasting, loss of visceral protein, and alterations in physiological functions including impaired immunity and a systemic inflammatory response) contributes to adverse outcomes through increased rates of infection, poor wound healing, pressure sores, reduced response to medical treatment, and increased risk of mortality.[10w5]

Weight loss in elderly people significantly increases the rate of hip bone loss and the risk of hip fracture. In a prospective cohort study of 6785 elderly women, weight loss—both intentional and unintentional—of 5% or more from baseline weight (regardless of whether baseline weight was low or normal) almost doubled the risk of subsequent hip fracture (odds ratio 1.8, 95% confidence interval 1.43 to 2.24) compared with those with stable or increasing weight.[11]

What can cause unintentional weight loss in older adults?

Although involuntary weight loss in younger adults often has a medical cause, in older patients causes are more diverse, with psychiatric and socioeconomic factors playing an important part.

Prospective and retrospective studies from Germany, Belgium, Israel, the United States, and Spain have looked at patients who were investigated for involuntary weight loss to determine the common causes and their relative frequency (table 1).[3] [4] [8] [12] [13w6] The studies varied considerably in terms of country, age of patients (most were not confined to the elderly), length of follow-up, and the type of patients recruited. However, cancer, non-malignant gastrointestinal disease, and psychiatric problems (particularly dementia

SUMMARY POINTS

- Unintentional weight loss is common in elderly people and is associated with considerable morbidity and mortality
- Weight loss is clinically relevant if more than 5% of body weight is lost over 6-12 months, although smaller losses may be important in frail elderly people
- Causes can be classified as organic (malignant and non-malignant), psychological, social, or unknown
- Drugs should be reviewed because side effects often contribute to weight loss
- All patients should be assessed by a dietitian and screened for depression and cognitive impairment
- If initial history, examination, and investigations are normal, three months of "watchful waiting" is preferable to further blind investigations

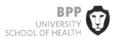

Table 1 Observational studies of causes of unintentional weight loss

Study	Follow-up (months)	Mean age of patients (years)	Most common cause of weight loss	Unknown cause of weight loss
Prospective German study of 158 men and women in secondary care[3]	25-36	68 (SD 14)	Cancer (24%) especially gastrointestinal (53% of cancers)	16%
			Non-malignant gastrointestinal disorders (19%)	
			Endocrine disease (11.4%)	
			Psychological (10.8%)	
			Cardiopulmonary disease (10.1%)	
Prospective Belgian study of 101 men and women in secondary care[4]	≥6	64 (SD 13)	Malignancy (22%) especially gastrointestinal (45% of cancers)	28%
			Psychological (16%)	
			Non-malignant GI disorders (15%)	
			Infectious diseases (8%)	
			Systemic inflammatory disorders (4%)	
Prospective study from the US of 91 men, mostly inpatients[8]	12	58 (SD 18)	Malignancy (19%)	26%
			Non-malignant gastrointestinal disorders (14%)	
			Psychiatric disorders (9%)	
			Cardiovascular disease (9%)	
			Alcohol related disease (8%)	
Retrospective Israeli study of 154 male and female inpatients[12]	30	64 (range 27-88)	Malignancy (36%)	23%
			Non-malignant gastrointestinal disorders (17%)	
			Psychiatric disorders (10%)	
			Endocrine disease, infectious disease, renal disease (4% each)	
Retrospective study of 50 male and female outpatients in the US[w6]	24	>63	Psychiatric (20%)	24%
			Malignancy (16%)	
			Non-malignant gastrointestinal disorders (11%)	
			Endocrine disease (9%)	
			Neurological disease (7%)	
Retrospective study of 236 inpatients and 92 outpatients in the US[13]	>12	65 (SD 17)	Malignancy (35%)	6% (although 30 patients were lost to follow-up)
			Psychiatric (24%)	
			Non-malignant gastrointestinal disorders (8.8%)	
			Endocrine disease (7%)	
			Rheumatic disease (7%)	

SD=standard deviation.

and depression) were consistently among the most common causes of unintentional weight loss).

Several aids have been devised to enable doctors to consider the many possible causes of unintentional weight loss in older patients. These include the "9 Ds of weight loss in the elderly"[14] and "meals on wheels"[15] mnemonics (box 1). Our approach is to group the possible causes of weight loss into organic (malignant and non-malignant), psychosocial, and unknown causes.

Organic causes
Organic causes of weight loss include cancer, non-malignant medical disorders, and side effects of drugs (table 2).

Psychosocial
Published observational studies (summarised in table 1) report that psychiatric problems, particularly dementia and depression, are the main cause of unexplained weight loss in 10-20% of elderly patients. This figure rises to 58% in nursing home residents.[17]

Cognitive impairment
Patients with cognitive impairment who are agitated or have a tendency to "wander" can expend substantial energy. Others may forget that they have to eat or become suspicious and paranoid about food.[1] Self feeding skills are lost with the progression of Alzheimer's disease and dysphagia may develop.[w9]

BOX 1 MNEMONICS FOR CAUSES OF UNINTENTIONAL WEIGHT LOSS IN ELDERLY PEOPLE

9 Ds of weight loss in elderly[14]
- Dementia
- Depression
- Disease (acute and chronic)
- Dysphagia
- Dysgeusia
- Diarrhoea
- Drugs
- Dentition
- Dysfunction (functional disability)
- (Don't know was later added as a 10th "D")[w7]

Meals on wheels[15]
- M: Medication effects
- E: Emotional problems (especially depression)
- A: Anorexia nervosa, alcoholism
- L: Late life paranoia
- S: Swallowing disorders
- O: Oral factors (such as poorly fitting dentures, caries)
- N: No money
- W: Wandering and other dementia related behaviours
- H: Hyperthyroidism, hypothyroidism, hyperparathyroidism, hypoadrenalism
- E: Enteric problems
- E: Eating problems (such as inability to feed self)
- L: Low salt, low cholesterol diet
- S: Stones, social problems (such as isolation, inability to obtain preferred foods)

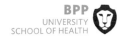

Table 2 Organic causes of unintentional weight loss in elderly people[1 3 4 8 12 13 w6]*

Causes	Comments
Cancer (16-36%)*	
Gastrointestinal malignancy	About 50% of cancers that present with weight loss are gastrointestinal in origin[3 4]
Other cancers (most often lung, lymphoma, prostate, ovarian, or bladder)	Non-gastrointestinal cancers present less commonly with involuntary weight loss, which tends to be a later feature
Non-malignant organic disorders	
Gastrointestinal disorders (11-19%):	
These include motility or swallowing disorders, peptic ulcers, gallstones, mesenteric ischaemia, and malabsorption disorders such as coeliac disease	Mechanisms contributing to weight loss include dysphagia, chronic nausea, pain related to eating (leading to food avoidance), and malabsorption
Other chronic diseases:	
These include congestive cardiac failure and other cardiac diseases (2-9%), chronic obstructive pulmonary disease and other respiratory diseases (6%), endocrine disease (4-11%), neurological disorders (2-7%), end stage renal failure (4%), connective tissue diseases (2-4%), and chronic or /recurrent infection (2-5%)	Any disease that increases metabolic demand or leads to a catabolic state can lead to weight loss despite a normal food intake; weight loss is often an indicator of disease severity in chronic disease[1]; elderly patients often do not fully regain weight lost because of acute stressful events, so a history of recurrent infections may lead to serious weight loss
Oral and dental problems:	
Poor dentition, ill fitting dentures, xerostomia (dry mouth)—often as a result of drugs	Often overlooked by the medical profession, but can lead to serious weight loss as a result of inadequate energy intake; the number of oral and dental problems has been shown to be an important predictor of weight loss at one year[w8]
Side effects of drugs†	
Anorexia (antibiotics, digoxin, opiates, selective serotonin reuptake inhibitors, anticonvulsants, antipsychotics, amantadine, metformin, benzodiazepines), nausea and vomiting (antibiotics, bisphosphonates, digoxin, dopamine agonists, levodopa, opiates, selective serotonin reuptake inhibitors, tricyclics), dry mouth (anticholinergics, loop diuretics, antihistamines), altered taste or smell (angiotensin converting enzyme inhibitors, calcium channel blockers, propranol, spironolactone, iron, anti-parkinsonian drugs (levodopa, pergolide, selegiline), opiates, gold, allopurinol), dysphagia (bisphosphonates, antibiotics, levodopa, gold, iron, non-steroidal anti-inflammatory drugs, potassium)	This is a particular problem in elderly patients because of the prevalence of polypharmacy, which in itself is known to interfere with taste and cause anorexia[16]; drugs such as sedatives and opiate analgesics may interfere with cognition and affect the patient's ability to eat

Percentages are based on the published studies referenced above.
†Drugs listed are only a few examples of commonly used drugs that cause these side effects and this is not intended to be a comprehensive list.

Depression
Depression can lead to weight loss because of loss of appetite or reduced motivation to buy and prepare food. Depression is more commonly associated with weight loss in elderly people than in younger adults,[w10] and it was associated with increased mortality in a systematic review of elderly patients (>65 years) living in the community (estimated odds ratio for mortality with depression of 1.73, 1.53 to 1.95).[18]

Reported rates of depression in the community vary dramatically according to a systematic review of 34 community based studies of the prevalence of depression in later life (>55 years), but they can be as high as 35%, depending on the criteria used to define depression.[19] Even higher prevalences have been reported in institutionalised elderly patients[w7 w10]

Socioeconomic factors
Poverty or social isolation may contribute to weight loss in elderly people through inadequate food intake and malnutrition.[20] Physical or cognitive impairment may prevent elderly people from shopping for themselves and may reduce the availability of preferred foods. Inability to cook or feed themselves may further contribute to insufficient food intake because they may rely on family members or carers, who may visit at erratic times.

Unknown
The cause of weight loss remained unknown in 16-28% of patients in published prospective and retrospective observational studies, despite extensive investigation over periods ranging from six months to three years.[3 4 8 12 13] This may be because elderly patients often have multiple comorbidities rather than one serious illness, are on multiple drugs, and may have psychological or social problems. Each individual factor might not be sufficient to cause substantial weight loss, but the cumulative effect of all the factors might result in clinically important weight loss.

All studies that have assessed prognosis in elderly patients with unintentional weight loss have found that patients who fall into this category of "unknown cause" have a much better prognosis than those diagnosed with cancer,[3 12] and no worse than that of patients diagnosed with non-malignant causes.[3] Cancers diagnosed in the setting of involuntary weight loss usually have a poor prognosis because they are often advanced by the time weight loss becomes apparent.[4]

How is unintentional weight loss in older adults investigated?
We present our approach to investigation, which is based on an extensive literature review (fig 1. We know of no clinical guidelines or standardised system for investigating this common and complex problem.

Initial evaluation of the patient involves a detailed history, clinical examination, and baseline investigations. The findings should be used to guide further investigation.

History
Try to establish the exact amount of weight loss over a specified time. Questions about appetite may help elucidate whether the weight loss is caused by inadequate energy intake or has occurred despite an adequate intake. A corroborative history from relatives or carers may help in patients with cognitive impairment.

Previous and current medical history may identify conditions that could have led to weight loss (see table 2) and drugs that may contribute via their side effects.

Social history may elicit information on alcohol intake (which might contribute to malnutrition or vitamin deficiency) and smoking (a risk factor for cancer and other organic diseases). It is important to elucidate the patient's social circumstances. Who does he or she live with? Who

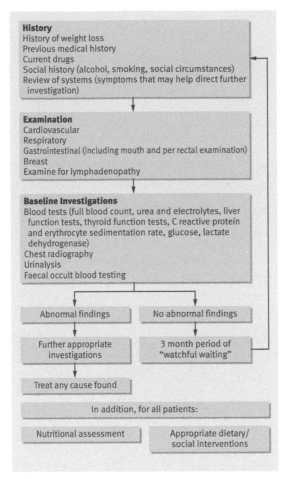

History
History of weight loss
Previous medical history
Current drugs
Social history (alcohol, smoking, social circumstances)
Review of systems (symptoms that may help direct further investigation)

Examination
Cardiovascular
Respiratory
Gastrointestinal (including mouth and per rectal examination)
Breast
Examine for lymphadenopathy

Baseline Investigations
Blood tests (full blood count, urea and electrolytes, liver function tests, thyroid function tests, C reactive protein and erythrocyte sedimentation rate, glucose, lactate dehydrogenase)
Chest radiography
Urinalysis
Faecal occult blood testing

Abnormal findings   No abnormal findings

Further appropriate investigations   3 month period of "watchful waiting"

Treat any cause found

In addition, for all patients:

Nutritional assessment   Appropriate dietary/social interventions

Evaluation of unintentional weight loss in elderly people

buys and prepares the food? Is there any home help or help from family members?

A history that includes a review of systems may elicit additional symptoms that might direct further investigation.

In addition, screen all patients for cognitive impairment and depression using standardised assessment tools.[21] [22W11]

Some authors recommend a nutritional assessment only when no evidence of organic disease is found.[1] [8] We believe, however, that all elderly patients presenting with unintentional weight loss should undergo nutritional assessment by a dietitian. This is because malnutrition has a high prevalence in elderly people and might still be present even when an organic cause of the weight loss is found.

We suggest that patients seen in primary care (by general practitioners)—where facilities (and time) for assessing cognitive function, mood, and nutritional status are not always readily available—should be referred to specialists in the care of older people.

Physical examination
In patients with unintentional weight loss a full physical examination should aim to exclude major cardiovascular and respiratory illnesses, as well as abdominal masses, organomegaly, prostate enlargement, and breast masses that may indicate cancer. Palpable lymphadenopathy could indicate infection, cancer, or haematological disease. Examine the mouth to exclude any obvious dental problems, poor oral hygiene, dry mouth, or lesions that may make chewing and swallowing difficult or painful.

Baseline investigations
Baseline investigations for all patients should include bloods tests (full blood count, urea and electrolytes, liver function tests, thyroid function tests, C reactive protein, glucose, and lactate dehydrogenase), chest radiography, urinalysis, and faecal occult blood testing.[1] [4] [12] [13] [23] The rationale behind these baseline tests is explained in box 2.

Tumour markers are not useful diagnostic tests; they should not be used as part of the initial evaluation and may be misleading.[1] [24] Their role is in monitoring response to treatment in patients with cancer or detecting tumour recurrence early after treatment. Abnormal findings on initial evaluation should be used to guide further investigations into the cause of the weight loss.

If the history, examination, and baseline investigations are all normal, published evidence suggests that further investigation is not warranted immediately and that three months' "watchful waiting" is advisable, rather than a blind pursuit of additional, more invasive or expensive investigations. Because organic disease is found only rarely in patients with normal results from physical examination and laboratory tests, this waiting period is unlikely to have an adverse outcome.[3] [4]

Although three scoring systems have been developed to help clinicians identify which patients with weight loss are likely to have a physical or malignant cause rather than a psychological or social cause,[8] [13] [23] none of these has been validated in independent populations presenting with weight loss.

Should a negative baseline reassure?
The claim that a negative baseline evaluation should reassure the clinician of the lack of serious underlying disease is based on only small non-randomised studies. Most of these are also not limited to elderly patients (in the UK defined as >70 years of age). However, most authors agree that in elderly patients with clinically relevant unintentional weight loss, major organic (and especially malignant) diseases are highly unlikely when a thorough baseline evaluation is normal, and that in this setting a watchful waiting approach may be preferable to undirected and invasive testing.[1] [3] [4] [13] [23]

There is currently no evidence that blind computed tomography scanning is helpful in investigating such patients. Disadvantages of blind computed tomography scanning include high costs (with low yield) and the likelihood of finding "incidental-omas."

Several studies have used abdominal ultrasound as part of their initial evaluation, although they did not comment on its usefulness in this role, noting only that 27% of patients with underlying cancer had hepatomegaly on examination and a similar percentage had palpable masses.[4] Abnormal findings on examination (or abnormal liver function tests) would have prompted further investigation anyway.

Gastrointestinal disorders (malignant and non-malignant) account for about a third of all causes of unexplained weight loss in studies of adults of all ages, so some authors advocate upper gastrointestinal endoscopy in patients as a first line investigation.[3] However, because endoscopy is invasive and not without risk (particularly for elderly patients), we think that it should be reserved for patients in whom it is indicated on the basis of history, examination, or baseline investigations (such as a history of gastrointestinal bleeding or evidence of iron deficiency anaemia).

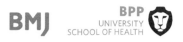

In one study where patients with a normal baseline evaluation underwent further investigations including computed tomography and endoscopy, only one additional diagnosis was made (a patient diagnosed with lactose intolerance).[4]

Managing unexplained weight loss in elderly people

The primary principle of management is to identify and treat any underlying causes. Optimal management often requires multidisciplinary assessment (doctors, dentists, dietitians, speech therapists, physiotherapists, occupational therapists, social services).[20W12] We strongly suggest reviewing drugs in an attempt to eliminate those whose side effects may contribute to weight loss.

If a psychiatric cause of weight loss, such as depression, is suspected we recommend assessment by a psychogeriatrician or psychologist. In such cases, consider treatment with an antidepressant because depression is a potentially reversible cause of weight loss.[W12]

If the initial baseline evaluation is negative, we suggest that patients are reassessed after three months to establish if any further symptoms or signs have developed and to check their weight. In the interim, because evidence to support any drug treatment is lacking,[1,20] a variety of non-drug based interventions can be used (outlined in box 3).

BOX 2 BASELINE TESTS FOR INVESTIGATING UNEXPLAINED WEIGHT LOSS IN OLDER PEOPLE

Blood tests

Full blood count

Anaemia is suggestive of an organic cause of weight loss,[13] and it should prompt further investigations, which will depend on the type of anaemia (microcytic, macrocytic, etc). A raised white cell count may also suggest organic disease (malignant, infectious, or inflammatory processes) and was felt to be an important variable in several observational studies that assessed likelihood of a malignant or other organic cause of unintentional weight loss[4,13]

Urea and electrolytes

Although the published studies do not seem to find this a particularly helpful test in predicting an organic versus non-organic cause for weight loss,[4,13] it is a reasonable investigation to perform at this stage and abnormal results may point towards an organic cause

Liver function tests, including γ-glutamyl transpeptidase and albumin

Normal liver function tests make serious organic causes for weight loss less likely, particularly cancer, which is usually advanced by the time weight loss occurs.[4] Alkaline phosphatase is particularly useful because it can be raised when liver or bone disease is present. One observational study found that alkaline phosphatase >300 IU/L increased the likelihood of a malignant cause of weight loss (odds ratio 14.7) and serum albumin >35 g/L reduced the likelihood (0.11)[13]

Thyroid function tests

Hyperthyroidism is a common endocrinal cause of weight loss

C reactive protein and erythrocyte sedimentation rate

Normal test results make a serious organic cause for the weight loss less likely. In one observational study, C reactive protein was raised in 91% of patients subsequently diagnosed with malignancy, and in 69% of patients with non-malignant organic disease.[4] In another study,[13] a raised erythrocyte sedimentation rate was associated with an increased likelihood of malignancy (2.9, 1.7 to 5.1). Erythrocyte sedimentation rate can also be raised in other organic disorders including systemic inflammatory disorders. A raised erythrocyte sedimentation rate or C reactive protein would therefore point towards a possible organic cause for the weight loss

Serum glucose

Uncontrolled diabetes is a common endocrinal cause of weight loss

Lactate dehydrogenase

Lactate dehydrogenase >500 IU/L is associated with an increased likelihood of a malignant cause of involuntary weight loss (26.9)[13]

Chest radiography

Chest radiography should be performed in all patients to identify respiratory disease, including malignant and non-malignant causes[1,4]

Urinalysis

Urinalysis is included in almost all studies as part of the initial evaluation and is non-invasive and inexpensive; however, the published studies do not specify its diagnostic benefit as part of the initial evaluation of elderly patients with unintentional weight loss, only that it is of less value than other investigations[4]

Faecal occult blood analysis

Because of the high proportion (about a third) of patients with an underlying gastrointestinal disorder,[3] whether malignant or non-malignant, such analysis is a reasonable first line investigation. It is non-invasive (compared with endoscopy), and although it is not particularly sensitive or specific, a positive result would prompt further investigation of the gastrointestinal tract (such as endoscopy or colonoscopy)

BOX 3 NON-DRUG BASED INTERVENTIONS FOR UNEXPLAINED WEIGHT LOSS IN ELDERLY PATIENTS

Optimise food intake

- Encourage the patient to eat smaller meals more often
- Encourage the patient to eating favourite foods and snacks, and minimise dietary restrictions (which are often energy poor and less palatable, therefore cause increased risk of weight loss in elderly patients)[2W13 W14]
- High energy foods should be eaten at the main meal of the day (elderly people, particularly those with dementia, tend to consume most of their daily energy at breakfast)[25]
- Optimise and vary dietary texture—this is of particular benefit in patients with dementia[26]
- Eating in company or with assistance is useful. Eating in company has been suggested to improve enjoyment of meals and therefore increase intake.[2] Many elderly people have physical or cognitive disabilities that impair their ability to feed themselves without assistance or prompting
- Community nutritional support services (such as "meals on wheels" programmes) are recommended for elderly patients in the community to improve dietary intake

Oral nutritional supplements if recommended by the dietitian

- Oral nutritional supplements (such as high energy drinks) have been shown to increase daily energy intake and weight gain, although evidence that they result in long term benefit in terms of health, functional ability, and survival in undernourished elderly patients is limited
- Supplements should be taken between meals to avoid appetite suppression and decreased intake of food at meal times[20]

Daily multivitamin tablet

- There is little evidence that this leads to a reduction in weight loss. However, it is recommended by some authors because of the high prevalence of nutritional deficiencies in elderly people

Ensure adequate oral health

- Problems with dentition and oral health are commonly overlooked causes of weight loss[W15]

Regular exercise or physiotherapy

- Regular exercise (particularly resistance training) is also recommended for frail elderly patients because it stimulates appetite and prevents sarcopenia. Physiotherapy may help achieve this in some patients

---

Contributors: AB had the idea for the article and is guarantor; JM and CS searched the literature; JM wrote the article, and AB and CS helped with editing.

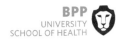

TIPS FOR NON-SPECIALISTS

- General practitioners and non-specialist hospital doctors should perform the initial history, examination, and baseline investigations
- Refer any abnormality suggesting a possible organic cause for the weight loss to the appropriate specialty
- If no obvious cause is found, the referrer can undertake the three months of watchful waiting or refer to secondary care (medicine for the elderly), where facilities for multidisciplinary assessment are often better
- If the initial evaluation and watchful waiting are undertaken by primary care, repeat the history, examination, and investigations at the end of this period. If no cause is identified and the patient is still losing weight, refer to secondary care

FURTHER RESEARCH AND UNANSWERED QUESTIONS

- Most published studies are based on small numbers of patients, focus on unintentional weight loss in adults of all ages, and many are more than 10 years old
- Studies focusing on elderly people are needed—ideally multicentre studies with large numbers of patients and with longer follow-up periods to see whether additional diagnoses are made and whether these patients continue to lose weight
- If the patient is referred to secondary care, weight loss persists or progresses but no cause has been identified after three months of watchful waiting, what then?
- Should we continue to assess at regular three monthly intervals? Should we consider blind investigations?

Competing interests: All authors have completed the Unified Competing Interest form at www.icmje.org/coi_disclosure.pdf (available on request from the corresponding author) and declare: no support from any organisation for the submitted work; no financial relationships with any organisations that might have an interest in the submitted work in the previous three years; no other relationships or activities that could appear to have influenced the submitted work.

Provenance and peer review: Not commissioned; externally peer reviewed.

1   Alibhai S.M.H, Greenwood C, Payette H. An approach to the management of unintentional weight loss in the elderly. *CMAJ* 2005:172:773-80.
2   Bouras EP, Lange SM, Scolapio JS. Rational approach to patients with unintentional weight loss, *Mayo Clin Proc*2001;76:923-9.
3   Lankish PG, Gerzmann M, Gerzmann JF, Lehnick D. Unintentional weight loss: diagnosis and prognosis. The first prospective follow-up study from a secondary referral centre. *J Intern Med*2001;249:41-6.
4   Metalidis C, Knockaert DC, Bobbaers H, Vanderschueren S. Involuntary weight loss. Does a negative baseline evaluation provide adequate reassurance? *Eur J Intern Med*2008;19:345-9.
5   Clarkston WK, Pantano MM, Morley JE, Horowitz M, Littlefield JM, Burton FR. Evidence for the anorexia of aging—gastrointestinal transit and hunger in healthy elderly vs young adults. *Am J Physiol*1997;41:R243-8.
6   Wallace JI, Schwartz RS. Epidemiology of weight loss in humans with special reference to wasting in the elderly. *Int J Cardiol*2002;85:15-21.
7   Newman A, Yanez D, Harris T, Duxbury A, Enright PL, Fried LP. Weight change in old age and its association with mortality. *J Am Geriatr Soc*2001:49:1309-18.
8   Marton KI, Sox HC Jr, Krupp JR. Involuntary weight loss: diagnostic and prognostic significance. *Ann Intern Med*1981;95:568.
9   Chapman KM, Nelson RA. Loss of appetite: managing unwanted weight loss in the older patient. *Geriatrics* 1994;49:54-9.
10 Ryan C, Bryant E, Eleazer P, Rhodes A, Guest K. Unintentional weight loss in long-term care: predictor of mortality in the elderly. *South Med J*1995;88:721-4.
11 Ensrud KE, Ewing SK, Stone KL, Cauley JA, Bowman PJ, Cummings SR. Intentional and unintentional weight loss increase bone loss and hip fracture risk in older women. *J Am Geriatr Soc*2003;51:1740-7.
12 Rabinovitz M, Pitlik SD, Leifer M, Garty M, Rosenfeld JB. Unintentional weight loss: a retrospective analysis of 154 cases. *Arch Intern Med*1986;146:186.
13 Hernandez JL, Riancho JA, Matorras P, Gonzalez-Macias J. Clinical evaluation for cancer in patients with involuntary weight loss without specific symptoms. *Am J Med*2003;114:631-7.
14 Robbins LJ. Evaluation of weight loss in the elderly. *Geriatrics*1989;44:31-4.
15 Morley JE, Silver AJ. Nutritional issues in nursing home care. *Ann Intern Med*1995;123:850-9.
16 Carr-Lopez SM, Phillips SK. The role of medications in geriatric failure to thrive. *Drugs Aging*1996;8:221-5.
17 Morley J.E, Kraenzie D. Causes of weight loss in a community nursing home. *J Am Geriatr Soc*1994;42:583-5.
18 Saz P, Dewey ME. Depression, depressive symptoms and mortality in persons aged 65 and over living in the community: a systematic review of the literature. *Int J Geriatr Psychiatry*2001;16:622-30.
19 Beekman AT, Copeland JR, Prince MJ. Review of community prevalence of depression in later life. *Br J Psychiatry* 1999;174:307-11.
20 Smith KL, Greenwood C, Payette H, Alibhai SMH. An approach to the nonpharmacologic and pharmacologic management of unintentional weight loss among older adults. *Geriatr Aging* 2007;10:91-8.
21 Folstein MF, Folstein SE, McHugh PR. "Mini-mental state". A practical method for grading the cognitive state of patients for the clinician. *J Psychiatr Res*1975;12:189-98.
22 Yesavage JA, Brink TL, Rose TL, Lum O, Huang V, Adey M, et al. Development and validation of a geriatric depression screening scale: a preliminary report. *J Psychiatr Res*1983;17:37-49.
23 Bilbao-Gara J, Barba R, Losa-Garcia JE, Martin H, Garcia de Casasola G, Castilla V. Assessing clinical probability of organic disease in patients with involuntary weight loss: a simple score. *Eur J Intern Med*2002;13:240-5.
24 Sturgeon CM, Lai LC, Duffy MJ. Serum tumour markers; how to order and interpret them. *BMJ*2009;339:b3527.
25 Young KW, Greenwood CE. Shift in diurnal feeding patterns in nursing home residents with Alzheimer's disease. *J Gerontol A Biol Sci Med Sci*2001;56:M656-61.
26 Boylston E, Ryan C, Brown C, Westfall B. Increasing oral intake in dementia patients by altering food texture. *Am J Alzheimer's Dis*1995;10:37-9.

Related links

bmj.com/archive
Previous articles in this series
- Managing adult patients who need home parenteral nutrition (2011;342:d1447)
- The management of abdominal aortic aneurysms (2011;342:d1384)
- The risks of radiation exposure related to diagnostic imaging and how to minimise them (2011; 342:d947)
- Pharmacological prevention of migraine (2011; 342:d583)

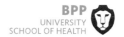
The changing epidemiology of lung cancer with a focus on screening

Gerard A Silvestri professor of medicine[1], Anthony J Alberg associate professor of epidemiology [2], James Ravenel associate professor of radiology[3]

[1]Division of Pulmonary and Critical Care Medicine, Medical University of South Carolina, Charleston, SC 29425, USA

[2]Hollings Cancer Center and Department of Biostatistics, Bioinformatics, and Epidemiology, Medical University of South Carolina

[3]Department of Radiology, Medical University of South Carolina

Correspondence to: G A Silvestri silvestri@musc.edu

Cite this as: BMJ 2009;339:b3053

‹DOI› 10.1136/bmj.b3053
http://www.bmj.com/content/339/bmj.b3053

Lung cancer is a global public health problem of epidemic proportions, and the number of people affected is expected to grow in the near future. Worldwide, in 2002 more than 1.3 million people were newly diagnosed with lung cancer.[1] It is the leading global cause of death from cancer, and it accounts for 18% of all deaths from cancer and more than one million deaths a year since as far back as 1993.[2] [3] Lung cancer is the 10th leading overall cause of death, and it is expected to move to fifth place as its incidence rises in developing countries. Lung cancer is a disease that seems to fit the profile for a successful screening programme. However, developing an efficacious screening test that meets the established criteria for screening has proved elusive, despite evidence from many screening trials, and screening remains controversial. This review aims to shed light on the questions surrounding screening for lung cancer.

What are the established causes of lung cancer?

Active cigarette smoking is the main cause—it accounts for 85-90% of all lung cancers.[2] [w1-w5] In addition, exposure to secondhand cigarette smoke; pipe and cigar smoking; occupational exposure to agents such as asbestos, nickel, chromium, and arsenic; exposure to radiation, including radon gas in homes; and exposure to air pollution are all established risk factors for lung cancer.[2] There has been longstanding interest in genetic susceptibility to lung cancer, and results of recent genome-wide association studies consistently point to the long arm of chromosome 15 as being linked to increased risk.[4] [5] [w6-w8]

What is the emerging global picture of lung cancer?

Whereas in the mid-1900s the lung cancer epidemic was largely confined to developed nations, by 2002 the absolute numbers of newly diagnosed lung cancers occurring in developed and developing countries were nearly equal.[1] [6]

Considerable geographical variation exists, with a greater than 20-fold variation in occurrence across countries (figure).[2] [7] As of 2002, the age adjusted annual incidence ranges from a high of 65.7 per 100 000 in Central and Eastern Europe to less than 25 per 100 000 in Africa, with most of that continent at less than five per 100 000 (figure).[1] [7]

The occurrence of lung cancer is so strongly determined by cigarette smoking that historical and current smoking prevalence data can help reliably forecast the future patterns of occurrence.

Countries where the lung cancer epidemic is in its infancy, or it is in full force without signs of coming under control, are of greatest public health concern. The hallmark characteristics of a country in transition from lower to higher rates of lung cancer are a low current incidence of lung cancer but a high current prevalence of cigarette smoking. The high prevalence of smoking in these countries foretells a future epidemic of lung cancer. Countries in the middle of an uncontrolled epidemic of lung cancer are those with high current mortality from lung cancer coupled with a high current prevalence of cigarette smoking. The populations of such countries are at the highest risk at present and for the foreseeable future. Korea, the Russian Federation, Kazakhstan, Poland, and Hungary fall into this last category as far as men are concerned, whereas in Venezuela, Germany, Norway, the United States, and Denmark women are at the greatest current and future risk.[8]

Populations may avoid the lung cancer epidemic entirely if cigarette smoking never becomes prevalent, as has historically been the case in many African countries. Unfortunately, several African countries have recently experienced a surge in cigarette smoking.[9] Conversely, the high burden of lung cancer currently seen in some countries will decrease because public health efforts have reduced the prevalence of smoking. Risks are now lower for men in Singapore, Canada, Germany, the United Kingdom, the US, the Netherlands, and Belgium, and for women in Malaysia, Korea, Bahrain, the Philippines, Canada, and Belgium.

Chinese men will strongly influence the global burden of lung cancer in the 21st century because they have a high prevalence of cigarette smoking and they form a large proportion of the world's population. Per capita cigarette consumption among Chinese men has risen from one cigarette per day in 1952, to four in 1972, to 10 in 1992.[10] The rate of smoking among Chinese men today is equivalent to the highest rates ever seen in developed countries. The incidence of lung cancer has already risen, with more substantial increases yet to come.[11] Socioeconomic status is inversely associated with the incidence of lung cancer and mortality. A recent study of nearly 400 000 Europeans found a higher risk of lung cancer in the least well educated populations (a proxy for socioeconomic status). Adjustment for smoking reduced the risk of lung cancer by 50% in men and women in all regions and for all histological types.[12]

With a sustained global burden of lung cancer projected for the coming decades, a method of early detection that could effectively reduce mortality from lung cancer would potentially have an enormous public health benefit.

SUMMARY POINTS

- Lung cancer is the most common cancer worldwide
- Incidence varies greatly between countries because of the varying prevalence of cigarette smoking
- The epidemic of lung cancer has just begun in developing countries, although a decrease is being seen in some developed countries
- Screening for lung cancer using low dose computed tomography has not been proved to be efficacious
- Several large randomised controlled trials to assess the efficacy of screening for lung cancer are under way
- Screening for lung cancer cannot be recommended outside a well designed clinical trial

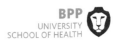

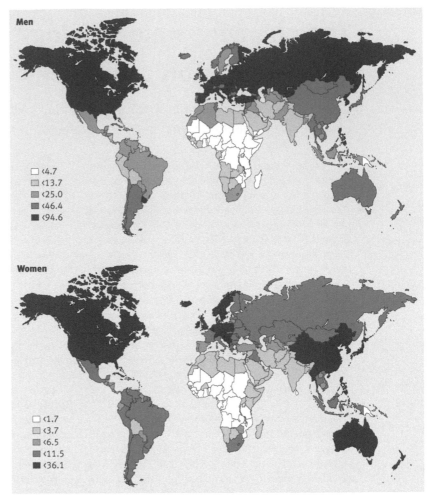

Global annual incidence (per 100 000) of lung cancer in men and women. Adapted, with permission, from GLOBOCAN 2002[7]

Why consider screening for lung cancer?

Three quarters of patients with lung cancer present with symptoms of advanced incurable disease.[13] Despite advances in treatment, the five year survival rate for all stages combined is around 16%.[14] Outcomes are significantly better in patients diagnosed at earlier stages, with a five year survival for stage I disease of 60-75%.[15] [w9-w11] An efficacious screening test that could result in early detection and reduced mortality would thus represent a major advance in combating mortality from lung cancer.

TEN CRITERIA FOR EFFECTIVE SCREENING

- The disease has serious consequences
- The screening population has a high prevalence of detectable preclinical disease
- The screening test detects little pseudodisease (overdiagnosis)
- The screening test has high accuracy for detecting preclinical disease
- The screening test detects disease before the critical point
- The screening test causes little morbidity
- The screening test is affordable and available
- Treatment exists
- Treatment is more effective when applied before symptomatic detection
- Treatment is not too risky or toxic

Does screening lead to reduced mortality from lung cancer?

Principles of a screening test

Screening is the process of detecting disease before it becomes symptomatic. For a screening test to be effective, certain criteria must be met regarding the disease, the proposed screening test, and treatment (box).[16] The disease must have serious consequences and be readily detectable in the preclinical phase. The test should have a high accuracy, detect the disease before a critical point, cause little morbidity, be available and affordable, and result in little overdiagnosis. Finally, treatment for the disease must exist, and it must be effective before symptoms occur, with little risk or morbidity. Both chest radiography and computed tomography have been evaluated as screening tests for lung cancer.

Findings from studies evaluating chest radiography

Several randomised trials in the 1960-1980s screened for lung cancer using chest radiography and found no difference in mortality between the screened and unscreened groups, even though more early stage cancers were identified in the screening group.[17] Late stage cancers were not reduced, and deaths from lung cancer were higher in the screened group after 20 years of follow-up, probably because of overdiagnosis.[18] [w12-w17]

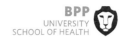

Findings from studies of screening using chest computed tomography

Low radiation dose computed tomography uses lower doses of radiation than standard techniques to generate an image. Nodules as small as 2-3 mm can be detected, which means that this method detects at least three times as many small lung nodules as a standard chest radiograph.[19] The only evidence on screening for lung cancer using this method is from observational cohort studies that provide information on the distribution of disease stage and survival of the screened population but do not measure efficacy of screening in reducing mortality.

Cohort studies conducted in Japan which included 15050 at risk participants detected 72 lung cancers during prevalence screening (0.5%), 57 of which were stage IA.[20][21][22] In 21762 annual incidence screens, 60 (0.3%) new cancers were detected, of which 50 were stage IA.

The Early Lung Cancer Action Project (ELCAP) screened 1000 asymptomatic volunteers with at least a 10 pack year (number of cigarettes smoked each day times number of years smoked) history of smoking with chest radiography and low radiation dose computed tomography.[23] Non-calcified lung nodules were detected in 23% using computed tomography and 7% using chest radiography. Malignant nodules were detected in 2.7% by computed tomography compared with 0.7% by chest radiography. Twenty seven lung cancers were identified and 23 were stage I.

This was followed by a prospective study at the Mayo Clinic of low radiation dose computed tomography screening in 1520 high risk subjects.[19] One year after baseline scanning, a total of 2244 non-calcified lung nodules were identified in 1000 of the 1520 participants (66%). Twenty five cases of lung cancer were diagnosed (22 prevalent cases and three incident cases), and 22 patients underwent surgical resection. Twelve of the 21 non-small cell cancers detected were stage IA at diagnosis. After five years of annual computed tomography scanning,[24] a total of 3356 non-calcified nodules were found in 73.5% of the cohort; about 95% of the nodules were found to be benign with clinical follow-up or surgical biopsy. Sixty eight primary lung tumours were documented in 66 participants, 34 on annual (incidence) studies and three interval lung cancers not detected through annual screening. Of the incident cancers, 21 were stage I and 11 presented at stage III or IV. The large proportion of non-calcified nodules found (5-51%) is problematic because most will turn out to be benign but will require further evaluation, including serial computed tomography scans, biopsy, or in some cases surgical resection, which can carry serious morbidity and a low but real risk of death.

A large multicentre multinational non-randomised trial, the International ELCAP (I-ELCAP) was recently reported.[25] This trial screened 31567 subjects using low radiation dose computed tomography. Lung cancer was detected in 484 patients (1.3%), 412 of whom had stage I disease. Estimated 10 year survival was 80% for all patients regardless of stage and treatment, and 88% for stage I cancer. This study confirmed earlier observations that lung cancers detected by computed tomography screening are at an early stage and are highly treatable.

This study provides a basis for optimism, but it cannot confirm the efficacy of screening for lung cancer with low radiation dose computed tomography because, although survival was higher in people diagnosed with early stage lung cancer, the study was not designed to assess whether screening reduces overall mortality in patients with lung cancer. A comment on the study gave four reasons why the findings did not make a persuasive case for screening.[26] Firstly, the lack of a control group precluded the study from investigating what would happen to a similar group of patients In the absence of screening. Secondly, lack of an unbiased outcome measure meant that the confounding features of lead time, length time, and overdiagnosis bias were not controlled for. Thirdly, the study did not take into account what is already known about lung cancer screening, particularly the evidence for overdiagnosis bias arising in single arm studies from Japan.[22] Finally, although the study emphasised the positive aspects of screening, it did not discuss potential harms, especially the unnecessary investigation or treatment of benign disease.

The positive findings of the I-ELCAP trial contrast with those from a longitudinal study that examined three populations of current or former smokers, one in Italy and two in the US. The study screened 3246 people annually with computed tomography and had a median follow-up of 3.9 years.[27] The numbers of observed new cases of lung cancer, resections for lung cancer, cases of advanced lung cancer, and deaths from lung cancer were compared with the numbers predicted using two validated models. One hundred and forty four people were diagnosed with lung cancer compared with 44.5 expected cases (relative risk 3.2, 95% confidence interval 2.7 to 3.8; P<0.001). The rate of lung cancer resection was 10 times higher than expected—109 compared with the 10.9 predicted for that cohort (10.0, 8.2 to 11.9; P<0.001). There were 42 cases of advanced lung cancer compared with 33.4 expected cases and 38 deaths, which is the number predicted for that cohort (1.0, 0.7 to 1.3; P=0.90). This study showed that screening with low radiation dose computed tomography increased the detection of lung cancers and the numbers of tumours resected, but it did not reduce the risk of advanced lung cancer or of overall mortality from lung cancer. The survival of patients with stage I tumours that were resected was similar to that seen by the I-ELCAP investigators.

What can we conclude?

Results from observational computed tomography studies show that low radiation dose computed tomography can detect early lung cancer in asymptomatic people. However, we still do not know whether early detection reduces mortality from lung cancer or is cost effective.[28] For this reason, the National Cancer Institute has instituted the National Lung Screening Trial (NLST; www.cancer.gov/nlst). The NLST is a randomised controlled trial that by 2004 recruited nearly 50000 current or former smokers and randomised them to screening with chest radiography (the control group) or helical computed tomography. Subjects were screened for three years and are now being followed up. The NLST is powered to detect a 20% reduction in mortality from lung cancer by screening with spiral computed tomography compared with chest radiography.

The NELSON trial is a European computed tomography based screening trial being conducted in the Netherlands and Denmark.[29] Almost 20000 at risk participants have been randomised to computed tomography screening versus no screening. It is designed to have 80% power to show at least a 25% reduction in mortality from lung cancer 10 years after randomisation.

Evidence based reviews have concluded that current evidence does not support computed tomography screening

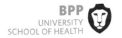

ONGOING RESEARCH AND UNANSWERED QUESTIONS

- Two large randomised controlled trials of more than 70000 people assessing the efficacy of screening with low radiation dose computed tomography for lung cancer are under way
- If lung cancer screening is found to be efficacious how would the health system implement mass screening?
- Would it be better to use scarce healthcare resources to prevent people starting to smoke or to provide better tools for smoking cessation?

TIPS FOR NON-SPECIALISTS

- Counselling patients about smoking cessation is the most effective way to reduce the risk of lung cancer
- Screening for lung cancer using chest radiography or low dose computed tomography of the chest is not currently recommended
- At risk patients who are interested in screening should be counselled about the potential harms of screening, including further unnecessary testing and complications associated with the evaluation of screen detected findings

ADDITIONAL EDUCATIONAL RESOURCES

Resources for healthcare professionals

- Manser R, Irving LB, Stone C, Byrnes G, Abramson MJ, Campbell D. Screening for lung cancer. *Cochrane Database Syst Rev* 2004;(1):CD001991.
- Bach BP, Silvestri GA, Hanger M, Jett JR. Screening for lung cancer: ACCP evidence-based clinical practice guidelines (2nd ed). *Chest* 2007;132 (supp):69S-77S.
- These two references provide an evidenced based review of screening for lung cancer

Resources for patients

- Welch HG. Should I be tested for cancer? Maybe not and here's why. Berkeley: University of California Press, 2004

for lung cancer outside the auspices of a well designed clinical trial.[30][31][w18] The upsurge in smoking in developing countries has thwarted the tremendous strides in tobacco control that have been made in many developed countries. The net result is that global mortality from lung cancer will rise in the short term.

Even if screening is found to be efficacious and new treatments are developed, global reductions in smoking initiation combined with effective smoking cessation strategies in those who currently smoke will have the biggest effect on mortality from lung cancer.

Contributors: All authors helped equally in researching and writing this article. GAS edited the final manuscript and responses to the critique and is guarantor.

Competing interests: None declared.

Provenance and peer review: Commissioned; externally peer reviewed.

1 Parkin DM, Bray F, Ferlay J, Pisani P. Global cancer statistics, 2002. *CA: Cancer J Clin* 2005;55:74-108.
2 Alberg AJ, Ford JG, Samet JM. Epidemiology of lung cancer: ACCP evidence-based clinical practice guidelines (2nd edition). *Chest* 2007;132:29S-55S.
3 Rosen G. *A history of public health. Expanded ed.* Baltimore, MD: Johns Hopkins University Press, 1993.
4 Amos CI, Wu X, Broderick P, Gorlov IP, Gu J, Eisen T, et al. Genome-wide association scan of tag SNPs identifies a susceptibility locus for lung cancer at 15q25.1. *Nat Genet* 2008;40:616-22.
5 Hung RJ, McKay JD, Gaborieau V, Boffetta P, Hashibe M, Zaridze D, et al. A susceptibility locus for lung cancer maps to nicotinic acetylcholine receptor subunit genes on 15q25. *Nature* 2008;452:633-7.
6 Ezzati M, Lopez AD. Estimates of global mortality attributable to smoking in 2000. *Lancet* 2003;362:847-52.
7 Ferlay J, Bray F, Pisani P, Parkin DM. *GLOBOCAN 2002: cancer incidence, mortality and prevalence worldwide.* IARC Cancer base no 5. version 2.0. IARC Press, 2004. www.dep.iarc.fr/.
8 Alberg AJ, Nonemaker J. Who is at high risk for lung cancer? Population-level and individual-level perspectives. *Semin Respir Crit Care Med* 2008;29:223-32.
9 Lam WK, White NW, Chan-Yeung MM. Lung cancer epidemiology and risk factors in Asia and Africa. *Int J Tuberc Lung Dis* 2004;8:1045-57.
10 Yang L, Parkin D, Ferlay J. Estimates of cancer incidence in China for 2000 and projections for 2005. *Cancer Epidemiol Biomarkers Prev* 2005;14:243-50.
11 Liu BQ, Peto R, Chen ZM, Boreham J, Wu YP, Li JY, et al. Emerging tobacco hazards in China: 1. Retrospective proportional mortality study of one million deaths. *BMJ* 1998;317:1411-22.
12 Menvielle G, Boshuizen H, Kunst AE, Dalton SO, Vineis P, Bergmann MM, et al. The role of smoking and diet in explaining educational inequalities in lung cancer incidence. *J Natl Cancer Inst* 2009;101:321-30.
13 Molina JR, Adjei AA, Jett JR. Advances in chemotherapy of non-small cell lung cancer. *Chest* 2006;130:1211-9.
14 American Cancer Society. *Cancer facts and figures 2007.* ACS, 2007.
15 Scott WJ, Howington J, Feigenberg S, Movsas B, Pisters K; American College of Chest Physicians. Treatment of non-small cell lung cancer stage I and stage II. *Chest* 2007;132:234S-42S.
16 Obuchowski NA, Graham RJ, Baker ME, Powell KA. Ten criteria for effective screening: their application to multislice CT screening for pulmonary and colorectal cancers. *AJR Am J Roentgenol* 2001;176:1357-62.
17 Bach PB, Niewoehner DE, Black WC. Screening for lung cancer: the guidelines. *Chest* 2003;123:83-8.
18 Marcus PM, Bergstralh EJ, Fagerstrom RM, Williams DE, Fontana R, Taylor WF, et al. Lung cancer mortality in the Mayo lung project: impact of extended follow-up. *J Natl Cancer Inst* 2000;92:1308-16.
19 Swensen SJ, Jett JR, Sloan JA, Midthun DE, Hartman TE, Sykes AM, et al. Screening for lung cancer with low-dose spiral computed tomography. *Am J Respir Crit Care Med* 2002;165:508-13.
20 Nawa T, Nakagawa T, Kusano S, Kawasaki Y, Sugawara Y, Nakata H. Lung cancer screening using low-dose spiral CT: results of baseline and 1-year follow-up studies. *Chest* 2002;122:15-20.
21 Sobue T, Moriyama N, Kaneko M. Screening for lung cancer with low-dose helical computed tomography: anti-lung cancer association project. *J Clin Oncol* 2002;20:911-20.
22 Sone S, Li F, Yang Z, Honda T, Maruyama Y, Takashima S, et al. Results of three-year mass screening programme for lung cancer using mobile low-dose spiral computed tomography scanner. *Br J Cancer* 2001;84:25-32.
23 Henschke CI, McCauley DI, Yankelevitz DF, Naidich DP, McGuinness G, Miettinen OS, et al. Early Lung Cancer Action Project: overall design and findings from baseline screening. *Lancet* 1999;354:99-105.
24 Swensen SJ, Jett JR, Hartman TE, Midthun DE, Mandrekar SJ, Hillman SL, et al. CT screening for lung cancer: five-year prospective experience. *Radiology* 2005;235:259-65.
25 Henschke CI, Yankelevitz DF, Libby DM, Pasmantier MW, Smith JP, Miettinen OS. Survival of patients with stage I lung cancer detected on CT screening. *N Engl J Med* 2006;355:1763-71.
26 Welch HG, Woloshin S, Schwartz LM, Gordis L, Gotzsche PC, Harris R, et al. Overstating the evidence for lung cancer screening: the International Early Lung Cancer Action Program (I-ELCAP) study. *Arch Int Med* 2007;167:2289-95.
27 Bach PB, Jett JR, Pastorino U, Tockman MS, Swensen SJ, Begg CB. Computed tomography screening and lung cancer outcomes. *JAMA* 2007;297:953-61.
28 Mahadevia PJ, Fleisher LA, Frick KD, Eng J, Goodman SN, Powe NR. Lung cancer screening with helical computed tomography in older adult smokers: a decision and cost-effectiveness analysis. *JAMA* 2003;289:313-22.
29 Van Iersel CA, de Koning HJ, Draisma G, Mali WP, Scholten ET, Nackaerts K, et al. Risk-based selection from the general population in a screening trial: selection criteria, recruitment and power for the Dutch-Belgian randomised lung cancer multi-slice CT screening trial (NELSON). *Int J Cancer* 2007;120:868-74.
30 Bach PB, Silvestri GA, Hanger M, Jett JR. Screening for lung cancer: ACCP evidence-based clinical practice guidelines (2nd edition). *Chest* 2007;132:69S-77S.
31 Manser R, Irving LB, Stone C, Byrnes G, Abramson MJ, Campbell D. Screening for lung cancer. *Cochrane Database Syst Rev* 2004;(1):CD001991.

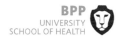

Screening for lung cancer using low dose computed tomography

Martin C Tammemagi professor[1], Stephen Lam professor[2]

[1]Department of Health Sciences, Brock University, St Catharines, ON, Canada

[2]British Columbia Cancer Agency and the University of British Columbia, Vancouver, BC, Canada V5Z 1L3

Correspondence to: S Lam slam2@bccancer.bc.ca

Cite this as: BMJ 2014;348:g2253

‹DOI› 10.1136/bmj.g2253

http://www.bmj.com/content/348/bmj.g2253

Screening for lung cancer with low dose computed tomography can reduce mortality from the disease by 20% in high risk smokers. This review covers the state of the art knowledge on several aspects of implementing a screening program. The most important are to identify people who are at high enough risk to warrant screening and the appropriate management of lung nodules found at screening. An accurate risk prediction model is more efficient than age and pack years of smoking alone at identifying those who will develop lung cancer and die from the disease. Algorithms are available for assessing people who screen positive to determine who needs additional imaging or invasive investigations. Concerns about low dose computed tomography screening include false positive results, overdiagnosis, radiation exposure, and costs. Further work is needed to define the frequency and duration of screening and to refine risk prediction models so that they can be used to assess the risk of lung cancer in special populations. Another important area is the use of computer vision software tools to facilitate high throughput interpretation of low dose computed tomography images so that costs can be reduced and the consistency of scan interpretation can be improved. Sufficient data are available to support the implementation of screening programs at the population level in stages that can be expanded when found to perform well to improve the outcome of patients with lung cancer.

Introduction

Worldwide, lung cancer is the leading cause of death from cancer, accounting for 1.6 million deaths a year.[1] Over the past four decades, clinical interventions have had only a minimal effect on reducing death from lung cancer.[2] The recent finding that lung cancer screening with low dose computed tomography can reduce death from lung cancer by 20% in high risk smokers provides an alternative strategy to improve outcomes in this group.[3] Many medical institutions and public health agencies worldwide are considering implementation of lung cancer screening.[4]

Effective implementation of lung cancer screening programs is complex and controversial, and it requires input from clinicians, researchers, public health officials, and the public. Major recent developments include lung cancer risk prediction tools to identify people at high risk who should be screened and a cancer risk calculator to guide clinical management of suspicious or indeterminate lung nodules found in a baseline computed tomogram. This review describes current understanding of low dose computed tomography lung cancer screening, the associated uncertainties, and future advances in the science of lung cancer screening. It also focuses on crucial aspects of screening that are not well covered in other reviews, including who should be screened and what to do when lung nodules are found at screening.

Epidemiology

In 2012, there were 1.8 million cases of lung cancer (13% of all new cases of cancer) and 1.6 million deaths from lung cancer (20% of all cancer deaths) worldwide.[1] It is projected that by 2030, lung cancer will be the third highest cause of death in high income countries and the fifth highest cause in middle income countries.[5] International variation and time trends of the incidence of lung cancer reflect smoking behaviors.[6] The incidence of lung cancer increased throughout most of the 20th century. It then began to decline in American men in the early 1980s and in women around 1999.[6] This pattern is similar in most developed countries, whereas in less developed countries smoking and lung cancer are on the rise.[6]

Most lung cancers are diagnosed at an advanced stage, so survival after lung cancer is generally poor even in developed countries, with five year survival rates of 18% or less.[7] Diagnosis of lung cancer at an early stage is associated with a much higher survival rate of more than 70%.[8] This indicates that early detection with low dose computed tomography could reduce mortality from lung cancer.

Lung cancer screening

Many recent reviews on lung cancer screening exist.[9] [10] Only key topics that are not well covered in previous publications are discussed here. Several lung cancer screening studies have been conducted since the 1950s using chest radiography with or without other modalities, such as sputum cytology.[11] Many of these studies were criticized as having methodological weaknesses and none produced encouraging results. The Prostate, Lung, Colorectal and Ovarian Cancer Screening Trial (PLCO) was the first large well designed and well conducted randomized controlled trial (RCT) to evaluate the effectiveness of annual screening with chest radiography. This trial found that chest radiography screening did not reduce lung cancer mortality.[14]

With rapid advances in imaging technology over the past two decades, it became possible to detect nodules as small as 1 mm by computed tomography using a radiation dose of no more than 1.5 mSv. With this came the hope that low dose computed tomography screening might reduce mortality from lung cancer by detecting early stage cancers while reducing exposure to radiation. Results from the Early Lung Cancer Action Project (ELCAP) suggested that lung cancer could be detected at an earlier stage and survival

SOURCES AND SELECTION CRITERIA

We searched PubMed, Medline, and the Cochrane Library from 1 January 1980 to 1 January 2014 using combinations of words or terms that included lung or pulmonary, cancer or neoplasm, epidemiology or risk factors, and screening or early detection. In addition, risk factors were searched individually by names and synonyms. Articles from the reference lists of articles and text chapters were reviewed and relevant articles were identified. Non-English language abstracts and articles were excluded. Weighting of evidence was commensurate with the appropriateness and quality of study design. We regarded randomized controlled trials as being most suitable for interventions; prospective cohort designs as most suitable for potentially injurious exposures and incidence data; and cross sectional population surveys as most suitable for prevalence data. In addition, results from well conducted meta-analyses were considered to provide strong evidence, especially when summarizing randomized controlled trials and cohort studies.

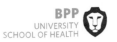

could be extended.[13] Subsequently, the National Lung Screening Trial (NLST) was the first well powered, designed, and conducted RCT to examine the effectiveness of such screening in reducing death from lung cancer.[10] It found that annual screening reduced death from lung cancer by 20% in high risk people aged 55-74 years who had smoked at least 30 pack years (a pack year is the equivalent of smoking one pack of 20 cigarettes a day for one year) and in former smokers who had quit 15 years ago or less.[3 14] This is the most definite finding regarding screening for lung cancer by low dose computed tomography available to date.

Other smaller RCTs have been conducted or are in progress in Europe:
- Detection and Screening of Early Lung Cancer by Novel Imaging Technology and Molecular Assays (DANTE)[15 16]
- Multicentric Italian Lung Detection (MILD) study[17]
- Danish Lung Cancer Screening Trial (DLCST)[18]
- Nederlands-Leuvens Longkanker Screenings Onderzoek (NELSON) trial, or Dutch-Belgian Lung Cancer Screening Trial[19]
- Italian Lung Cancer Computed Tomography Screening Trial (ITALUNG)[20 21]
- Depiscan]–a French pilot lung screening RCT[22]
- German lung cancer screening intervention study (LUSI)[23]
- United Kingdom Lung Screening Trial (UKLS).[24]

The study designs of European lung screening trials have been reviewed.[10 25] To date, published interim results from the DANTE trial,[16] MILD trial,[17] and DLCST[18] have not suggested a protective effect for computed tomography screening, possibly because of small sample sizes, inadequate randomization, unclear allocation, differences in baseline demographic characteristics, differential follow-up, or relatively short duration of follow-up.[10]

Results of the NELSON trial, the second largest trial after the NLST, are awaited in 2015. It is hoped that it will more clearly quantify the effects of screening with low dose computed tomography. Lung cancer screening is more effective when enrollment of screenees is based on accurate risk prediction.[26] It is most effective in people with a high risk,[27] and when performed annually.[28] Also, subset analysis of NLST has shown that screening is more effective in women (overall mortality relative risk: 0.92 in men and 0.73 in women; interaction P=0.08).[29] These associations were all unknown when the NELSON trial was designed. The NELSON trial enrolled fewer participants than the NLST (7557 v 26314 in the screening arm) and more men (84% v 59%). Participants had also smoked fewer pack years (38 v 48 median pack years), and the second to third and third to fourth screenings were spaced 2 and 2.5 years apart, so the study may lack sufficient power and the design may be suboptimal to demonstrate an effect. The European trials, even combined, will probably not have enough statistical power to change the conclusions drawn from the NLST.

As a result of the findings of NLST, several organizations have recommended low dose computed tomography lung cancer screening of high risk people when high quality follow-up and healthcare are available. Recommendations have come from the following organizations:
- American Association of Thoracic Surgery[30 31]
- American College of Chest Physicians, American Society for Clinical Oncology[9]
- American Cancer Society[32]
- American Lung Association[33]
- Cancer Care Ontario[34]
- National Comprehensive Cancer Network[35]

- French Inter-/Oncology Group[36]
- United States Preventive Services Task Force (USPSTF).[37 38]

Most of these recommendations base their definition of high risk on the NLST criteria of age 55-74 years, smoking history of 30 pack years or more (or smokers who had quit no more than 15 years ago), or some variant of the NLST criteria. For the purposes of a screening trial, this definition of risk was practical. However, it is not as useful for selecting people for screening. Because these criteria dichotomize continuous variables, they lose information.[39] Many valuable predictors are omitted, and non-linear effects are ignored.

Recently the USPSTF published recommendations on low dose computed tomography screening for lung cancer.[37 40] It recommended annual screening of people aged 55-80 years who had smoked at least 30 pack years (or smokers who had quit only in the past 15 years). Some USPSTF conclusions were based on microsimulation modeling by the Cancer Intervention and Surveillance Modeling Network (CISNET) Lung Group, which was based on summarizing models prepared by five separate modeling teams.[28] CISNET modeling found that screening was most efficient when conducted every year (versus biennial or triennial screening) and the age range was extended to 80 years.

Over the past few years many institutions have initiated computed tomography lung cancer screening programs and others are planning them. A non-comprehensive list of institutions providing such screening identified by an internet search on 7 February 2014 provides a sense of where screening is being done in the US (box). Variations between selected programs have been documented.[4]

EXAMPLES OF US INSTITUTIONS PROVIDING LUNG SCREENING

University of Alabama at Birmingham, Columbia University Medical Center, Duke Raleigh Hospital in North Carolina, Oklahoma Heart Hospital, University Hospital Seidman Cancer Center in Cleveland Ohio, University of Kansas Cancer Centre, Virginia Hospital Center, Beverly Hospital in Massachusetts, Huntsman Cancer Institute at University of Utah, University of Illinois, University of Southern California Norris Cancer Hospital, MD Anderson at Orlando, Yale Cancer Center.

Disadvantages of screening

The NLST population was healthier and better educated than expected for the general US population. The quality of medical care and outcomes in the NLST were also better. Consequently, computed tomography screening may not perform as well in the general population as in the NLST.[41] Countering this view is the belief that screening extended beyond three annual rounds may be more efficient than observed in the NLST and may lead to greater than 20% mortality reduction.[28] Several screening guidelines emphasize that screening be undertaken only by centers with multidisciplinary specialized teams capable of providing high quality care and follow-up.[9 34]

False positives

As well as causing psychological distress, false positive results can cause unnecessary expense, exposure to radiation, biopsies, and surgery, which can result in pain, disability, and, rarely, death. It is important to minimize false positive results, which are 20% or more in the baseline screen and 3% or more in subsequent screens,[3 14 19] while still having a high sensitivity for lung cancer.

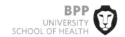

Psychological stress

Some studies have found that lung cancer screening or false positive results are associated with distress or loss of health related quality of life.[42] [43] Others, however, did not detect distress or found that when it was present it was of small magnitude or transient.[44] [45] [46] [47] [48]

Overdiagnosis

This refers to cancers that would not have become clinically significant and led to death if left untreated.[49] Such tumors may be relatively common in some cancers that are screened for, such as breast and prostate cancer. Overdiagnosis can result in the same harms as false positive test results. The extent of overdiagnosis in computed tomography lung cancer screening is unknown. A review of the literature found little evidence of substantial numbers of overdiagnosed lung cancers and concluded that overdiagnosis in lung cancer screening is mostly limited to in situ adenocarcinomas (formally called bronchioloalveolar adenocarcinomas), which appear on computed tomograms as non-solid nodules.[50] To reduce overdiagnosis, Grannis suggests "clear evidence of progression in the form of growth or transition from non-solid to part-solid or solid nodules" before recommending a biopsy or surgical resection.[50] Although most pure non-solid nodules seem to be slow growing, a recent study, which retrospectively reviewed resected and pathologically examined non-solid nodules, showed that 12% of pure non-solid nodules were invasive adenocarcinoma and another 16% were minimally invasive adenocarcinoma.[51] The study suggests that the criteria for "evidence of progression" require a clearer definition and further research.

On the basis of CISNET modeling, the USPSTF estimated overdiagnosis to occur in 10-12% of lung cancers.[38] An analysis of overdiagnosis in the NLST estimated an overdiagnosis rate with three annual screens of 19% (95% confidence interval 16% to 23%) versus chest radiography with seven years of follow-up and 9% (5% to 13%) with lifetime follow-up.[52] Another study assessed overdiagnosis using volume doubling time.[53] It found that 25% of the lung cancers detected on screening were slow growing or indolent, and that many of them may have been overdiagnosed. Further research is needed to help understand and estimate the extent of overdiagnosis. For example, we need to understand the differing and interacting roles played by indolence and death not caused by lung cancer in overdiagnosis and how they change with age.

Exposure to excess radiation

It has been estimated that one death from cancer per 2500 people screened may be caused by radiation from three low dose computed tomography screens plus related diagnostic imaging.[9] A contrasting view is presented in the 2011 American Association of Physicists in Medicine policy statement: "Risks of medical imaging at effective doses below 50 mSv for single procedures or 100 mSv for multiple procedures over short time periods are too low to be detectable and may be nonexistent."[54] However, this could underestimate the effect of repeated screens, especially in those who are screened annually until 74 or 80 years of age.

The potential for harm is shown by a study in children under the age of 15, which showed a significant excess relative risk of 0.036 per mGy of radiation (95% confidence interval 0.005 to 0.120; P=0.0097) from computed tomography for leukemia and 0·023 per mGy of radiation

(0.010 to 0.049; P<0.0001) for brain cancer.[55] Technology is rapidly changing, and lung cancer screening can now be done with as little as 0.1 mSv using the new generation of dual source computed tomography scanners with selective photon shields. However, ongoing research into the harmful effects of radiation is needed, and several large cohort studies of adults exposed to diagnostic imaging are in progress worldwide.

Harris and colleagues reviewed the literature on screening harms and proposed a taxonomy for classifying harms, in particular for lung cancer screening.[56] The review concluded that decisions to screen are more often based on evidence of benefits, and that data on harms are less available and when available are given less weighting.[56]

Cost effectiveness

Cost effectiveness analyses have assessed whether the benefits of computed tomography lung cancer screening outweigh the hazards and whether the costs to society and the medical system are affordable.[57] [58] [59] [60] [61] [62] [63] [64] [65] [66] [67] [68] These studies' methods, perspectives, assumptions, data sources, outcomes, subset analyses, and findings differ. Their outcomes have ranged widely, from a low of $2500 (£1500; €1812) for an incremental cost effectiveness ratio per one year of life saved for one baseline screen,[60] to a high of $2 322 700 per one quality adjusted life year saved in former smokers.[59] However, none of these studies was based on real world RCT data. The cost effectiveness analysis based on NLST data estimated $67 000 per quality adjusted life year gained.

Preliminary analysis from the Pan-Canadian Early Detection of Lung Cancer study suggested that the cost of a screening program could be cost neutral to healthcare providers.[69] This is because low dose computed tomography screening led to the detection of mostly early stage (I and II) cancers, which can be treated with surgical resection and cost around half as much to treat as stage III and IV lung cancers.[69] Targeted therapies, such as tyrosine kinase inhibitors, cost much more than chemotherapy.[70] In addition, compared with surgical treatment with curative intent for early stage lung cancer, chemotherapy and targeted therapy for advanced disease are largely palliative.

Several factors influence the cost of a screening program. Costs are highly sensitive to the risk of lung cancer, the number of follow-up computed tomograms and other imaging studies, complications from diagnostic procedures, and treatment.

Smoking cessation rates among current smokers also affect cost effectiveness. In the general population, the annual spontaneous smoking cessation rate is 3-7%.[71] In observational computed tomography studies, cessation rates vary from 7% to 23%. In the Danish Lung Screening Trial, smoking cessation rates in participants with and without positive computed tomography results were 17.7% and 11.9%, respectively.[72] In the Lung Screening Study component of the NLST, the probability of subsequent smoking was inversely associated with the abnormality of the screening result in a dose-response fashion (P<0.001).[73] Other studies have also found higher smoking cessation rates in those who have abnormal results on computed tomography.[74] [75] These findings suggest that lung cancer screening may help reduce smoking in current smokers, and hence reduce all cause mortality.

The cost effectiveness of lung cancer screening can be improved by screening high risk people selected by an

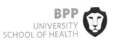

accurate risk prediction tool, optimization of lung nodule management protocols, and integration of effective smoking cessation programs within screening programs.

Predicting the risk of lung cancer

Lung cancer screening is most effective when applied to people at high risk.[26] [27] To identify these people and improve lung cancer risk prediction models, which can be used to select potential screenees, it is useful to understand the risk factors for lung cancer (summarized in web table). The use of an accurate risk prediction model that incorporates risk factors besides age and smoking history is more efficient at identifying people who will develop lung cancer and die from the disease and leads to more efficient screening (lung cancers deaths averted per screen) compared with NLST criteria.[26] [27] When the Tammemagi 2012 prediction model[26] used with the same number of smokers from the PLCO trial as the NLST criteria, it had 11.9% (P<0.001) greater sensitivity in identifying those who would be diagnosed with lung cancer in six years of follow-up. It also had a significantly higher positive predictive value (PPV) than the NLST criteria (4.0% v 3.4%; P<0.01).

Another prediction model showed that the number of deaths from lung cancer averted per 10 000 person years in the computed tomography screening group, compared with the radiography group, increased with risk (0.2 in the lowest fifth, then 3.5, 5.1, 11.0, and 12.0 in the highest fifth; P=0.01 for trend).[27]

The use of accurate risk prediction models to identify people at high risk should improve cost effectiveness and reduce the numbers of false positive screens. The International Association for the Study of Lung Cancer high risk working group has recommended that lung cancer screening be based on high risk, and that risk prediction models are most useful for this purpose.[76]

To be useful in lung cancer screening, prediction models need to show high predictive performance as measured by discrimination or ability to classify disease status and by calibration—that is, does the model predicted probability match the observed probability. The receiver operator characteristic area under the curve (AUC) or its equivalent, the C-statistic, are often used to evaluate discriminations.

Specific risk prediction models

Currently, at least 15 lung cancer risk prediction models exist. They differ in the populations that they can be used in, requirements for patient contact and clinical information, and study designs used in modeling and evaluating predictive performance. Some models have been developed in special populations and apply only to that population. The Etzel model is for African-Americans, and the Li and Park models apply to Chinese and Korean men, respectively.[77] [78] [79] Maisonneuve presented two models. The first is a version of the Bach model recalibrated in an Italian population for identifying those at high risk who would be suitable for screening; the second model uses initial screening results so is not applicable for pre-screening use.[80] The Spitz expanded model, Young, Hippisley-Cox, Li, and Iyen-Omofoman models use biomarker, genetic, or clinical data that require patient contact, biosampling, and testing or they use medical record data.[78] [81] [82] [83] [84] These models are therefore not useful for population sampling based on self report and non-personal contact. The Kovalchik model is the only one that is primarily modeled on death from lung cancer using NLST data.[27] However, the NLST selected

high risk people for screening so the trial's sample was representative of only about 40% of all smokers. In addition, the follow-up periods in many NLST lung cancer cases were not long enough to identify mortality. Hence, this model was based on less than 50% of the lung cancer deaths expected in a population of smokers.

The Cassidy (Liverpool Lung Projects) and Spitz models are based on matched case-control data so were unable to evaluate important variables including age and some smoking variables.[85] [86] They also did not work directly with incidence data, which best estimates risk, so are vulnerable to calibration problems. They show only moderate discrimination when compared with other models that are based on prospective data in smokers. The Bach model was based on a high risk population of smokers or people exposed to asbestos (or both) from the Beta-Carotene and Retinol Efficacy Trial (CARET). The Tammemagi 2011 and 2012 PLCO models and the Hoggart European Prospective Investigation into Cancer and Nutrition (EPIC) model were based on large prospectively followed population based samples not limited to people at high risk of lung cancer,[26] [87] [88] and they show high discrimination in smokers.

Population and medical system based approaches

Implementation of lung cancer screening may be population based or medical system based, and this will determine how the risk of potential screenees is assessed. Population based approaches can use an existing model and do not require direct contact—risk can be assessed by telephone or online. This approach is relatively simple, has broad coverage, and is less time consuming and costly than the medical system based approach.

The medical system based approach works through direct contact with patients. It can therefore make use of clinical data and data from validated biomarker testing in risk prediction models. Currently, no biomarkers have been shown to help detect early stage lung cancer or select high risk people for screening. However, in the future, validated biomarkers may be measured using assays on airway epithelium, sputum, exhaled breath, and blood.[89] Medical system based enrollment into screening is expected to be more time consuming and costly than the population based approach, but it may be more effective in enrolling some sectors of society. Relevant data from clinical evaluation, medical records, and biomarker assays can be incorporated into novel risk models.

Several problems remain regarding the integration of model based risk prediction into lung screening programs. These include how best to select people for screening to optimize sensitivity, specificity, and cost effectiveness compared with the USPSTF criteria, and whether risk should be revised on the basis of findings in previous screens, increasing age, and duration of smoking cessation. In the next year, ongoing research is likely to provide improvements in the application of risk prediction models to the selection of screenees.

Management of screen detected lung nodules

Other considerations when implementing computed tomography screening at the population level include the definition of a positive screen and the appropriate management of screen detected lung nodules. The first round of screening generates the greatest number of diagnostic investigations because there are no previous imaging studies to help decide whether lung nodules are

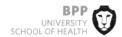

Table 1 Management thresholds for pulmonary nodules found on first (baseline) low dose computed tomography (LDCT) screen

Guideline or study protocol	Annual or next scheduled scan	Repeat LDCT before next scheduled annual LDCT	Biopsy or surgery with or without prior PET-CT or LDCT in 3 months
Solid nodules			
NCCN[35 94]	<6 mm	6-8 mm	>8 mm, hypermetabolism†, or interval growth
Fleischner Society[95]	≤4 mm	>4 to 8 mm	>8 mm, hypermetabolism, or interval growth
ACCP[96]	≤4 mm	>4-8 mm and pretest probability <5%; nodule >8 mm, pretest probability <30%, and negative PET	Biopsy for nodule >8 mm, pretest probability 5% to 65%, and hypermetabolism or interval growth; surgery for nodule >8 mm and pretest probability >65% or hypermetabolism
NLST (ACRIN)[3 14 97]	<4 mm	4-10 mm	>10 mm
NELSON[19 98]	Benign or nodule <50 mm³	50-500 mm³ (diameter 4.6-9.8 mm); pleural based 5-10 mm minimum diameter	>500 mm³ (diameter >9.8 mm); pleural based >10 mm minimum diameter
I-ELCAP[99 100]	<5 mm	≥5-14 mm	>15 mm
Part solid nodules			
NCCN[35 94]	<6 mm	6-8 mm	>8 mm with interval growth or increased in solid component
Fleischner Society[101]		Solid component <5 mm	Solid component .5 mm or nodule >10 mm
ACCP[96]		≤8 mm	>8 mm with interval growth or increase in solid component; nodule >15 mm
NLST (ACRIN)[3 14 97]	<4 mm	4-10 mm	>10 mm
NELSON[19 98]	<8 mm and solid component <50 mm³	Non-solid component .8 mm and solid component 50-500 mm³	Solid component >500 mm³
I-ELCAP[99 100]	<5 mm	≥5-14 mm	>15 mm
Non-solid nodules			
NCCN[35 94]	≤5 mm	>5-10 mm	>10 mm with interval growth or increased attenuation
Fleischner Society[101]	None	>5 mm	>10 mm with interval growth or increased attenuation
ACCP[96]	>5 mm		>10 mm and persistent, interval growth, or development of solid component
NLST (ACRIN)[3, 14 97]	≤10 mm		
NELSON[19 98]	<8 mm	≥8 mm mean diameter	
I-ELCAP[99 100]	<5 mm	≥8 mm	≥15 mm

*ACCP=American College of Chest Physicians; I-ELCAP=International Early Lung Cancer Action Program; NCCN=National Comprehensive Cancer Network; NELSON=Dutch-Belgium randomized lung screening trial; NLST=National Lung Screening Trial; PET-CT=positron emission tomography-computed tomography.
†Hypermetabolism=increased FDG uptake.

Table 2 Implication for resource utilization of different clinical follow-up pathways*

Screen	NLST[14 90]	NELSON[19 91]
Baseline screen		
Number screened	26 309	7557
Repeat chest computed tomography	5153 (19.6%)	1438 (19%)
PET-CT	728 (2.8%)	0
Biopsy	461 (1.8%)	162 (2.1%)
Surgery	297 (1.1%)	92 (1.2%)
Lung cancer diagnosed	270 (1%)	70 (0.9%)
Surgery for benign disease	30%	35%
First annual repeat screen		
Number screened	24 715	7289
Repeat chest computed tomography	2046 (8.3%)	275 (3.8%)
PET-CT	350 (1.4%)	0
Biopsy	238 (0.96%)	101 (1.39%)
Surgery	197 (0.8%)	61 (0.8%)
Lung cancer diagnosed	168 (0.7%)	55 (0.8%)
Surgery for benign disease	26%	21%

*NELSON=Dutch-Belgium randomized lung screening trial; NLST=National Lung Screening Trial; PET-CT=positron emission tomography-computed tomography.

new or to determine their growth behaviors.[15 19 90 91 92 93] To minimize downstream investigations—such as repeat chest imaging, biopsy, or even surgical resection, which can harm the participant and increase costs—RCTs, cohort studies, and practice guidelines use action thresholds based on nodule type and nodule size (table 1).[3 14 35 19 94 95 96 97 98 99 100 101]

Different size cut-offs points (from 4 mm to 15 mm) are used for solid, partly solid, or non-solid nodules. Nodule diameter is used in some protocols, whereas others use volume measurements. Some guidelines use a combination of nodule size, nodule type, and malignancy pre-test probability.[96] Positron emission tomography-computed tomography (PET-CT) is an integral part of the diagnostic algorithm in some guidelines but not in others.

All RCTs defined what a positive screen is. Some trials, such as NELSON, have a formal diagnostic regimen for investigating patients with a positive screen. In NLST, the decision about how to proceed was left to the referring physician owing to variation in clinical practice and local expertise. Nevertheless, resource utilization was similar in NLST and NELSON with regard to repeat imaging studies before the next annual repeat screen, biopsy or surgery rates, and proportion of surgical procedures for benign disease (table 2).[14 19 90 91] After the first annual repeat screen, when the new images could be compared with baseline images to look for new nodules or evidence of growth of pre-existing lung nodules, the proportion of repeat imaging requests was lower in the NELSON study. However, the proportion of lung biopsies was slightly higher in the NELSON study, although a similar proportion of lung cancer cases was diagnosed. Thus, while the volumetric measurement and volume doubling time used in NELSON are theoretically more accurate than two dimensional measurements to monitor growth in subsequent screens, the two methods have similar resource utilization for the first (baseline) scan.

The corresponding data on the I-ELCAP protocol (1.7% biopsy rate, 1.3% surgery rate, and 1.3% lung cancer diagnosed) were similar, although the study does not allow an analysis of frequency of repeat chest computed tomography, the frequency of diagnostic PET-CT, or the proportion of biopsies or surgery performed for benign disease.[102] Depending on the frequency of biopsy to confirm the diagnosis of lung cancer before surgery, 6-43% of surgical procedures were performed for a benign diagnosis.[9]

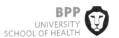

Category	Low dose computed tomography finding	Action plan
CAT1	Normal finding, benign calcification, perifissural nodule, hamartoma, nodule risk index <1.5%	Consider biennial screening
CAT2	Low risk of malignancy: Nodule risk index 1.5% to <6%	Schedule annual repeat screening
CAT3	Moderate risk of malignancy: Nodule risk index 6% to <30%	Rescreen in 3 months: • If no growth, annual screening • If interval growth, refer for definitive diagnosis • May consider definitive diagnosis for nodule risk index between 10% and <30% after discussion between the clinician and patient
CAT4	High risk of malignancy: Nodule risk index ≥30%	Refer for definitive diagnosis
CAT5	Suspicious for lung cancer: Mass lesion with a non-infectious cause; mediastinal or hilar lymphadenopathy irrespective of nodule size	Refer for definitive diagnosis

Fig 1 Probabilistic approach to guide clinical decisions using the Pan Canadian model

Table 3 Accuracy measurements for pulmonary cancer at different risk score thresholds using the Pan Canadian prediction model[92]*

Measurement	Risk score (%)								
	1.5	6	10	20	30	40	50	60	70
Sensitivity (%)	89.1	73.9	60.9	47.83	32.6	23.9	12.0	7.6	2.2
Specificity (%)	88.4	96.4	97.7	98.8	99.3	99.7	99.9	99.9	100.0
Positive predictive value (%)	9.9	22.7	27.1	37.0	40.0	55.0	55.0	63.6	50.0
Negative predictive value (%)	99.8	99.6	99.4	99.3	99.0	98.9	98.8	98.7	98.6
Accuracy (%)	88.4	96.1	97.2	98.1	98.4	98.7	98.6	98.6	98.6
Nodules positive (%)	12.7	4.6	3.2	1.8	1.14	0.61	0.31	0.17	0.06

*Using the parsimonious model without spiculation.

Table 4 Lung cancer risk in relation to baseline low dose computed tomography finding

Baseline finding	Participants (%)	Lung cancer risk (%)
NELSON criteria*		
Negative (<50 mm³)	79.2	1
Indeterminate (50-500 mm³)	19.2	5.7
Positive (>500 mm³)	1.6	48.3
Pan Canadian criteria†		
CAT 1: No nodule or nodule risk <1.5%	80	0.7
CAT 2: Nodule risk 1.5% to <6%	12	6
CAT 3: Nodule risk 6% to <30%	6	24
CAT 4: Nodule risk ≥30%	2	57

*Lung cancer risk over 5.5 years.[91]
†From 4360 participants with median follow-up of 4.7 years including those without lung nodules not in reference 92. None of the participants in the CAT 1 group was diagnosed as having lung cancer within 12 months of the baseline scan.

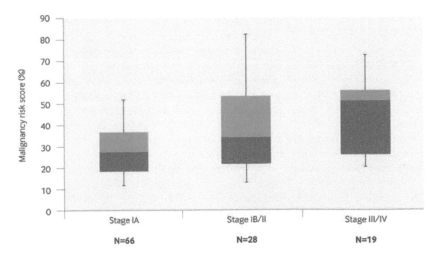

Fig 2 Box and whisker plot showing the distribution of nodule risk scores according to tumor stage in the Pan Canadian study.[92] The boxes represent the 25th to 75th centiles, with the medians indicated by the horizontal lines. The whiskers represent the 5th to 95th centiles

External validation

An externally validated probabilistic approach to guide clinical decisions at the first (baseline) screen without information on growth or density change was recently reported.[92] This Pan Canadian prediction model and calculator (www.brocku.ca/lung-cancer-risk-calculator) simplifies decision management by not having separate models for solid versus non-solid and partly solid nodules.[35 95 96 101] Previous lung nodule prediction models were retrospective in design, hospital or clinic based, and were based on people with a high prevalence of lung cancer (23-54%) compared with the general high risk population screening setting (≤5%).[104 105 106 107]

When externally validated, other models have modest accuracy.[107 108 109] Models based on lung nodules detected by chest radiography may not be applicable to the screening setting,[104 105 106] where more than half of lung cancers are 2 cm or less and about 25% of lung nodules are non-solid or partly solid and rarely visible on chest radiography.[80 92] When the full Pan Canadian model without spiculation (irregular margins) of the lung nodule was applied to an external validation dataset, the AUC was 0.97 (0.947 to 0.986).[92] Even when the model was limited to nodules 10 mm or less, or to non-solid nodules alone or non-solid plus part solid nodules, the AUC was 0.936 (0.872 to 0.978), 0.918 (0.835 to 0.968), and 0.933 (0.882 to 0.968), respectively.[92 110]

Table 3 shows the Pan Canadian model's prediction accuracies by probability cut-off points. These cut-off points may serve as a framework to guide clinical investigations (fig 1).[92] For example, screenees with no lung nodules or nodules with a risk score of less than 1.5% have a less than 0.7% chance of lung cancer with a median follow-up of 4.7 years (table 4).[92]

In the NELSONa study, the risk of lung cancer was 1% over 5.5 years in people with no nodules or nodules 50 mm³ or less (table 4).[91] A similarly low risk of lung cancer was found in other studies in people with no nodules or nodules of 3 mm or less.[14 17 111] Annual screening may not be needed in this very low risk group. The thresholds for biopsy or surgery with or without a previous repeat low dose computed tomography scan or PET-CT scan can be determined by the nodule risk score, physician's assessment, and patient preference.

Figure 2 shows the distribution of the risk scores versus tumor stage using the raw data in the Pan Canadian study.[92] Stage IA tumors had a risk score of 10% or more. A risk score of 30% has a PPV of 40% (table 3). Only 1.14% of the nodules have a risk score of 30% or more (table 3).[92] In other studies, the PPV of abnormal screening results using

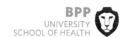

nodule diameter or volume ranges from 2.2% to 36%.[10] In the NLST study, the PPV for nodules larger than 30 mm was 41.3%.[10][90]

A Pan Canadian nodule risk score of 30% or more suggests that a diagnostic biopsy is needed. In people with a Pan Canadian risk score of 6-30%, a repeat scan can be done in three months to look for evidence of interval growth before deciding on a biopsy. This lower limit has a PPV of 22.7 and an NPV of 99.6 for malignancy. Those with risk scores of 1.5% to less than 6% can have their scheduled annual repeat scan. This probabilistic approach (fig 1) can greatly reduce costs and the risk of morbidity and mortality associated with clinical diagnostic investigations. Algorithms like this can be prospectively evaluated by monitoring the frequency of additional imaging studies, non-surgical biopsies, surgical resection, and the outcome of these procedures.

Tumor volume

The management of lung nodules identified after the first screen is simplified by having a previous scan for comparison to determine whether a nodule is new or whether the size or density of a pre-existing nodule have changed. For new nodules detected in the second or subsequent screening rounds, criteria similar to the baseline scan are often used, although some studies use a more aggressive follow-up protocol, with shorter intervals between repeat scans.[100]

For pre-existing nodules, a greater than 25% increase in volume or a tumor volume doubling time of less than 400 days is considered to be a positive test result if volumetric analysis is used. If nodule diameter is used, a minimum of more than 1 mm increase in the maximum diameter or at least a 10% increase is considered positive.[97][112] For non-solid or semi-solid nodules, the development of a solid component or an increase in the size of the solid component, respectively, are suspicious for malignancy (table 1). Positive nodules would then undergo clinical diagnostic investigations.

Although volumetric analysis is theoretically more accurate for measuring growth in non-spherical nodules,[113][114][115][116] two dimensional diameter measurement is commonly used because of its simplicity. Semi-automated or fully automated three dimensional volume measurement requires specially provided software and measurement variability is still too high for non-solid and semi-solid nodules,[114][117] although the technology is improving rapidly.[118][119][120]

Tumor volume doubling time is often misunderstood. Because small nodules are not usually biopsied, it is not possible to tell whether a long volume doubling time reflects the growth behavior of preinvasive lesions (atypical adenomatous hyperplasia or adenocarcinoma in situ) before it becomes invasive versus the true tumor growth rate. In a surgical series, 66% of the pure ground glass nodules suspicious enough to be removed by surgery were atypical adenomatous hyperplasia or adenocarcinoma in situ.[51]

Tumor volume doubling time can increase, decrease, or both during the course of disease.[121][122] The fact that a preinvasive or minimally invasive lesion is growing slowly does not mean that it cannot evolve into a lethal cancer. In addition, it is not possible to determine prospectively, at an individual level, which lung cancers are overdiagnosed because it is not known which patients would have died from lung cancer if they had not been treated.[121] The International Association for the Study of Lung Cancer and other organizations are working to clarify a pathway for the

management of lung nodules on the basis of best available evidence.[123]

Frequency of screening

CISNET microsimulation modeling assessed annual, biennial, and triennial screening intervals and concluded that annual screening was most efficient.[28] In contrast, a small Italian pilot RCT comparing annual and biennial CT screening with regular care found no significant difference in lung cancer mortality between annual and biennial screening.[17] However, it also found that screening did not reduce death from lung cancer compared with controls, so the results do not provide strong evidence in favor of biennial screening. The optimum frequency of screening requires further research. In low risk groups, such as those with no nodules on the baseline screen or nodules with a lung cancer risk of 1.5% or less, annual screening may not be needed (table 4).

Duration of screening

The optimum duration of screening is also yet to be defined. The longest duration of screening in an RCT is five years. The benefits of annual screening for up to 25 years are unknown. The potential harm of radiation and the discovery of new nodules that are not malignant should not be underestimated. There are insufficient data to recommend repeat screening annually until age 80 for everyone after participation in the first round of screening. For example, the individual risk of lung cancer may need to be revised downward for those with a negative baseline screen (table 4), those with repeat normal screens, and long term former smokers.[80][91][124] Those at low risk may not benefit from a repeat scan for two or more years. Studying the variability of risk by birth cohorts using pooled data from studies with long term follow-up will shed light on this.

If the duration of smoking cessation is used as an exclusion criterion, a screening program needs to specify that screening would eventually stop in former smokers. However, recent analyses indicate that some increased risks that warranting screening remain long after the 15 years since quitting threshold (MC Tammemagi, unpublished data, 2014).

Evaluation of lung cancer screening programs

It is generally accepted that systematic cancer screening is more effective than ad hoc screening. Quality assurance measures should be in place to evaluate the performance of the program. For lung cancer screening, such measures have not been well defined. However, they may include whether there was a stage shift to earlier stage at detection and a reduction in lung cancer mortality in the screened population compared with the unscreened target population, as well as the proportion of the target population that was contacted and participated.

Future directions

The reading and interpretation of low dose computed tomograms are time consuming because the scans contain 200-400 high resolution sections. Reading involves slowly scrolling through thin slab maximum intensity projections to detect pulmonary nodules. This task requires around 10 minutes per scan, which is substantially more than the amount of time needed to inspect four mammograms in breast cancer screening. Reader variability is substantial.[125]

In the NLST trial, the mean false positive rate for radiologists was estimated at 28.7% (standard deviation

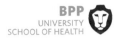

13.7%), with a range of 3.8-69.0%.[126] Quality assurance of the interpretation of diagnostic and screening computed tomograms is a hot topic. Computer vision software tools that interpret such scans to determine whether nodule(s) are present and to identify scans that do not require further formal reading by a chest radiologist are being developed. When they have high accuracy for true negativity, they could be used to process large numbers of lung screening images at reduced costs.

Diagnostic biomarkers using blood or other non-invasively obtained specimens such as exhaled breath may have a role in sub-centimeter nodules or people whose scans are negative. A major advance in lung cancer screening would be the ability to identify people who are at risk of developing interval lung cancer that is more likely to be aggressive. Promising predictive biomarkers of the risk of lung cancer, such as spirometry, micro-RNA and pro-surfactant protein B,[127] [128] [129] need to be evaluated to determine their incremental value and cost implication versus clinical, demographic, and imaging parameters that are readily obtained without laboratory testing. Quantitative analysis of the nodule and the adjacent lung parenchyma, vessels, and airways may provide valuable information on risk of cancer. The accuracy of an individual's overall risk of lung cancer can also be increased by using information about environmental and occupational exposures as well as validated biomarkers.

Conclusion

Lung cancer screening with low dose computed tomography in high risk smokers can reduce lung cancer mortality by about 20%. Currently, no new treatment modality can reduce death from lung cancer to this extent. The development of lung cancer risk prediction tools to identify people at high risk is a major advance in lung cancer screening. In addition, accurate lung nodule malignancy risk calculators can reduce the number of people who need follow-up scans and other

investigations for suspicious or indeterminate lung nodules found in a baseline computed tomogram from over 20% to less than 8%. Sufficient data exist to support implementation of trial screening programs, which if successful and made efficient can be expanded to widespread population based screening programs to improve the outcome of patients with lung cancer. Staged programs will provide the framework to refine the screening parameters to incorporate new data and ideas as they emerge.

Contributors: Both authors substantially contributed to the conception and design of the work; the acquisition, analysis, and interpretation of the data; and drafting the work and revising it critically for important intellectual content. They both approved the final version for publication. MCT is accountable for epidemiologic aspects of the work and SL is accountable for clinical aspects of the work. SL is guarantor.

Competing interests: We have read and understood the BMJ Group policy on declaration of interests and declare the following interests: None.

Provenance and peer review: Commissioned; externally peer reviewed.

1   Brambilla E, Travis WD, Brennan P, Harris CC, Padilla JRP. Lung cancer. In: Stewart BW, Wild CP, eds. World cancer report 2014. International Agency for Research on Cancer, 2014:350-61.
2   Siegel R, Naishadham D, Jemal A. Cancer statistics, 2013. CA Cancer J Clin2013;63:11-30.
3   Aberle DR, Adams AM, Berg CD, Black WC, Clapp JD, Fagerstrom RM, et al. Reduced lung-cancer mortality with low-dose computed tomographic screening. N Engl J Med2011;365:395-409.
4   Boiselle PM, White CS, Ravenel JG. Computed tomographic screening for lung cancer: current practice patterns at leading academic medical centers. JAMA Intern Med2014;174:286-7.
5   Mathers CD, Loncar D. Projections of global mortality and burden of disease from 2002 to 2030. PLoS Med2006;11:e442.
6   Youlden DR, Cramb SM, Baade PD. The international epidemiology of lung cancer: geographical distribution and secular trends. J Thorac Oncol2008;3:819-31.
7   Coleman MP, Forman D, Bryant H, Butler J, Rachet B, Maringe C, et al. Cancer survival in Australia, Canada, Denmark, Norway, Sweden, and the UK, 1995-2007 (the International Cancer Benchmarking Partnership): an analysis of population-based cancer registry data. Lancet2011;377:127-38.
8   Goldstraw P, Crowley J, Chansky K, Giroux DJ, Groome PA, Rami-Porta R, et al. The IASLC Lung Cancer Staging Project: proposals for the revision of the TNM stage groupings in the forthcoming (seventh) edition of the TNM classification of malignant tumours. J Thorac Oncol2007;2:706-14.
9   Bach PB, Mirkin JN, Oliver TK, Azzoli CG, Berry DA, Brawley OW, et al. Benefits and harms of CT screening for lung cancer: a systematic reviewbenefits and harms of ct screening for lung cancer. JAMA 2012;307:2418-29.
10 Humphrey LL, Deffebach M, Pappas M, Baumann C, Artis K, Mitchell JP, et al. Screening for lung cancer with low-dose computed tomography: a systematic review to update the US Preventive Services Task Force recommendation. Ann Intern Med2013;159:411-20.
11 Manser RL, Irving LB, Byrnes G, Abramson MJ, Stone CA, Campbell DA. Screening for lung cancer: a systematic review and meta-analysis of controlled trials. Thorax 2003;58:784-9.
12 Oken MM, Hocking WG, Kvale PA, Andriole GL, Buys SS, Church TR, et al. Screening by chest radiograph and lung cancer mortality: the Prostate, Lung, Colorectal, and Ovarian (PLCO) randomized trial. JAMA2011;306:1865-73.
13 Henschke CI. Early lung cancer action project: overall design and findings from baseline screening. Cancer 2000;89:2474-82.
14 Aberle DR, DeMello S, Berg CD, Black WC, Brewer B, Church TR, et al. Results of the two incidence screenings in the National Lung Screening Trial. N Engl J Med2013;369:920-31.
15 Infante M, Lutman FR, Cavuto S, Brambilla G, Chiesa G, Passera E, et al. Lung cancer screening with spiral CT: baseline results of the randomized DANTE trial. Lung Cancer2008;59:355-63.
16 Infante M, Cavuto S, Lutman FR, Brambilla G, Chiesa G, Ceresoli G, et al. A randomized study of lung cancer screening with spiral computed tomography: three-year results from the DANTE trial. Am J Respir Crit Care Med2009;180:445-53.
17 Pastorino U, Rossi M, Rosato V, Marchianò A, Sverzellati N, Morosi C, et al. Annual or biennial CT screening versus observation in heavy smokers: 5-year results of the MILD trial. Eur J Cancer Prev2012;21:308-15.
18 Saghir Z, Dirksen A, Ashraf H, Bach KS, Brodersen J, Clementsen PF, et al. CT screening for lung cancer brings forward early disease. The randomised Danish Lung Cancer Screening trial: status after five annual screening rounds with low-dose CT. Thorax2012;67:296-301.
19 Van Klaveren RJ, Oudkerk M, Prokop M, Scholten ET, Nackaerts K, Vernhout R, et al. Management of lung nodules detected by volume CT scanning. N Engl J Med2009;361:2221-9.

TRIAL ACRONYMS

- CISNET: Cancer Intervention and Surveillance Modeling Network
- DANTE: Detection and Screening of Early Lung Cancer by Novel Imaging Technology and Molecular Assays
- DLCST: Danish Lung Cancer Screening Trial
- I-ELCAP: International Early Lung Cancer Action Project
- MILD: Multicentric Italian Lung Detection study
- NELSON: Nederlands-Leuvens Longkanker Screenings Onderzoek
- NLST: National Lung Screening Trial
- PLCO: Prostate, Lung, Colorectal and Ovarian Cancer Screening Trial
- USPSTF: United States Preventive Services Task Force

FUTURE RESEARCH AREAS

- The accurate measurement of the harmful effects of low dose computed tomography screening radiation
- Several problems remain regarding the integration of model based risk prediction into lung screening programs:
- At what model estimated risk should people be selected for screening to optimize sensitivity, specificity, and cost effectiveness compared with the US Preventive Services Task Force criteria?
- For which populations do we need unique risk prediction models? For example, are they needed for those who are exposed to specific occupational lung carcinogens, or populations which may have unique indoor and outdoor environmental exposures and genetic predispositions, such as Asian people? How can this be accomplished in the absence of complete quality data?
- Do repeat normal lung cancer screens revise a person's baseline risk downward?

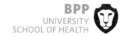

20 Lopes Pegna A, Picozzi G, Mascalchi M, Maria Carozzi F, Carrozzi L, Comin C, et al. Design, recruitment and baseline results of the ITALUNG trial for lung cancer screening with low-dose CT. *Lung Cancer* 2009;64:34-40.

21 Lopes Pegna A, Picozzi G, Falaschi F, Carrozzi L, Falchini M, Carozzi FM, et al. Four-year results of low-dose CT screening and nodule management in the ITALUNG trial. *J Thorac Oncol* 2013;8:866-75.

22 Blanchon T, Brechot JM, Grenier PA, Ferretti GR, Lemarie F, Milleron B, et al. Baseline results of the Depiscan study: a French randomized pilot trial of lung cancer screening comparing low dose CT scan (LDCT) and chest X-ray (CXR). *Lung Cancer* 2007;58:50-8.

23 Becker N, Motsch E, Gross ML, Eigentopf A, Heussel CP, Dienemann H, et al. Randomized study on early detection of lung cancer with MSCT in Germany: study design and results of the first screening round. *J Cancer Res Clin Oncol* 2012;138:1475-86.

24 Baldwin DR, Duffy SW, Wald NJ, Page R, Hansell DM, Field JK. UK Lung Screen (UKLS) nodule management protocol: modelling of a single screen randomised controlled trial of low-dose CT screening for lung cancer. *Thorax* 2011;66:308-13.

25 Field JK, van Klaveren R, Pedersen JH, JH, Pastorino U, Paci E, Becker N, et al. European randomized lung cancer screening trials: post NLST. *J Surg Oncol* 2013;108:280-6.

26 Tammemagi MC, Katki HA, Hocking WG, Church T, Caporaso N, Kvale P, et al. Selection criteria for lung-cancer screening. *N Engl J Med* 2013;368:728-36.

27 Kovalchik SA, Tammemagi M, Berg CD, Caporaso NE, Riley TL, Korch M, et al. Targeting of low-dose CT screening according to the risk of lung-cancer death. *N Engl J Med* 2013;369:245-54.

28 De Koning H, Meza R, Plevritis S, ten Haaf K, Munshi VN, Jeon J, et al. Benefits and harms of computed tomography lung cancer screening programs for high-risk populations. Agency for Healthcare Research and Quality, 2013. www.uspreventiveservicestaskforce.org/uspstf13/lungcan/lungcanmodeling.htm.

29 Pinsky PF, Church TR, Izmirlian G, Kramer BS. The national lung screening trial: results stratified by demographics, smoking history, and lung cancer histology. *Cancer* 2013;119:3976-83.

30 Jacobson FL, Austin JH, Field JK, Jett JR, Keshavjee S, Macmahon H, et al. Development of the American Association for Thoracic Surgery guidelines for low-dose computed tomography scans to screen for lung cancer in North America: recommendations of the American Association for Thoracic Surgery task force for lung cancer screening and surveillance. *J Thorac Cardiovasc Surg* 2012;144:25-32.

31 Jaklitsch MT, Jacobson FL, Austin JH, Field JK, Jett JR, Keshavjee S, et al. The American Association for Thoracic Surgery guidelines for lung cancer screening using low-dose computed tomography scans for lung cancer survivors and other high-risk groups. *J Thorac Cardiovasc Surg* 2012;144:33-8.

32 Wender R, Fontham ET, Barrera E Jr, Colditz GA, Church TR, Ettinger DS, et al. American Cancer Society lung cancer screening guidelines. *CA Cancer J Clin* 2013;63:106-17.

33 American Lung Association. American Lung Association provides guidance on lung cancer screening. 2012. www.lung.org/lung-disease/lung-cancer/lung-cancer-screening-guidelines.

34 Roberts H, Walker Dilks C, Sivjee K, Ung Y, Yasufuku K, Hey A, et al. Screening high-risk populations for lung cancer—guideline recommendations. *J Thorac Oncol* 2013;8:1232-7.

35 National Comprehensive Cancer Network clinical practice guidelines for detection, prevention and risk reduction. Version 1.2014. Lung cancer screening. 2014. www.nccn.org/professionals/physician_gls/f_guidelines.asp#lung_screening.

36 Couraud S, Cortot AB, Greillier L, Gounant V, Mennecier B, Girard N, et al. From randomized trials to the clinic: is it time to implement individual lung-cancer screening in clinical practice? A multidisciplinary statement from French experts on behalf of the french intergroup (IFCT) and the groupe d'Oncologie de langue francaise (GOLF). *Ann Oncol* 2013;24:586-97.

37 US Preventive Services Task Force. Screening for lung cancer: US Preventive Services Task Force draft. 2013. www.uspreventiveservicestaskforce.org/draftrec.htm.

38 Moyer VA. Screening for lung cancer: US Preventive Services Task Force recommendation statement. *Ann Intern Med* 2013; published online 31 Dec.

39 Royston P, Altman DG, Sauerbrei W. Dichotomizing continuous predictors in multiple regression: a bad idea. *Stat Med* 2006;25:127-41.

40 Humphrey L, Deffebach M, Pappas M, Baumann C, Artis K, Mitchell JP, et al. Screening for lung cancer: systematic review to update the US Preventive Services Task Force recommendation. Evidence synthesis no 105. Agency for Healthcare Research and Quality. 2013. www.uspreventiveservicestaskforce.org/uspstf13/lungcan/lungcanes103.pdf.

41 Bach PB. Perilous potential: the chance to save lives, or lose them, through low dose computed tomography screening for lung cancer. *J Surg Oncol* 2013;108:287-8.

42 Bunge EM, van den Bergh KA, Essink-Bot ML, van Klaveren RJ, de Koning HJ. High affective risk perception is associated with more lung cancer-specific distress in CT screening for lung cancer. *Lung Cancer* 2008;62:385-90.

43 Byrne MM, Weissfeld J, Roberts MS. Anxiety, fear of cancer, and perceived risk of cancer following lung cancer screening. *Med Decis Making* 2008;28:917-25.

44 McGovern PM, Gross CR, Krueger RA, Engelhard DA, Cordes JE, Church TR. False-positive cancer screens and health-related quality of life. *Cancer Nurs* 2004;27:347-52.

45 Vierikko T, Kivisto S, Jarvenpaa R, Uitti J, Oksa P, Virtema P, et al. Psychological impact of computed tomography screening for lung cancer and occupational pulmonary disease among asbestos-exposed workers. *Eur J Cancer Prev* 2009;18:203-6.

46 Van den Bergh KA, Essink-Bot ML, Borsboom GJ, Th Scholten E, Prokop M, de Koning HJ, et al. Short-term health-related quality of life consequences in a lung cancer CT screening trial (NELSON). *Br J Cancer* 2010;102:27-34.

47 Van den Bergh KA, Essink-Bot ML, Borsboom GJ, Scholten ET, van Klaveren RJ, de Koning HJ. Long-term effects of lung cancer computed tomography screening on health-related quality of life: the NELSON trial. *Eur Respir J* 2011;38:154-61.

48 Kaerlev L, Iachina M, Pedersen JH, Green A, Norgard BM. CT-screening for lung cancer does not increase the use of anxiolytic or antidepressant medication. *BMC Cancer* 2012;12:188.

49 Detterbeck FC. Cancer, concepts, cohorts and complexity: avoiding oversimplification of overdiagnosis. *Thorax* 2012;67:842-5.

50 Grannis FW Jr. Minimizing over-diagnosis in lung cancer screening. *J Surg Oncol* 2013;108:289-93.

51 Ichinose J, Kohno T, Fujimori S, Harano T, Suzuki S, Fujii T. Invasiveness and malignant potential of pulmonary lesions presenting as pure ground-glass opacities. *Ann Thorac Cardiovasc Surg* 2013; published online 3 Oct.

52 Patz EF Jr, Pinsky P, Gatsonis C, Sicks JD4, Kramer BS2, Tammemägi MC, et al. Overdiagnosis in low-dose computed tomography screening for lung cancer. *JAMA Intern Med* 2014;174:269-74.

53 Veronesi G, Maisonneuve P, Bellomi M, Rampinelli C, Durli I, Bertolotti R, et al. Estimating overdiagnosis in low-dose computed tomography screening for lung cancer: a cohort study. *Ann Intern Med* 2012;157:776-84.

54 American Association of Physicists in Medicine. AAPM position statement on radiation risks from medical imaging procedures. 2011. www.aapm.org/org/policies/details.asp?id=318&type=PP&current=true.

55 Pearce MS, Salotti JA, Little MP, McHugh K, Lee C, Kim KP, et al. Radiation exposure from CT scans in childhood and subsequent risk of leukaemia and brain tumours: a retrospective cohort study. *Lancet* 2012;380:499-505.

56 Harris RP, Sheridan SL, Lewis CL, Barclay C, Vu MB, Kistler CE, et al. The harms of screening: a proposed taxonomy and application to lung cancer screening. *JAMA Intern Med* 2014;174:281-5.

57 Marshall D, Simpson KN, Earle CC, Chu C. Potential cost-effectiveness of one-time screening for lung cancer (LC) in a high risk cohort. *Lung Cancer* 2001;32:227-36.

58 Chirikos TN, Hazelton T, Tockman M, Clark R. Screening for lung cancer with CT: a preliminary cost-effectiveness analysis. *Ch est* 2002;121:1507-14.

59 Mahadevia PJ, Fleisher LA, Frick KD, Eng J, Goodman SN, Powe NR. Lung cancer screening with helical computed tomography in older adult smokers: a decision and cost-effectiveness analysis. *JAMA* 2003;289:313-22.

60 Wisnivesky JP, Mushlin AI, Sicherman N, Henschke C. The cost-effectiveness of low-dose CT screening for lung cancer: preliminary results of baseline screening. *Chest* 2003;124:614-21.

61 Manser R, Dalton A, Carter R, Byrnes G, Elwood M, Campbell DA. Cost-effectiveness analysis of screening for lung cancer with low dose spiral CT (computed tomography) in the Australian setting. *Lung Cancer* 2005;48:171-85.

62 Black C, Bagust A, Boland A, Walker S, McLeod C, De Verteuil R, et al. The clinical effectiveness and cost-effectiveness of computed tomography screening for lung cancer: systematic reviews. *Health Technol Assess* 2006;10:iii-iv, ix-x, 1-90.

63 Castleberry AW, Smith D, Anderson C, Rotter AJ, Grannis FW Jr. Cost of a 5-year lung cancer survivor: symptomatic tumour identification vs proactive computed tomography screening. *Br J Cancer* 2009;101:882-96.

64 Reich JM. Cost-effectiveness of computed tomography lung cancer screening. *Br J Cancer* 2009;101:879-80.

65 McMahon PM, Kong CY, Bouzan C, Weinstein MC, Cipriano LE, Tramontano AC, et al. Cost-effectiveness of computed tomography screening for lung cancer in the United States. *J Thorac Oncol* 2011;6:1841-8.

66 Goulart BH, Bensink ME, Mummy DG, Ramsey SD. Lung cancer screening with low-dose computed tomography: costs, national expenditures, and cost-effectiveness. *J Natl Compr Canc Netw* 2012;10:267-75.

67 Pyenson BS, Sander MS, Jiang Y, Kahn H, Mulshine JL. An actuarial analysis shows that offering lung cancer screening as an insurance benefit would save lives at relatively low cost. *Health Aff (Millwood)* 2012;31:770-9.

68 Shmueli A, Fraifeld S, Peretz T, Gutfeld O, Gips M, Sosna J, et al. Cost-effectiveness of baseline low-dose computed tomography screening for lung cancer: the Israeli experience. *Value Health* 2013;16:922-31.

69 Cressman S, Peacock S, Cromwell I. Resource utilization and costs of screening high-risk individuals for lung cancer in Canada. *J Thorac Oncol* 2013;8 (suppl):S150.

70 Kantarjian HM, Fojo T, Mathisen M, Zwelling LA. Cancer drugs in the United States: Justum Pretium—the just price. *J Clin Oncol* 2013;31:3600-4.

71 Fiore M, Jaen C, Baker T, Bailey W, Benowitz N, Curry S, et al. Treating tobacco use and dependence. Clinical practice guideline: Update 2008. US Department of Health and Human Services. Public Health Service; 2008. www.ncbi.nlm.nih.gov/books/NBK63952/.

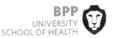

72 Ashraf H, Tonnesen P, Holst Pedersen J, Dirksen A, Thorsen H, Dossing M. Effect of CT screening on smoking habits at 1-year follow-up in the Danish Lung Cancer Screening Trial (DLCST). Thorax2009;64:388-92.

73 Tammemagi MC, Berg CD, Riley TL, Cunningham CR, Taylor KL. Impact of lung cancer screening results on smoking cessation. J Natl Cancer Inst [forthcoming].

74 Townsend CO, Clark MM, Jett JR, Patten CA, Schroeder DR, Nirelli LM, et al. Relation between smoking cessation and receiving results from three annual spiral chest computed tomography scans for lung carcinoma screening. Cancer2005;103:2154-62.

75 Styn MA, Land SR, Perkins KA, Wilson DO, Romkes M, Weissfeld JL. Smoking behavior 1 year after computed tomography screening for lung cancer: Effect of physician referral for abnormal CT findings. Cancer Epidemiol Biomarkers Prev2009;18:3484-9.

76 International Association for the Study of Lung Cancer (IASLC). Lung Cancer Computed Tomography Screening Workshop 2013 Report. Sydney, Australia, 26-27 October, 2013. J Thorac Oncol [forthcoming].

77 Etzel CJ, Kachroo S, Liu M, D'Amelio A, Dong Q, Cote ML, et al. Development and validation of a lung cancer risk prediction model for African-Americans. Cancer Prev Res (Phila)2008;1:255-65.

78 Li H, Yang L, Zhao X, Wang J, Qian J, Chen H, et al. Prediction of lung cancer risk in a Chinese population using a multifactorial genetic model. BMC Med Genet2012;13:118.

79 Park S, Nam BH, Yang HR, Lee JA, Lim H, Han JT, et al. Individualized risk prediction model for lung cancer in Korean men. PLoS One2013;8:e54823.

80 Maisonneuve P, Bagnardi V, Bellomi M, Spaggiari L, Pelosi G, Rampinelli C, et al. Lung cancer risk prediction to select smokers for screening CT—a model based on the Italian COSMOS trial. Cancer Prev Res (Phila) 2011;4:1778-89.

81 Spitz MR, Etzel CJ, Dong Q, Amos CI, Wei Q, Wu X, et al. An expanded risk prediction model for lung cancer. Cancer Prev Res (Phila)2008;1:250-4.

82 Young RP, Hopkins RJ, Hay BA, Epton MJ, Mills GD, Black PN, et al. A gene-based risk score for lung cancer susceptibility in smokers and ex-smokers. Postgrad Med J 2009;85:515-24.

83 Hippisley-Cox J, Coupland C. Identifying patients with suspected lung cancer in primary care: derivation and validation of an algorithm. Br J Gen Pract2011;61:e715-23.

84 Iyen-Omofoman B, Tata LJ, Baldwin DR, Smith CJ, Hubbard RB. Using socio-demographic and early clinical features in general practice to identify people with lung cancer earlier. Thorax2013;68:451-9.

85 Spitz MR, Hong WK, Amos CI, Wu X, Schabath MB, Dong Q, et al. A risk model for prediction of lung cancer. J Natl Cancer Inst2007;99:715-26.

86 Cassidy A, Myles JP, van Tongeren M, Page RD, Liloglou T, Duffy SW, et al. The LLP risk model: an individual risk prediction model for lung cancer. Br J Cancer2008;98:270-6.

87 Tammemagi CM, Pinsky PF, Caporaso NE, Kvale PA, Hocking WG, Church TR,et al. Lung cancer risk prediction: prostate, lung, colorectal and ovarian cancer screening trial models and validation. J Natl Cancer Inst2011;103:1058-68.

88 Hoggart C, Brennan P, Tjonneland A, Vogel U, Overvad K, Ostergaard JN, et al. A risk model for lung cancer incidence. Cancer Prev Res (Phila)2012;5:834-46.

89 Hensing TA, Salgia R. Molecular biomarkers for future screening of lung cancer. J Surg Oncol 2013;108:327-33.

90 Church TR, Black WC, Aberle DR, Berg CD, Clingan KL, Duan F, et al. Results of initial low-dose computed tomographic screening for lung cancer. N Engl J Med2013;368:1980-91.

91 Horeweg N, van der Aalst CM, Vliegenthart R, Zhao Y, Xie X, Scholten ET, et al. Volumetric computer tomography screening for lung cancer: three rounds of the NELSON trial. Eur Respir J2013;42:1659-67.

92 McWilliams A, Tammemagi MC, Mayo JR, Roberts H, Liu G, Soghrati K, et al. Probability of cancer in pulmonary nodules detected on first screening CT. N Engl J Med2013;369:910-9.

93 Pedersen JH, Ashraf H, Dirksen A, Bach K, Hansen H, Toennesen P, et al. The Danish randomized lung cancer CT screening trial—overall design and results of the prevalence round. J Thorac Oncol2009;4:608-14.

94 Wood DE, Eapen GA, Ettinger DS, Hou L, Jackman D, Kazerooni E, et al. Lung cancer screening. J Natl Comprehens Cancer Netw2012;10:240-65.

95 MacMahon H, Austin JH, Gamsu G, Herold CJ, Jett JR, Naidich DP, et al. Guidelines for management of small pulmonary nodules detected on CT scans: a statement from the Fleischner Society. Radiology2005;237:395-400.

96 Gould MK, Donington J, Lynch WR, Mazzone PJ, Midthun DE, Naidich DP, et al. Evaluation of individuals with pulmonary nodules: when is it lung cancer? Diagnosis and management of lung cancer. 3rd ed. American College of Chest Physicians evidence-based clinical practice guidelines. Chest2013;143:e93S-120S.

97 American College of Radiology Imaging Network. Contemporary screening for the detection of lung cancer. 2013. www.acrin.org/6654_protocol.aspx.

98 Xu DM, Gietema H, de Koning H, Vernhout R, Nackaerts K, Prokop M, et al. Nodule management protocol of the NELSON randomised lung cancer screening trial. Lung Cancer2006;54:177-84.

99 Henschke CI, Yip R, Yankelevitz DF, Smith JP; International Early Lung Cancer Action Program Investigators. Definition of a positive test result in computed tomography screening for lung cancer: a cohort study. Ann Intern Med2013;158:246-52.

100 Henschke CI, Yip R, Yankelevitz DF, Smith JP. Computed tomography screening for lung cancer. Ann Intern Med2013;159:156-7.

101 Naidich DP, Bankier AA, MacMahon H, Schaefer-Prokop CM, Pistolesi M, Goo JM, et al. Recommendations for the management of subsolid pulmonary nodules detected at CT: a statement from the Fleischner Society. Radiology2013;266:304-17.

102 International Early Lung Cancer Action Program Investigators; Henschke CI, Yankelevitz DF, Libby DM, Pasmantier MW, Smith JP, Miettinen OS. Survival of patients with stage I lung cancer detected on CT screening. N Engl J Med2006;355:1763-71.

103 Lam S, McWilliams A, Mayo J, Tammemagi M. Computed tomography screening for lung cancer: what is a positive screen? Ann Intern Med2013;158:289-90.

104 Swensen SJ, Silverstein MD, Ilstrup DM, Schleck CD, Edell ES. The probability of malignancy in solitary pulmonary nodules. Application to small radiologically indeterminate nodules. Arch Intern Med1997;157:849-55.

105 Gurney JW, Lyddon DM, McKay JA. Determining the likelihood of malignancy in solitary pulmonary nodules with Bayesian analysis. Part II. Application. Radiology 1993;186:415-22.

106 Gould MK, Ananth L, Barnett PG. A clinical model to estimate the pretest probability of lung cancer in patients with solitary pulmonary nodules. Chest2007;131:383-8.

107 Schultz EM, Sanders GD, Trotter PR, Patz EF, Jr., Silvestri GA, Owens DK, et al. Validation of two models to estimate the probability of malignancy in patients with solitary pulmonary nodules. Thorax 2008;63:335-41.

108 Balekian AA, Silvestri GA, Simkovich SM, Mestaz PJ, Sanders GD, Daniel J, et al. Accuracy of clinicians and models for estimating the probability that a pulmonary nodule is malignant. Ann Am Thorac Soc2013;10:629-35.

109 Isbell JM, Deppen S, Putnam JB Jr, Nesbitt JC, Lambright ES, Dawes A, et al. Existing general population models inaccurately predict lung cancer risk in patients referred for surgical evaluation. Ann Thorac Surg2011;91:227-33; discussion 33.

110 Tammemagi M, Mayo J, Lam S. Cancer in pulmonary nodules detected on first screening CT—reply to correspondence to the editor. N Engl J Med2013;369:2061-2.

111 Swensen SJ, Jett JR, Hartman TE, Midthun DE, Mandrekar SJ, Hillman SL, et al. CT screening for lung cancer: five-year prospective experience. Radiology2005;235:259-65.

112 McWilliams AM, Mayo JR, Ahn MI, MacDonald SL, Lam SC. Lung cancer screening using multi-slice thin-section computed tomography and autofluorescence bronchoscopy. J Thorac Oncol2006;1:61-8.

113 Field JK, Oudkerk M, Pedersen JH, Duffy SW. Prospects for population screening and diagnosis of lung cancer. Lancet2013;382:732-41.

114 Heuvelmans MA, Oudkerk M, de Bock GH, de Koning HJ, Xie X, van Ooijen PM, et al. Optimisation of volume-doubling time cutoff for fast-growing lung nodules in CT lung cancer screening reduces false-positive referrals. Eur Radiol2013;23:1836-45.

115 Mehta HJ, Ravenel JG, Shaftman SR, Tanner NT, Paoletti L, Taylor KK, et al. The utility of nodule volume in the context of malignancy prediction for small pulmonary nodules. Chest 2014;145:464-72.

116 Xie X, Zhao Y, Snijder RA, van Ooijen PM, de Jong PA, Oudkerk M, et al. Sensitivity and accuracy of volumetry of pulmonary nodules on low-dose 16- and 64-row multi-detector CT: an anthropomorphic phantom study. Eur Radiol2013;23:139-47.

117 Lim HJ, Ahn S, Lee KS, et al. Persistent pure ground-glass opacity lung nodules .10 mm in diameter at CT scan: histopathologic comparisons and prognostic implications. Chest 2013;144:1291-9.

118 Lassen B, van Rikxoort EM, Schmidt M, Kerkstra S, van Ginneken B, Kuhnigk JM. Automatic segmentation of the pulmonary lobes from chest CT scans based on fissures, vessels, and bronchi. IEEE Trans Med Imaging2013;32:210-22.

119 Jacobs C, Sanchez CI, Saur SC, Twellmann T, de Jong PA, van Ginneken B. Computer-aided detection of ground glass nodules in thoracic CT images using shape, intensity and context features. Med Image Comput Comput Assist Interv2011;14:207-14.

120 Jacobs C, van Rikxoort EM, Twellmann T, Scholtenet ET, et al. Automatic detection of subsolid pulmonary nodules in thoracic computed tomography images. Med Image Anal2014;18:374-84.

121 Horeweg N, de Koning HJ. Reply: Stage distribution of lung cancers detected by computed tomography screening in the NELSON trial. Am J Respir Crit Care Med2013;188:1035-6.

122 Lindell RM, Hartman TE, Swensen SJ, Jett JR, Midthun DE, Mandrekar JN. 5-year lung cancer screening experience: growth curves of 18 lung cancers compared to histologic type, CT attenuation, stage, survival, and size. Chest2009;136:1586-95.

123 Field JK, Smith RA, Aberle DR, Oudkerk M, Baldwin DR, Yankelevitz D, et al. International Association for the Study of Lung Cancer computed tomography screening workshop 2011 report. J Thorac Oncol2012;7:10-9.

124 Veronesi G, Maisonneuve P, Rampinelli C, Bertolotti R, Petrella F, Spaggiari L, et al. Computed tomography screening for lung cancer: results of ten years of annual screening and validation of cosmos prediction model. Lung Cancer2013;82:426-30.

125 Armato SG, 3rd, Roberts RY, Kocherginsky M, Aberle DR, Kazerooni EA, Macmahon H, et al. Assessment of radiologist performance in the detection of lung nodules: dependence on the definition of "truth." Acad Radiol2009;16:28-38.

126 Pinsky PF, Gierada DS, Nath PH, Kazerooni E, Amorosa J. National lung screening trial: variability in nodule detection rates in chest CT studies. Radiology2013;268:865-73.

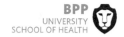

127 Tammemagi MC, Lam SC, McWilliams AM, Sin DD. Incremental value of
     pulmonary function and sputum DNA image cytometry in lung cancer
     risk prediction. *Cancer Prev Res (Phila)*2011;4:552-61.
128 Sin D, Tammemagi MC, Lam S, Barnett MJ, Duan X, Tam A, et al. Pro-
     surfactant protein B as a biomarker for lung cancer prediction. *J Clin
     Oncol*2013;31:4536-43.
129 Sozzi G, Boeri M, Rossi M, Verri C, Suatoni P, Bravi F, et al. Clinical
     utility of a plasma-based miRNA signature classifier within computed
     tomography lung cancer screening: a correlative MILD trial study. *J
     Clin Oncol*2014; published online Jan 13.

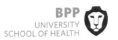

Serum tumour markers: how to order and interpret them

C M Sturgeon consultant clinical scientist[1], L C Lai professor of clinical biochemistry and metabolic medicine[2], M J Duffy professor of pathology and laboratory medicine[3] [4]

[1]Department of Clinical Biochemistry, Royal Infirmary of Edinburgh, Edinburgh EH16 4SA

[2]Faculty of Medicine, International Medical University, Bukit Jalil, 57000 Kuala Lumpur, Malaysia

[3]Department of Pathology and Laboratory Medicine, St Vincent's University Hospital, Dublin 4, Ireland

[4]UCD School of Medicine and Medical Science, Conway Institute of Biomolecular and Biomedical Research, University College Dublin, Dublin 4, Ireland

Correspondence to: C M Sturgeon
C.Sturgeon@ed.ac.uk

Cite this as: BMJ 2009;339:b3527

‹DOI› 10.1136/bmj.b3527
http://www.bmj.com/content/339/
bmj.b3527

Tumour markers are molecules that may be present in higher than usual concentrations in the tissue, serum, urine, or other body fluids of patients with cancer.[1] [2] [3] Serum tumour markers may aid cancer diagnosis, assess prognosis, guide choice of treatment, monitor progress during and after treatment, and/or be used as screening tests. Conservative estimates suggest that in the United Kingdom alone close to 15 million such measurements are made each year.

If tumour markers are requested and interpreted correctly, they undoubtedly help clinical management. Somewhat alarmingly, however, a recent audit in a single Greek hospital found that only about 10% of requests for tumour markers were appropriate.[4] The cost of inappropriate testing of tumour markers was estimated to be about €23 974 (£21 000; $35 000) a month, even without including the cost of unnecessary second level follow-up investigations such as colonoscopy and ultrasonography.[4] However, awareness of the limitations of tumour markers is crucial not only because of the economic implications of their misuse but even more importantly because inappropriately used tumour marker results can cause patients additional anxiety and distress. Unnecessary investigations (such as biopsy) may be associated with serious side effects and may delaying correct diagnosis and treatment.

Here we focus on more commonly used serum tumour markers, reviewing recommendations for their optimal application.

Which are the most clinically useful serum tumour markers and how should they be used?

Serum tumour markers may be used in screening, to help in diagnosis, or to monitor response to treatment. Although routinely available, tumour markers are specialised tests, ideally measured only after consideration of the likelihood that results will improve patient outcome, increase quality of life, or reduce overall cost of care.[5] Table 1 lists the 10 serum tumour markers most likely to be requested by non-specialists, with current recommendations for their use. PSA (prostate specific antigen) is the marker most often requested, and the increased incidence of prostate cancer in the United States during the past two decades is attributed largely to its widespread measurement.[6]

When are tumour markers helpful for diagnosis?

With a few important exceptions (such as α fetoprotein and human chorionic gonadotrophin in germ cell tumours), measuring more than one serum tumour marker is unlikely to be helpful when trying to establish a diagnosis. Table 2 outlines typical clinical presentations that would prompt requests for each of the seven most commonly requested tumour markers. The National Academy of Clinical Biochemistry recommends that requests for panels of tumour markers are actively discouraged, as are requests for prostate specific antigen in women or CA125 in men.[1] The likely benefit of the result to the individual patient must be considered before requesting any tumour marker. If decisions about treatment depend solely on the result of a single tumour marker, the result should be confirmed on a repeat specimen.

In carefully selected undiagnosed patients who are at medium to high risk of malignancy, highly raised levels of the appropriate tumour marker may provide helpful information—for example, in a patient unable or unwilling to have further, invasive investigations such as colonoscopy. Major recent improvements in the speed of access to ultrasonography in UK general practice may reduce the number of unfocused requests for tumour markers, which previously may have been made pragmatically while awaiting more definitive radiological testing.

Together with radiological testing, measurement of both human chorionic gonadotrophin and α fetoprotein is mandatory in patients in whom testicular or other germ cell cancers are strongly suspected, although these markers are not raised in all such patients.[6]

A recently developed UK consensus statement on ovarian cancer recommends measurement of CA125 and pelvic ultrasonography in women aged over 50 years presenting with persistent, continuous, or worsening unexplained abdominal or urinary symptoms and in whom abdominal palpation gives cause for concern.[9] The rationale is to reduce the risk of delaying diagnosis if women with ovarian cancer are referred to non-gynaecological specialists.

Inadequate sensitivity and specificity limit the use of CA 19-9 measurement in the early diagnosis of pancreatic cancer.[10] In patients without jaundice, however, CA19-9 measurement may complement other diagnostic procedures, especially in the absence of cholestasis.

In conjunction with abdominal ultrasonography, the National Comprehensive Cancer Network, like other expert groups, recommends α fetoprotein measurements at six-monthly intervals in patients at high risk of hepatocellular carcinoma (especially those with liver cirrhosis related

SUMMARY POINTS

- Tumour markers can contribute usefully to patient management, but awareness of their limitations is essential
- The main application of tumour markers is in monitoring
- Measurement of α fetoprotein and human chorionic gonadotrophin is mandatory in the management of germ cell tumours
- Carcinoembryonic antigen (CEA) is recommended for postoperative follow-up of patients with stage II and III colorectal cancer if further surgery or chemotherapy is an option
- Prostate specific antigen (PSA) may be used for detecting disease recurrence and monitoring treatment in patients with prostate cancer
- In some high risk patients, measurement of α fetoprotein, CA125, or CA19-9 may aid early detection of hepatocellular carcinoma, ovarian cancer, or pancreatic cancer, respectively
- Opportunistic screening with panels of tumour markers is not helpful, nor is measurement of CA125 in men or PSA in women

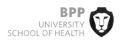

Table 1 Most frequently requested serum tumour markers and the current recommendations of the National Academy of Clinical Biochemistry for the appropriate clinical use of these markers[6]

Tumour marker	Relevant cancer	Currently recommended clinical recommendations				
		Screening or early detection	Diagnosis or case finding	Prognosis (with other factors)	Detecting recurrence	Monitoring treatment
α fetoprotein	Germ cell/testicular tumour	No	Yes	Yes	Yes	Yes
	Hepatocellular carcinoma	Yes*	Yes†	Yes	Yes	Yes‡
Calcitonin	Medullary thyroid carcinoma	No	Yes	No	Yes	Yes
Cancer antigen 125 (CA125)	Ovarian cancer	Under evaluation§	Yes¶	Yes	Yes	Yes**
Cancer antigen 15-3 (CA15-3)	Breast cancer	No	No	No	Yes††	Yes‡‡
Cancer antigen 19-9 (CA19-9)	Pancreatic cancer	No	Yes§§	Yes	Yes	Yes¶¶
Carcinoembryonic antigen (CEA)	Colorectal cancer	No	No	Yes	Yes‡	Yes‡
Human chorionic gonadotrophin	Germ cell and testicular cancers; gestational trophoblastic neoplasia***	No	Yes	Yes	Yes	Yes
Paraproteins (M protein/Bence Jones protein); also measured in urine[8]	B cell proliferative disorders (such as multiple myeloma)	No	Yes	No	Yes	Yes
Prostate specific antigen	Prostate cancer	No	Yes	Yes	Yes	Yes
Thyroglobulin	Thyroid cancer (follicular or papillary)	No	No	No	Yes	Yes

*Only for subjects in high risk groups (such as those with chronic hepatitis B or C, or cirrhosis) and only in conjunction with ultrasonography (impact on mortality unclear).

†In conjunction with liver imaging, α fetoprotein levels >200 µg/l are regarded as virtually diagnostic of hepatocellular carcinoma in patients with hypervascular lesions.

‡Especially for disease that cannot be evaluated by other means.

§Through the UK Collaborative Trial of Ovarian Cancer Screening[19] (see text) and (for women at high familial risk of ovarian cancer and in conjunction with genetic studies and transvaginal ultrasonography) through the UK Familial Ovarian Cancer Screening Study.

¶Only for differential diagnosis of pelvic masses, especially in post-menopausal women.

**Preliminary results of a randomised trial show no survival benefit from early treatment based on a raised serum CA125 level alone,[7] so this recommendation may be modified to exclude asymptomatic patients.

††After surgery, when it may provide lead time for early detection of metastasis, but the clinical value is unclear.

‡‡Especially in patients with non-evaluable disease (for which carcinoembryonic antigen is also recommended in carefully selected patients).

§§In patients in whom pancreatic disease is strongly suspected CA19-9 may complement other diagnostic procedures.

¶¶Especially after chemotherapy and combined with imaging.

*** Use of human chorionic gonadotrophin in screening for gestational trophoblastic neoplasia, a rare malignancy which develops most often after a molar pregnancy, provides an excellent example of "best practice" in screening. Further information is available from the Trophoblastic Tumour Screening and Treatment Centre, Department of Medical Oncology, Charing Cross Hospital, London W6 8RF (www.hmole-chorio.org.uk/).

Table 2 The most frequently used tumour markers and typical clinical presentations that might prompt a request for them. Other cancers in which each marker is often raised are also listed

Tumour marker	Relevant cancer	Typical clinical presentation	Other cancers in which marker may be raised*
α fetoprotein	Germ cell/testicular tumour	Diffuse testicular swelling; hardness	Colorectal; gastric; hepatobiliary; hepatocellular; lung; pulmonary
	Hepatocellular carcinoma	Ascites; encephalopathy; jaundice; upper abdominal pain; weight loss; early satiety in high risk subjects (that is, cirrhosis related to hepatitis B or C)	Colorectal; gastric; germ cell/testicular; lung; pulmonary
Cancer antigen 125 (CA125)	Ovarian cancer	Pelvic mass; persistent, continuous or worsening unexplained abdominal or urinary symptoms; bloating	Breast; cervical; endometrial; hepatocellular; lung; non-Hodgkin's lymphoma; pancreas; peritoneal; uterus
Cancer antigen 19-9 (CA19-9)	Pancreatic cancer	Progressive obstructive jaundice with profound weight loss and/or pain in the abdomen or mid-back	Colorectal; gastric; hepatocellular; oesophageal; ovarian
Carcinoembryonic antigen (CEA)	Colorectal cancer	Intermittent abdominal pain, nausea, vomiting or bleeding; palpable abdominal mass	Breast; gastric; lung; mesothelioma; oesophageal; pancreatic
Human chorionic gonadotrophin	Germ cell/testicular tumour	Diffuse testicular swelling, hardness, and pain	Gestational trophoblastic neoplasia; lung
	Gestational trophoblastic neoplasia†	Symptoms leading to radiography showing cannon ball secondaries; history of hydatidiform mole/molar pregnancy†	Germ cell/testicular; lung
Paraproteins (M protein/Bence Jones protein); also measured in urine[8]	B cell proliferative disorders (such as multiple myeloma)	Combination of symptoms including some/all of the following: anaemia; back pain; weakness or fatigue; osteopenia; osteolytic lesions; raised erythrocyte sedimentation rate or raised or lowered globulins; spontaneous fractures; recurrent infections	None known
Prostate specific antigen (PSA)	Prostate cancer	Frequency, urgency, nocturia, dysuria; acute retention; back pain, weight loss, anaemia	None known

* Not a comprehensive list. All markers listed in this table are not specific for malignancy but may also be raised in patients with certain benign diseases (see box).

†Use of human chorionic gonadotrophin in screening for gestational trophoblastic neoplasia, a rare malignancy which develops most often after a molar pregnancy, provides an excellent example of "best practice" in screening. Further information is available from the Trophoblastic Tumour Screening and Treatment Centre, Department of Medical Oncology, Charing Cross Hospital, London W6 8RF (www.hmole-chorio.org.uk/).

to hepatitis B or hepatitis C) and further investigation if increases in α fetoprotein persist.[11] The effectiveness of such testing will reflect prevalence of disease in the screened population.

Although PSA is essentially organ specific (table 2), it is not cancer specific (box). Sustained high levels of PSA occur in benign prostatic hyperplasia, and transient increases may occur in some patients with urinary tract infections, in prostatitis, and after catheterisation (table 3). Provided these latter conditions are excluded, the higher the PSA level, the greater the probability of prostate cancer. About 15% of men with a PSA <4 µg/l will have cancer on biopsy, as will about 25% with a PSA 4-10 µg/l and 50% with a PSA >10 µg/l.[13] Confirmed levels >100 µg/l are usually consistent with metastatic disease. Prostatic biopsy or radiological evidence

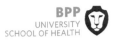

BENIGN CONDITIONS THAT MAY CAUSE RISES (SOME TRANSIENT) IN SERUM TUMOUR MARKER LEVELS THAT MAY LEAD TO INCORRECT INTERPRETATION*

- Acute cholangitis (CA19-9)
- Acute hepatitis (CA125, CA15-3)
- Acute and/or chronic pancreatitis (CA125, CA19-9)
- Acute urinary retention (CA125, PSA†)
- Arthritis/osteoarthritis/rheumatoid arthritis (CA125)
- Benign prostatic hyperplasia (PSA)
- Cholestasis (CA19-9)
- Chronic liver diseases—such as cirrhosis, chronic active hepatitis (CA125, CA15-3, CA19-9, carcinoembryonic antigen (CEA))
- Chronic renal failure (CA125, CA15-3, CEA, human chorionic gonadotrophin)
- Colitis (CA125, CA15-3, CEA)
- Congestive heart failure (CA125)
- Cystic fibrosis (CA125)
- Dermatological conditions (CA15-3)
- Diabetes (CA125, CA19-9)
- Diverticulitis (CA125, CEA)
- Endometriosis (CA125)
- Heart failure (CA125)
- Irritable bowel syndrome (CA125, CA19-9, CEA)
- Jaundice (CA19-9, CEA)
- Leiomyoma (CA125)
- Liver regeneration (α fetoprotein)
- Menopause (human chorionic gonadotrophin)
- Menstruation (CA125)
- Non-malignant ascites (CA125)
- Ovarian hyperstimulation (CA125)
- Pancreatitis (CA125, CA19-9)
- Pericarditis (CA125)
- Peritoneal inflammation (CA125)
- Pregnancy (α fetoprotein, CA125, human chorionic gonadotrophin)
- Prostatitis (PSA)
- Recurrent ischaemic strokes in patients with metastatic cancer (CA125)
- Respiratory diseases—such as pleural inflammation, pneumonia (CA125, CEA)
- Sarcoidosis (CA125)
- Systemic lupus erythematosus (CA125)
- Urinary tract infection (PSA‡)

*Not a comprehensive list of conditions.
†Delay PSA measurement for at least two weeks.[12]
‡Repeat PSA no earlier than two to four weeks after urinary tract infection.[12]

Table 3 Factors that may influence interpretation of tumour markers*

Factor	Tumour marker
Lifestyle	
Smoking	CEA—minor increase in some assays
Cannabis use	Human chorionic gonadotrophin—transient increase
Medication	
5 α reductase inhibitors (such as finasteride, dutasteride)	PSA—median decrease of about 50%
Medical investigation/intervention	
Catheterisation	PSA†
Chemotherapy	Most tumour markers, especially with bulk disease, transient
Cystoscopy	PSA‡
Digital rectal examination	PSA (in some men)‡
Laparoscopy	CA125
Prostatic needle biopsy	PSA§
Prostatic massage	PSA‡
Prostate ultrasonography	PSA‡
Transurethral prostatic biopsy	PSA§

*Not comprehensive; other factors may be relevant for some of these markers.
†Measure PSA before catheterisation.
‡Measure PSA before or one week after the investigation or intervention.
§Measure PSA before biopsy or >6 weeks after the investigation.[12]

of bone metastases is generally required for definitive diagnosis.

Are tumour markers helpful for diagnosis in patients with non-specific symptoms?

Tumour markers are not helpful for diagnosis in patients with non-specific symptoms. Many tumour markers (particularly carcinoembryonic antigen (CEA), CA125, CA15-3, and CA19-9) are raised in several cancers (table 2) but may also be raised in certain benign diseases (box). They therefore cannot either identify or exclude suspected malignancy (especially early stage disease) reliably, owing to low diagnostic sensitivity (the ability to identify the true cases of a particular cancer type) and low specificity (the ability not to identify people as having a particular cancer type when they do not have it).

For example, the proportion of patients with early stage (Dukes's type A) colorectal cancer who have CEA levels >5 µg/l is only 3%, compared with 25%, 45%, and 65% for Dukes's type B, C, and D respectively.[14] Measurement of these markers is therefore not recommended in patients with non-specific symptoms (a presentation most likely to be encountered in primary care) before imaging or a definitive diagnosis of malignancy by biopsy.

Are tumour markers effective for screening asymptomatic populations?

Population based screening of asymptomatic people with most serum tumour markers is not recommended owing to low diagnostic sensitivity and specificity. Screening for prostate cancer with PSA has the potential to detect malignancy at least five years before clinical evidence of disease but remains controversial, with some expert groups in favour and others not.[6] Interim results of two large prospective trials of PSA screening are contradictory, one suggesting no mortality benefit[15] and the other concluding that 1410 men would need to be offered screening and 48 men treated to prevent one death from prostate cancer during a 10 year period,[16] a benefit achieved only at the cost of substantial overdiagnosis and overtreatment.[17] Until these studies finally report their findings, asymptomatic men should be informed of the benefits and limitations of PSA screening before deciding whether to have the test.[6] [18] The Prostate Cancer Risk Management Programme (part of the NHS Cancer Screening Programmes) provides helpful information packs intended for distribution through primary care (www.cancerscreening.nhs.uk/prostate/informationpack.html).

Serial measurements of CA125 are included in a UK collaborative trial of ovarian cancer screening involving 208 638 women aged 50-74 years.[19] The final results of this trial will not be known until 2015, and in the meantime the National Academy of Clinical Biochemistry does not recommend opportunistic screening of asymptomatic women with CA125.[6]

What are the pros and cons of monitoring response to treatment?

Serial monitoring of patients after treatment is the most appropriate use of tumour markers (table 1), but its effect on outcome varies. In patients with a diagnosis of cancer, measurement of markers before and after treatment can provide evidence of efficacy of treatment and identify recurrence some months before clinically evident. Whether the latter benefits an individual patient depends on the

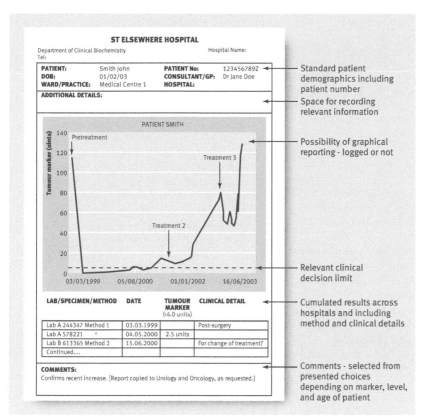

ST ELSEWHERE HOSPITAL

Department of Clinical Biochemistry
Tel: Hospital Name:

PATIENT:	Smith John	PATIENT No:	123456789Z
DOB:	01/02/03	CONSULTANT/GP:	Dr Jane Doe
WARD/PRACTICE:	Medical Centre 1	HOSPITAL:	

ADDITIONAL DETAILS:

PATIENT SMITH

→ Standard patient demographics including patient number

→ Space for recording relevant information

→ Possibility of graphical reporting - logged or not

→ Relevant clinical decision limit

LAB/SPECIMEN/METHOD	DATE	TUMOUR MARKER (<4.0 units)	CLINICAL DETAIL
Lab A 244347 Method 1	03.03.1999		Post-surgery
Lab A 578221 "	04.05.2000	2.5 units	
Lab B 613365 Method 2	15.06.2000		For change of treatment?
Continued....			

→ Cumulated results across hospitals and including method and clinical details

COMMENTS:
Confirms recent increase. [Report copied to Urology and Oncology, as requested.]

→ Comments - selected from presented choices depending on marker, level, and age of patient

Possible template for a clinical laboratory report for tumour markers that fulfils current reporting recommendations.[1] Close collaboration between clinical and laboratory staff together with provision of relevant clinical details allows laboratory staff to provide advice on further action (such as referral) on the basis of the most recent result and/or on the rate at which marker level is increasing

availability of further treatment (such as chemotherapy or resection).

For patients with germ cell tumours, all guidelines recommend measurement of α fetoprotein and human chorionic gonadotrophin according to well established protocols,[20] as further treatment can be started after a confirmed increase in markers even without radiological evidence of progression.

Similar benefit in monitoring can be achieved in patients with colorectal cancer by measuring CEA; serial measurement as part of an intensive surveillance programme improves survival when compared with less intensive follow-up.[6] Most expert groups recommend measurement of CEA at three-monthly intervals for at least three years in patients with stage II or III colorectal cancer who are candidates for surgery or systemic treatment of metastatic disease.[6] Current trials are investigating whether intervention (such as chemotherapy) is similarly beneficial after a rise in CA125 in patients with ovarian cancer. Results of one such trial suggest not, probably reflecting the current lack of curative treatments.[7]

The National Academy of Clinical Biochemistry recommends monitoring with PSA measurements after treatment for prostate cancer but cautions that the clinical utility varies depending on the disease stage of the individual patient.[6] Importantly, cancer progression may occur without increases in the concentration of the relevant tumour marker, and a tumour may occasionally lose its ability to produce a marker, perhaps as a result of dedifferentiation.

Sustained decreases in marker concentrations provide reassuring and objective evidence of tumour regression. However, as rising levels provide early evidence of progression, if alternative treatment is not available then monitoring with marker measurements can cause psychological distress without much clinical benefit. The ultimate decision about whether to monitor with tumour markers requires close cooperation between clinicians and patients.[6] A recent article provides insight into these issues from the perspective of a patient with ovarian cancer monitored with CA125 measurement.[21]

Why is non-selective requesting of tumour markers undesirable?

If they are inappropriately requested, tumour marker measurements may lead to additional and unnecessary investigations, as recently illustrated for a cirrhotic patient extensively investigated for ovarian cancer because her serum CA125 was raised.[22] Raised markers may lead to suspicion of disease in organs not relevant to the patient's presentation, potentially causing undue alarm, while normal levels may provide false reassurance. Either scenario can result in additional cost (such as admission to hospital), risk of side effects (such as endoscopy, which carries a small risk of mortality), and/or delayed diagnosis.

What evidence exists that tumour markers are often requested inappropriately?

A recent audit of practice in Northern Ireland found that, although 80% of tumour marker requests were associated with the relevant organ, 54% of clinicians used tumour markers to screen for malignancy, with a low index of suspicion in 35% of these requests.[23] Another audit in a single UK hospital found that 26% of all tests for the marker of breast cancer CA15-3 were for men—even though none of these men had breast biopsies in the year of the study or in the two years before—as were 17% of requests for the marker of ovarian cancer CA125.[24] In the Greek study mentioned earlier, only 20% of 10 291 retrospectively reviewed tumour marker results for 1944 patients were for patients with cancer.[4] The lowest level of appropriate requesting was for the pancreatic marker CA19-9 (1.9%), and 26% of CA125 requests were for men.[4] The colorectal cancer marker CEA was most often correctly requested (27%).[4]

Is the method by which tumour markers are measured important?

When interpreting results, particularly serial results, clinicians need to be aware that results obtained using different methods are not necessarily comparable.[25] The National Academy of Clinical Biochemistry recommends that laboratories indicate the method used when reporting the results for tumour markers, provide cumulative (ideally graphical) reporting, and append an interpretative comment, especially if there have been intervening method changes (figure).[1] Early discussion with laboratory staff about any results that do not accord with the clinical picture facilitates early identification of analytical errors.[1 12] Such identification is helped by the provision of relevant clinical information when tests are ordered, which is strongly recommended by the National Academy of Clinical Biochemistry.[1]

How can the process of requesting tumour markers be improved?

Guidelines provide a helpful framework for initiatives to promote best practice, with local ownership being essential for successful implementation.[26] Encouraging effective communication between clinical and laboratory staff—such

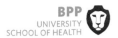

SOURCES AND SELECTION CRITERIA

This review is based on recently published guidelines for tumour markers from the National Academy of Clinical Biochemistry, which include summaries of relevant recommendations of other clinical organisations including the American Society for Clinical Oncology, the European Group on Tumour Markers, the National Comprehensive Cancer Network, the National Institute for Health and Clinical Excellence, and the Scottish Intercollegiate Guideline Network. We also searched PubMed and the Cochrane database to identify the best available evidence using search words including "tumour marker", "guidelines", and the names of relevant tumour markers. We supplemented these sources with our own knowledge of the literature and relevant authoritative reviews

TIPS FOR NON-SPECIALISTS

- Tumour marker results are rarely diagnostic and cannot replace biopsy for establishing the primary diagnosis of cancer. A raised tumour marker result does not necessarily indicate a particular malignancy but may provide some indication of its likelihood. Results within normal limits do not exclude malignancy or progression
- Measurements of tumour markers are not recommended for patients with vague symptoms when the population likelihood of cancer is low, as in general practice
- The main clinical use of existing serum tumour markers is in postoperative surveillance and in monitoring after chemotherapy, endocrine therapy, or radiotherapy
- Tumour marker results are often method dependent—patients should, ideally, be monitored using the same method and its name indicated on the report form
- Tumour marker results should always be interpreted in the context of all available information including clinical findings, imaging investigations, and other blood tests (such as renal and liver function and haematological tests). The possible influence of other factors (such as medication) should be carefully considered
- Laboratory staff should be alerted to any results that are unexpected or do not accord with the clinical picture in order to minimise the risk of clinical error or misinterpretation. Where doubt exists about a result a confirmatory specimen is usually desirable

A PATIENT'S PERSPECTIVE

In an area of medicine with conflicting views about at what point it is even necessary to investigate if a patient has prostate cancer, and with similar conflicting claims about the efficacy or even desirability of different forms of treatment, two words sum up the experience of the average male patient—uncertain and vulnerable.

In this situation one thing men have to cling on to is their PSA reading. It appeals to men, or at least to those men who wish to know the detail of what is happening to them. It is something tangible, non-conceptual. We're also used to scouring the football or rugby results for the measurable minutiae of progress, decline, movement, and the like.

I doubt that my own case is particularly exceptional. A PSA reading of 7 µg/l was identified through the ProtecT Study (a randomised controlled trial evaluating treatments for localised prostate cancer, comparing surgery (radical prostatectomy), radiotherapy (radical conformal), and monitoring with regular check-ups). My GP told me that with that particular reading he would have said not to worry and to come back to the surgery the following year. (I subsequently talked to other men who visited their GPs only to be told it was not the policy of the practice to do PSA tests unless there were "symptoms" and that PSA readings were often inaccurate and could create unnecessary anxiety for patients.)

I did extensive research and felt my PSA was high enough to warrant a biopsy. The PSA reading was the definitive catalyst for my action. It was also all I really had, and still have, even though it would seem to be a test that's been around a long time by current medical standards.

My biopsy gave a Gleason reading of 7 (3+4). On that basis, in consultation with my urologist, I had a laparoscopic prostatectomy. The subsequent laboratory report showed a Gleason reading of 7, but 4+3, with a 50% chance of spread. After two and four months my PSA was 0.1 µg/l, but after a further four months it had risen to 0.2 µg/l. Is this a "blip," or a sign that cancer cells are active and thus requiring more treatment? I will find out at my next appointment. So believe me, my PSA reading is very important to me. It does dominate my thinking and I have little doubt that it will be a factor for the rest of my life.

ONGOING AND FUTURE RESEARCH

- Prospective trials to evaluate utility of tumour markers in screening for early malignancy are in progress for α fetoprotein, CA125, and PSA
- Prospective trials to evaluate whether early intervention based on tumour marker increases in the absence of other clinical evidence of progression benefits outcome are about to report for CA125; similar trials are needed for CA15-3 in patients with breast cancer
- Validation is needed of emerging promising markers. Studies are currently in progress to evaluate PCA-3 in prostate cancer, epididymis 4 protein in ovarian cancer, and progastrin releasing peptide in small cell lung cancer
- New markers are needed for certain cancers—such as cervical and gastric malignancies (currently, serum markers are lacking for these cancers)
- Development of predictive markers are needed for cytotoxic therapies and the new biological therapies. Predictive markers are particularly important for the latter, as these agents are usually effective in only a small proportion of patients and are also expensive. Emerging predictive markers include the mutational status of k-ras for predicting benefit from cetuximab and panitumumab in patients with advanced colorectal cancer and the mutational status of epidermal growth factor receptor in predicting benefit from gefitinib (still being tested in research trials) or erlotinib in patients with advanced non-small cell lung cancer

of PCA-3 in urine may help to stratify patients according to their risk of prostate cancer before biopsy, although large scale validation studies are needed.[28] Similar studies are needed to assess the utility of methylated genes in the management of patients with cancer.[29]

Serum tumour markers currently contribute relatively little to treatment decisions, often owing to the lack of effective second line treatment. As treatments improve, predictive serum tests may help to identify patients most likely to benefit from new and expensive drugs. Personalised treatment is most advanced for breast cancer, with tissue markers such as oestrogen receptor and HER-2 (human epidermal growth factor receptor 2) predicting response to endocrine therapy and trastuzumab respectively.[30]

We thank Sheila Liggat, Ranjit Manchanda, Orest Mulka, Julietta Patnick, Carole Shahin, and Simon Walker for their careful reading of the manuscript and most helpful comments.

Contributors: All authors contributed to the preparation of this paper. Orest P Mulka read the manuscript at an early stage and commented on it from a general practice perspective. CMS is the guarantor.

Competing interests: None declared.

Provenance and peer review: Commissioned; externally peer reviewed.

Patient consent obtained.

1   Sturgeon CM, Hoffman BR, Chan DW, Ch'ng SL, Hammond E, Hayes DF, et al. National Academy of Clinical Biochemistry Laboratory Medicine Practice Guidelines for use of tumor markers in clinical practice: quality requirements. *Clin Chem*2008;54(8):e1-10.
2   Lai LC, Cheong SK, Goh KL, Leong CF, Loh CS, Lopez JB, et al. Clinical usefulness of tumour markers. *Malays J Pathol*2003;25(2):83-105.
3   Duffy MJ. Role of tumor markers in patients with solid cancers: a critical review. *Eur J Intern Med*2007;18:175-84.
4   Ntaios G, Hatzitolios A, Chatzinikolaou A, Karalazou P, Savopoulos C, Karamouzis M, et al. An audit of tumour marker utilization in Greece. *Eur J Intern Med*2009;20(3):e66-9.
5   Duffy MJ. Evidence for the clinical use of tumour markers. *Ann Clin Biochem*2004;41(pt 5):370-7.
6   Sturgeon CM, Duffy MJ, Stenman UH, Lilja H, Brunner N, Chan DW, et al. National Academy of Clinical Biochemistry laboratory medicine practice guidelines for use of tumor markers in testicular, prostate, colorectal, breast, and ovarian cancers. *Clin Chem*2008;54(12):e11-79.
7   Rustin GJ, van der Burg ME. A randomized trial in ovarian cancer (OC) of early treatment of relapse based on CA125 level alone versus

as through laboratory provision of more informative reports (figure)—is likely to improve test requesting, particularly if underpinned by audit.

What new tumour markers are emerging?

New tumour markers may complement existing markers.[6] The gene product human epidymis 4 protein has been cleared by the US Food and Drug Administration as an aid for monitoring patients with ovarian cancer.[27] Measurement

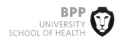

ADDITIONAL EDUCATIONAL RESOURCES

Resources for healthcare professionals

- European Group on Tumour Markers (www.egtm.eu/)—The group's website provides information about tumour markers for several cancer sites

- McAllister EJ, Sturgeon CM. Tumour markers. In: Marshall WJ, Bangert SK, eds. *Clinical biochemistry. Metabolic and clinical aspects.* 2nd ed. Edinburgh: Churchill Livingstone Elsevier, 2008:891-913.

- National Academy of Clinical Biochemistry (www.aacc.org/members/nacb/Pages/default.aspx)—This part of the American Association of Clinical Chemistry and Laboratory Medicine provides consensus based guidelines for the laboratory evaluation and monitoring of patients with specified disorders, including those with cancer

- National Comprehensive Cancer Network (www.nccn.org)—The network, an alliance of 20 of the world's foremost cancer centres, provides detailed clinical practice guidelines for most malignancies

- Scottish Intercollegiate Guideline Network (http://sign.ac.uk)—Provides summaries of evidence based guidelines for more than 12 cancer sites, together with guidelines related to other aspects of medicine

Resources for patients

- Labs Are Vital (www.labsarevital.com)—Provides information about how laboratories contribute to the healthcare community with up to date bulletins on new tests, including tumour markers

- Lab Tests Online UK (www.labtestsonline.org.uk/)—Provides information about how clinical laboratory tests contribute to diagnosis and treatment of all diseases, including cancer. Facility for searching for tests or for specific conditions and diseases

- National Institute for Health and Clinical Excellence (www.nice.org.uk/)—Provides national guidance on the promotion of good health and the prevention and treatment of ill health, including guidance relating to several cancer sites

- NHS Choices: Your health, your choices (www.nhs.uk/Livewell/cancer/Pages/Cancerhome.aspx)—Includes advice about prevention, diagnosis, and treatment for several cancers

- NHS National Cancer Screening Programmes (www.cancerscreening.nhs.uk/prostate/informationpack.html)—An updated information pack (July 2009) about PSA testing and the UK Prostate Cancer Risk Management Informed Choice programme

delayed treatment based on conventional clinical indicators (MRC OV05/EORTC 55955 trials). *J Clin Oncol*2009;27:18s:abstract 1.

8   Smith A, Wisloff F, Samson D. Guidelines on the diagnosis and management of multiple myeloma 2005. *Br J Haematol*2006;132:410-51.

9   Department of Health. *Key messages for ovarian cancer for health professionals.* 2009. www.dh.gov.uk/en/Healthcare/Cancer/DH_095624.

10 Duffy MJ, Sturgeon C, Lamerz R, Haglund C, Holbec VL, Klapdor R, et al. Tumor markers in pancreatic cancer: a European Group on Tumor Markers (EGTM) status report. *Ann Oncol*2009; advance access, 18 Aug, doi:10.1093/annonc/mdp332.

11 National Comprehensive Cancer Network. *NCCN clinical practice guidelines in oncology.* Hepatobiliary cancers. Version 2. 2009. www.nccn.org/professionals/physician_gls/f_guidelines.asp

12 Sturgeon C. Quality assurance of PSA testing. In: Schmeller N, ed. *Clinical value of PSA.* Bremen, Germany: Uni-Med, 2005:28-39.

13 American Cancer Society. *Can prostate cancer be found early?*2009. www.cancer.org/.

14 Wanebo HJ, Rao B, Pinsky CM, Hoffman RG, Stearns M, Schwartz MK, et al. Preoperative carcinoembryonic antigen level as a prognostic indicator in colorectal cancer. *N Engl J Med*1978;299:448-51.

15 Andriole GL, Crawford ED, Grubb RL 3rd, Buys SS, Chia D, Church TR, et al. Mortality results from a randomized prostate-cancer screening trial. *N Engl J Med*2009;360:1310-9.

16 Schroder FH, Hugosson J, Roobol MJ, Tammela TL, Ciatto S, Nelen V, et al. Screening and prostate-cancer mortality in a randomized European study. *N Engl J Med*2009;360:1320-8.

17 Barry MJ. Screening for prostate cancer—the controversy that refuses to die. *N Engl J Med*2009;360:1351-4.

18 Graham J, Baker M, Macbeth F, Titshall V. Diagnosis and treatment of prostate cancer: summary of NICE guidance. *BMJ*2008;336:610-2.

19 Menon U, Gentry-Maharaj A, Hallett R, Ryan A, Burnell M, Sharma A, et al. Sensitivity and specificity of multimodal and ultrasound screening for ovarian cancer, and stage distribution of detected cancers: results of the prevalence screen of the UK Collaborative Trial of Ovarian Cancer Screening (UKCTOCS). *Lancet Oncol*2009;10:327-40.

20 Krege S, Beyer J, Souchon R, Albers P, Albrecht W, Algaba F, et al. European consensus conference on diagnosis and treatment of germ cell cancer: a report of the second meeting of the European Germ Cell Cancer Consensus Group (EGCCCG): part I. *Eur Urol*2008;53:478-96.

21 Fleming LW. Playing the waiting game . . . the asymptomatic patient with recurrent ovarian cancer detected only by rising Ca125 levels. *Scott Med J*2001;46(3):81-3.

22 Kilpatrick ES, Lind MJ. Appropriate requesting of serum tumour markers. *BMJ*2009;339:b3111.

23 McDonnell M. An audit of tumour marker requests in Northern Ireland. *Ann Clin Biochem*2004;41(pt 5):378-84.

24 McGinley PJ, Kilpatrick ES. Tumour markers: their use and misuse by clinicians. *Ann Clin Biochem*2003;40(pt 6):643-7.

25 Sturgeon CM, Seth J. Why do immunoassays for tumour markers give differing results? A view from the UK national external quality assessment schemes. *Eur J Clin Chem Clin Biochem*1996;34:755-9.

26 Sturgeon C. Practice guidelines for tumor marker use in the clinic. *Clin Chem*2002;48:1151-9.

27 Hellstrom I, Raycraft J, Hayden-Ledbetter M, Ledbetter JA, Schummer M, McIntosh M, et al. The HE4 (WFDC2) protein is a biomarker for ovarian carcinoma. *Cancer Res*2003;63:3695-700.

28 Wang R, Chinnaiyan AM, Dunn RL, Wojno KJ, Wei JT. Rational approach to implementation of prostate cancer antigen 3 into clinical care. *Cancer*2009;115:3879-86.

29 Duffy MJ, Napieralski R, Martens JW, Span PN, Spyratos F, Sweep FC, et al. Methylated genes as new cancer biomarkers. *Eur J Cancer*2009;45:335-46.

30 Duffy MJ, Crown J. A personalized approach to cancer treatment: how biomarkers can help. *Clin Chem*2008;54:1770-9.

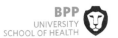
Testicular germ cell tumours

Alan Horwich professor of radiotherapy and honorary consultant in clinical oncology[1],
David Nicol consultant urological surgeon[2], Robert Huddart reader in urological oncology
and honorary consultant in clinical oncology[1]

[1]Royal Marsden Hospital and Institute of Cancer Research, Sutton SM2 5PT, UK

[2]Royal Marsden Hospital, London, UK

Correspondence to: A Horwich, Division of Radiotherapy and Imaging, Royal Marsden Hospital and Institute of Cancer Research, Sutton SM2 5PT, UK alan.horwich@icr.ac.uk

Cite this as: BMJ 2013;347:f5526

‹DOI› 10.1136/bmj.f5526
http://www.bmj.com/content/347/bmj.f5526

Testicular germ cell cancer affects mainly young men, with 85% presenting between 15 and 44 years of age. The incidence of this disease is increasing—the lifetime risk for a man is now about one in 200 in the United Kingdom.[1] Presentation is usually with a painless lump. If the tumour is diagnosed early, more than 95% of men are cured and treatment can be less intensive. Recent management changes include avoidance of radiotherapy, although cured patients still have increased risk of cardiac problems and second cancers. Some patients also experience chronic side effects of chemotherapy, such as neuropathy, hearing loss, renal impairment, and borderline hypogonadism. This article will review how testicular cancer presents, how it is diagnosed, and what treatments are available, including recent management changes to minimise toxicity.

What kinds of cancer arise in the testis?

This review covers germ cell cancers, which make up almost all testicular cancers seen in young men. Germ cell tumours are classified as pure seminomas or non-seminomas, which include variants such as embryonal carcinoma, teratocarcinoma, yolk sac tumour, choriocarcinoma, and teratoma. Tumours may contain one or more of these elements; those with both seminoma and non-seminoma components are managed as non-seminomas. Spermatocytic seminoma tends to occur in older men and is rarely, if ever, malignant.

In older patients, primary lymphomas of the testis become more common; a study from the Danish population based non-Hodgkin's lymphoma registry found that the median age at presentation was 71 years.[2] Tumours arising from endocrine structures, such as Leydig cell tumours or Sertoli cell tumours, can occur at various ages but are uncommon and usually benign. Rare tumours arising in paratesticular structures include rhabdomyosarcomas in children and liposarcomas in older men.

How does testicular germ cell cancer present?

More than 95% of these cancers present with a lump in the body of the testis.[3] The lump is usually painless but may cause episodic pains, possibly due to haemorrhage, and occasionally may mimic epididymo-orchitis or cause a hydrocele. Rarely, these cancers present with symptoms from metastases, such as backache from enlarging abdominal lymph nodes or chest symptoms from lung metastases such as cough, pain, or haemoptysis. Human chorionic gonadotrophin (HCG) production by the tumour can cause nipple tenderness and gynaecomastia. Less than 5% of germ cell tumours arise from an extragonadal primary site, such as the retroperitoneum or mediastinum.[4] Germ cell cancers are more common in men who have had a germ cell cancer of the contralateral testis, men with a first degree relative who has had testicular germ cell cancer, and those with a history of testicular maldescent.[5]

The testicular lump is usually noticed by the patient. Because of the lack of pain, medical consultation is often delayed, typically for several months.[6] Delay can influence the stage of the cancer and survival in men with non-seminomas. The diagnosis is suspected on physical examination of the testis when a discrete lump is palpable within the body of the testis. Differential diagnoses include cysts and inflammatory swellings of the epididymis, which may be tender and separable from the body of the testis. Analysis of 1017 patients seen at a rapid access testicular clinic included 203 referred because of "testicular lump" and 41 referred using a two week wait proforma because of suspected cancer. Eleven radical orchidectomies were performed and 10 of these men had malignant disease.[7]

How should a testicular lump be investigated?

National Institute for Health and Care Excellence (NICE) guidelines recommend that any patient with a swelling or mass in the body of the testis should be referred urgently for investigation. Consider urgent ultrasound in men with a scrotal mass that does not transilluminate or when the body of the testis cannot be palpated, such as when there is a reactive hydrocele. Suspected tumours can be confirmed by scrotal ultrasound (fig 1), which is the modality of choice for evaluating scrotal disease and has a sensitivity of almost 100% in diagnosing testicular cancer.[8]

Tumour markers, such as HCG or α fetoprotein, are often detectable on blood tests. The combination of a testicular lump and an increased concentration of HCG or α fetoprotein indicates a germ cell tumour. However, α fetoprotein is not increased in seminomas and HCG is raised in less than a quarter of cases[9]; in addition, about a third of non-seminomas are marker negative.[9] Because normal marker levels do not exclude testicular cancer and these markers are raised in other cancers and some benign conditions, they are not clinically useful in community practice.

METHODS

We searched our personal archives of references relating to the epidemiology, diagnosis, and management of testicular germ cell cancers as well as the Cochrane Database for reviews or meta-analyses. We also reviewed guideline publications from the European Society of Medical Oncology and the European Germ Cell Cancer Collaborative Group.

SUMMARY POINTS

- Testicular germ cell cancers occur mainly in young men
- Presentation is usually painless and the diagnosis can be confirmed by ultrasound
- Inguinal orchidectomy may be sufficient treatment in those with no evidence of metastases
- These tumours are sensitive to chemotherapy and radiotherapy, and even men with metastases are usually cured
- Men cured of metastatic disease have an increased risk of cardiac events and of second non-germ cell cancers

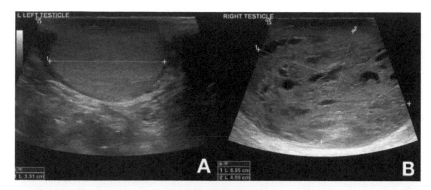

Fig 1 Testicular ultrasound scan of patient with normal left testis (A) and a germ cell tumour in the right testis (B)

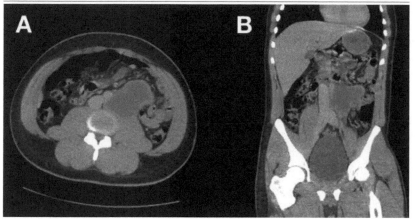

Fig 2 Axial (A) and coronal (B) computed tomograms showing a left sided retroperitoneal metastasis, which was causing backache

How is the diagnosis of testicular cancer confirmed?

Testicular cancer is diagnosed on the basis of the results from the above tests. The diagnosis is not confirmed by a biopsy, and standard initial management is orchidectomy in continuity with the spermatic cord, performed with an inguinal approach. It is a day case procedure performed under general anaesthesia. Normal testosterone concentrations are usually maintained by the contralateral testis. Partial orchidectomy may be considered in a patient with only one testis or in the rare circumstance of bilateral tumours at presentation.

What needs to be discussed before orchidectomy?

In the context of a normal contralateral testis, a unilateral orchidectomy should not cause infertility or abnormally low testosterone concentrations. If there is particular concern, and especially if chemotherapy may be needed, men can be referred for sperm cryopreservation. Testosterone concentrations can be monitored after orchidectomy and replacement testosterone products, such as three monthly depot testosterone undecanoate, can be prescribed.

Scottish Intercollegiate Guidelines Network (SIGN) guidelines suggest that a prosthesis should be offered.[10] A retrospective questionnaire review of 424 men post-orchidectomy included 71 who had received a prosthesis[11];

about 70% were satisfied, but 30% were unhappy about the shape or size of the implant and 25% were unhappy with the position or weight. Of those who had not been offered an implant, 64% said they would have accepted one, but two thirds of them did not feel this wish was strong enough to merit a second surgical intervention.

How is testicular cancer staged?

Staging is undertaken after orchidectomy and requires a computed tomogram of the thorax, abdomen, and pelvis (fig 2) and repeat tumour markers (table 1).[9] Raised markers should fall after orchidectomy—HCG and α fetoprotein have half lives of less than two days and about five days, respectively. Persisting or rising concentrations indicate metastasis even if a computed tomogram is normal. A positive positron emission tomography scan or retroperitoneal node biopsy can clarify equivocal lymph nodes, although these are not part of standard staging.

Germ cell cancers are now being diagnosed at an earlier stage and about 75% of patients present without evidence of metastases—that is, at stage I.[12] The first site of metastasis is typically the para-aortic lymph nodes. Tumour staging influences prognosis and treatment. Seminomas rarely present with metastasis beyond the retroperitoneal lymph nodes, whereas lung metastases are seen in about 15% of non-seminomas at presentation, and less commonly liver and brain metastases are found.

Who needs adjuvant treatment?

The risk in stage I patients is that they may harbour microscopic metastases. There are two main strategies to manage this risk—adjuvant chemotherapy or surveillance (reserving treatment for relapse).[13] [14]

Non-seminoma

In a minority of centres in some countries a staging lymph node dissection is considered, but it has the perceived disadvantage of being major surgery followed by the need

---

Table 1 Staging classification[10]

Stage	Characteristics
Stage I	No disease outside testis
Stage IM	No disease found outside testis but rising post-orchidectomy tumour markers
Stage II	Infradiaphragmatic nodes
Stage III	Supradiaphragmatic nodes
Stage IV	Extranodal metastases

The American Joint Committee on Cancer staging system, commonly used internationally, includes both supradiaphragmatic node metastasis and extranodal metastases as stage III and has no stage IV.

> **A PATIENT'S PERSPECTIVE**
>
> I discovered a swelling in my right testicle after falling on a rugby ball, and although I thought it was unlikely to be testicular cancer, I visited my general practitioner and was sent for an ultrasound. I had an orchidectomy as a day case and had no serious discomfort. Histological analysis showed that the testicle was cancerous.
>
> I was sent to a specialist hospital for further treatment. This involved having a positron emission tomography scan, which I was worried about. Thankfully the results came back quickly and showed that I was fit and well. However, I was asked if I wanted chemotherapy as a precaution. After further discussion, I decided to have my abdominal lymph nodes removed to identify any secondary tumours. Although a major operation, I was in hospital for only five days and recovered quickly.
>
> I received chemotherapy over the next three months and was fine until the third course, which took about four weeks to get over. I am now in remission and feeling fine, a bit achy with some loss of feeling in my toes. The tinnitus I was warned about was well managed by spreading the chemotherapy and doesn't cause any real problems. I feel "lucky'" to have had this form of cancer—from the outset the doctors were confident of cure, which gave me confidence. After my first surveillance check all seems well thanks to the care and professionalism of the team who looked after me and the fantastic support of my family.

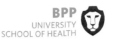

for surveillance or adjuvant chemotherapy. A prospective randomised trial compared retroperitoneal node dissection with adjuvant chemotherapy in 382 patients and found recurrence rates within two years of 8% and 1%, respectively.[15]

With stage I non-seminoma, an overview analysis of multiple surveillance studies found an overall relapse risk of about 30% or 50% in men with lymphovascular invasion.[16] Relapse can be treated successfully by chemotherapy, with cure rates close to 100%.[17] Surveillance avoids unnecessary treatment in the 70% of men who will not need it, but it must be continued for five years, which some men find stressful. Others do not adhere to the surveillance protocol, risking recurrence with advanced disease.

An argument for the alternative strategy of adjuvant chemotherapy is that less chemotherapy is needed in the adjuvant setting than when patients relapse. A multicentre prospective Medical Research Council study established the efficacy of two cycles of bleomycin, etoposide, cisplatinum in the adjuvant setting, with a relapse risk of less than 2%.[13] However, recent studies suggest that a single cycle may be equally effective. A large prospective randomised German multicentre trial reported a relapse risk of only 1% after one cycle of bleomycin, etoposide, cisplatinum.[18]

Seminoma

Several large prospective cohort studies in men with stage I seminoma show that the relapse rate on surveillance is about 18%,[19] higher in larger tumours. Seminomas are more indolent than non-seminomas, and radiological surveillance must continue for more than five years. The Royal Marsden Hospital surveillance regimen (fig 3) includes three monthly outpatient visits for the first two years after orchidectomy, four monthly visits in the third year, and six monthly visits until five years. However, as for non-seminoma tumours, there are concerns that those who relapse require more anticancer treatment than with the adjuvant approach.

An alternative adjuvant strategy for stage I seminoma has also been investigated—a single dose of the low toxicity drug carboplatin, to which seminomas are particularly sensitive. Carboplatin at the moderate dose needed does not cause alopecia, nephrotoxocity, neuropathy, or hearing loss. Follow-up from a large randomised trial showed that the relapse-free rate at five years was 94.7% with carboplatin compared with 96% for adjuvant radiotherapy.[20] Thus, patients with stage I seminoma can be advised that surveillance is associated with a relapse risk of one in six compared with one in 25 after a single cycle of carboplatin. Agreed guidelines, such as those from the European Society of Medical Oncology or SIGN, recommend that management choice is based on discussion of these issues between the clinician and patient with both surveillance and adjuvant therapy curing about 99%. Many centres use a risk based approach, with adjuvant chemotherapy reserved for those with highest risk, such as those with larger tumours. The Spanish Germ Cell Group evaluated such an approach in a prospective multicentre study and found a recurrence rate of 7% in low risk patients on surveillance compared with 1% in high risk patients after adjuvant carboplatin.[21]

Reducing radiation

Until recently, standard adjuvant treatment for stage I testicular seminoma comprised abdominal radiotherapy, which achieved cure in 95% of men. Worries about the carcinogenic effects of radiation led to prospective multicentre trials that evaluated the impact of reducing the dose of radiation and the extent of the radiation field.[22] These established the efficacy of only 20 Gy in 10 fractions over two weeks, confined to a field that included the para-aortic nodes but spared the pelvic organs.[23] [24]

What problems are associated with surveillance?

Failure to adhere to rigorous surveillance protocols may result in recurrence with advanced stage disease. A prospective UK study of 184 men who completed a range of questionnaires initially, and whose clinic attendance was subsequently analysed,[25] found no significant differences between attenders and non-attenders in most psychosocial and medical variables. However, a highly significant association was seen between non-attendance and a patient's perception of an unsatisfactory affective relationship with his clinician (P=0.005; hazard ratio 3.1, 95% confidence interval 1.4 to 6.6). This was shown by the level of agreement with statements in the medical interview satisfaction scale such as "The doctors are people I would trust with my life."

How effective is chemotherapy in metastatic disease?

More than 80% of men with metastatic germ cell cancer are cured.[26] This is due to exquisite sensitivity to cisplatinum based combination chemotherapy. The standard regimen for metastatic disease is three or four cycles of cisplatinum, etoposide, and bleomycin repeated every 21 days. If scans show any residual masses, surgery is considered. The high dose of cisplatinum requires intensive saline hydration to prevent nephrotoxicity. Previously this involved inpatient care for three to five days. Nowadays, in suitable patients, administration is on an outpatient basis with hydration supplemented orally.

Using a database of more than 5800 patients, relapse rates of 18-33% and 11-59% were found in seminoma and non-seminoma, respectively, after initial chemotherapy.[26] An international prognostic classification based on this information is now used to guide the intensity of chemotherapy for patients with metastatic disease. Prognostic groupings are based on serum concentrations of the tumour markers, α fetoprotein, HCG, and lactate dehydrogenase, as well as the presence of non-pulmonary visceral metastases or a mediastinal primary. Patients are classified into good, intermediate, and poor prognostic groups (table 2) and 48-99% can expect to survive. Patients who do not respond to first line chemotherapy may still be cured, so overall survival is higher than progression-free survival.

What if there are residual masses after chemotherapy?

Residual masses after chemotherapy for non-seminoma may consist of necrotic or fibrotic tissue, but may also contain residual active cancer cells or teratoma (differentiated). Removal is recommended, because current imaging modalities cannot reliably differentiate between these diseases. Teratoma is chemoresistant and resection

Table 2 Cure rates in testicular germ cell cancers

Type of disease	Seminoma	Non-seminoma
Stage	99%	99%
Metastatic:		
Good	86%	92%
Intermediate	72%	80%
Poor	—	48%

Month	Clinical	Markers	Chest radiography	CT abdomen
3	O	O		
6	O	O	O	O
9	O	O		
12	O	O	O	O
15	O	O		
18	O	O	O	O
21	O	O		
24	O	O	O	O
28	O	O		
32	O	O		
36	O	O	O	O
42	O	O		
48	O	O	O	O
54	O	O		
60	O	O	O	O
72	O	O		
84	O	O		
96	O	O		
108	O	O		
120	O	O		

Fig 3 Surveillance follow-up schedule after orchidectomy for seminoma. Computed tomography (CT) scans should be of the abdomen only unless the pelvis at risk. Markers: α fetoprotein, β human chorionic gonadotrophin, lactate dehydrogenase

prevents growth and risk of carcinomatous or sarcomatous transformation. The operation—generally referred to as a retroperitoneal lymph node dissection—requires a laparotomy, is a complex procedure, and patients must be referred to a specialist centre. A specific complication of this operation is retrograde (or dry) ejaculation. This can sometimes be avoided by a nerve sparing procedure. The operation can be performed in selected cases by laparoscopic or robotic surgery, but not when major vascular structures (such as the aorta, vena cava, and renal vessels) are involved. Residual masses at sites other than the abdominal lymph nodes (such as the chest) require similar management.

In seminoma, surgery is not usually recommended for residual masses, which are usually benign and associated with a dense fibrotic process obscuring anatomical planes.

How are patients who do not respond to initial chemotherapy treated?

Second line chemotherapy, often with surgery, can salvage about half of recurrences.[27] The chance of cure depends on the extent of disease at relapse and initial sensitivity of the disease. A recent multivariate analysis identified five prognostic groups with a chance of cure, varying from less than 10% to over 70%.[28] Relapses are challenging, requiring referral to specialist centres. Salvage chemotherapy usually involves further cisplatin, so the risk of chronic toxicities is high. The usefulness of high dose chemotherapy with autologous stem cell support is the subject of much debate and controversy. It has not yet been established in a prospective randomised trial, but pilot and retrospective studies have reported promising results.[29] Recent studies have shown that a small number of patients relapse late (defined as after two years, but sometimes after 10 years or more).[30] These relapses tend to be chemoresistant and surgical resection is recommended as primary treatment.

What are the side effects of combination chemotherapy?

Side effects depend on the choice of anticancer drug and total dose. For the standard germ cell regimen of bleomycin, etoposide, and cisplatinum, the side effects include nausea and vomiting, alopecia, fatigue, rashes and skin pigmentation, and neutropenia and thrombocytopenia.

Gastrointestinal side effects are less problematic since the development of neurokinin antagonists (such as aprepitant) and serotonin antagonists, usually given together with steroids.[31]

Bleomycin may cause pneumonitis in some patients (during or within a few months of completing chemotherapy), so chest symptoms require urgent specialist assessment.[32] This drug can also affect the vasculature and lead to Raynaud's phenomenon.[33]

Cisplatinum can cause a peripheral neuropathy and ototoxicity, characteristically a loss of high tone sensitivity, both of which can persist and require specialist referral. Standard chemotherapy causes azoospermia, although men treated with no more than four cycles usually recover spermatogenesis,[34] and as a precaution men can be offered sperm cryopreservation before chemotherapy. An analysis of 170 patients who were re-assessed at least one year after chemotherapy showed that of 89 patients whose pre-chemotherapy sperm counts were normal, the post-chemotherapy count was normal in 64%, reduced in 16%, and zero in 20%. There was clear evidence for continued recovery beyond one year; the probability of spermatogenesis increased to 48% by two years and 80% by five.[34]

These concerns have led to studies aimed at maintaining cure rate with less toxicity.[35] A large prospective trial showed that for metastatic disease with a good prognosis, three cycles of bleomycin, etoposide, and cisplatinum are as effective as four.[36] For men who present with advanced disease and a poor prognosis, more intensive chemotherapy schedules have been evaluated,[37] [38] although high dose treatments have not been proved to be beneficial.[39]

What are the long term health consequences in testicular cancer survivors?

Most survivors of testicular cancer regain a normal quality of life. A proportion of patients become hypogonadal after orchidectomy,[40] and this is likely to affect quality of life.[41] Testosterone concentrations clearly below the normal range should be treated, but the benefit of correcting borderline low values (7-12 nmol/L; 1 nmol/L=28.82 ng/dL) is uncertain and the subject of a current UK trial (TRYMS). Fertility may be reduced after chemotherapy, with risk depending on dose and type of chemotherapy.[34] Peripheral neuropathy, Raynaud's phenomenon, and hearing loss as a result of chemotherapy may persist for years.[33]

The risk of developing a second (non-germ cell) cancer is doubled in those who were treated in the past with standard chemotherapy regimens or radiotherapy.[42] For those who had radiotherapy the risk is to organs in the radiation field. After chemotherapy the risk includes leukaemias, lung cancer, and melanoma.[43] There is also an increased risk of cardiac events. A cohort study of UK survivors found a relative risk of cardiovascular disease of 2.6 after chemotherapy and 2.4 after radiotherapy.[44] The cause of this increase is not clear, but an increased rate of metabolic syndrome has been noted after treatment.

The increased risk of cardiovascular disease and a second cancer is similar to the risk seen from long term smoking. More comprehensive studies of the health of survivors of testicular cancer are needed.[45] Patients should be counselled with respect to lifestyle, strongly advised not to smoke, and screened for other cardiac risk factors.

A review of reports on problems encountered by survivors of testicular cancer found overall quality of life scores

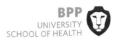

similar to those in the general population, but that anxiety associated with fear of recurrence, economic worries, alcohol misuse, and sexual difficulties were more common in survivors.[46]

This work was undertaken in the Royal Marsden NHS Foundation Trust, which received a proportion of its funding from the NHS Executive; we acknowledge NHS funding to the NIHR Biomedical Research Centre. The views expressed in this publication are those of the authors and not necessarily those of the NHS Executive. This work was supported by the Institute of Cancer Research (ICR).

Contributors: All three authors collaborated in identifying clinical evidence and writing this review. AH is guarantor.

Competing interests: We have read and understood the BMJ Group policy on declaration of interests and declare the following interests: None.

Provenance and peer review: Commissioned; externally peer reviewed.

1 Cancer Research UK. Testicular cancer incidence statistics. 2011. www.cancerresearchuk.org/cancer-info/cancerstats/types/testis/incidence/uk-testicular-cancer-incidence-statistics#source29.
2 Møller MB, d'Amore F, Christensen BE. Testicular lymphoma: a population-based study of incidence, clinicopathological correlations

and prognosis. The Danish Lymphoma Study Group, LYFO. *Eur J Cancer*1994;30A:1760-4.
3 Trama A, Mallone S, Nicolai N, Necchi A, Schaapveld M, Gietema J, et al; RARECARE Working Group. Burden of testicular, paratesticular and extragonadal germ cell tumours in Europe. *Eur J Cancer*2012;48:159-69.
4 Bokemeyer C, Nichols CR, Droz JP, Schmoll H J, Horwich A, Gerl A, et al. Extragonadal germ cell tumors of the mediastinum and retroperitoneum: results from an international analysis. *J Clin Oncol*2002;20:1864-73.
5 McGlynne KA, Cook MB. Etiologic factors in testicular germ cell tumors. *Future Oncol*2009;5:1389-402.
6 Huyghe E, Muller A, Mieusset R, Bujan L, Bachaud JM, Chevreau C, et al. Impact of diagnostic delay in testis cancer: results of a large population-based study. *Eur Urol* 2007;52:1710-6.
7 Rochester M, Scurrell S, Parry JR. Prospective evaluation of a novel one-stop testicular clinic. *Ann R Coll Surg Engl*2008;90:565-70.
8 Dogra VS, Gottlieb RH, Oka M, Rubens DJ. Sonography of the scrotum. *Radiology*2003;227:18-36.
9 Gilligan TD, Seidenfeld J, Basch EM, Einhorn L H, Fancher T, Smith D C, et al. American Society of Clinical Oncology Clinical Practice guideline on uses of serum tumor markers in adult males with germ cell tumors. *J Clin Oncol*2010;28:3388-494.
10 Scottish Intercollegiate Guidelines Network. Management of adult testicular germ cell tumours. 2011. www.sign.ac.uk/pdf/sign124.pdf.
11 Adshead J, Khoubehi B, Wood J, Rustin G. Testicular implants and patient satisfaction: a questionnaire-based study of men after orchidectomy for testicular cancer. *BJU Int*2001;88:559-62.
12 Horwich A, Shipley J, Huddart R. Testicular germ-cell cancer. *Lancet*2006;367:754-65.
13 Cullen MH, Stenning SP, Parkinson MC, Fossa S D, Kaye S B, Horwich A, et al. Short-course adjuvant chemotherapy in high-risk stage I nonseminomatous germ cell tumors of the testis: a Medical Research Council report. *J Clin Oncol*1996;14:1106-13.
14 Read G, Stenning SP, Cullen MH, Parkinson MC, Horwich A, Kaye SB, et al. Medical Research Council prospective study of surveillance for stage I testicular teratoma. Medical Research Council testicular tumors working party. *J Clin Oncol*1992;10:1762-8.
15 Albers P, Siener R, Krege S, Schmelz HU, Dieckmann KP, Heidenreich A, et al. German Testicular Cancer Study Group randomized phase III trial comparing retroperitoneal lymph node dissection with one course of bleomycin and etoposide plus cisplatin chemotherapy in the adjuvant treatment of clinical stage I Nonseminomatous testicular germ cell tumors: AUO trial AH 01/94 by the German Testicular Cancer Study Group. *J Clin Oncol*2008;26:2966-72.
16 Vergouwe Y, Steyerberg EW, Eijkemans MJ, Albers P, Habberna JD. Predictors of occult metastasis in clinical stage I non-seminoma: a systematic review. *J Clin Oncol*2003;21:4092-9.
17 Kollmannsberger C, Moore C, Chi KN, Murray N, Daneshmand S, Gleave M, et al. Non risk-adapted surveillance for patients with stage I nonseminomatous testicular germ-cell tumors: diminishing treatment-related morbidity while maintaining efficacy. *Ann Oncol*2010;21:1296-301.
18 Albers P, Siener R, Krege S, Schmelz HU, Dieckmann KP, Heidenreich A, et al. Randomised phase III trial comparing retroperitoneal lymph node dissection with one course of bleomycin and etopside plus cisplatin chemotherapy in the adjuvant treatment of clinical stage I nonseminomatous testicular germ cell tumors. AUO trial AH 01/94 by the German Testicular Cancer Study Group. *J Clin Oncol*2008;26:2966-72.
19 Cummins S, Yau T, Huddart R, Dearnaley D, Horwich A. Surveillance in stage I seminoma patients: a long-term assessment. *Eur Urol*2010;57:673-8.
20 Oliver RT, Mead GM, Rustin GJ, Joffe JK, Aass N, Coleman R, et al. Randomized trial of carboplatin versus radiotherapy for stage I seminoma: mature results on relapse and contralateral testis cancer rates in MRC TE19/EORTC 30982 study (ISRCTN27163214). *J Clin Oncol*2011;29:957-62.
21 Aparicio J, Maroto P, del Muro XG, Gumà J, Sánchez-Muñoz A, Margelí M, et al. Risk-adapted treatment in clinical stage I testicular seminoma: the third Spanish Germ Cell Cancer Group study. *J Clin Oncol*2011;29:4677-81.
22 Zagars GK, Ballo MT, Lee AK, Strom SS. Mortality after cure of testicular seminoma. *J Clin Oncol*2004;22:640-7.
23 Jones WG, Fossa SD, Mead GM, Roberts JT, Sokal M, Horwich A, et al. Randomised trial of 30 versus 20 Gy in the adjuvant treatment of stage I testicular seminoma: a report on Medical Research Council Trial TE18, European Organisation for the Research and Treatment of Cancer Trial 30942. *J Clin Oncol*2005;23:1200-8.
24 Fossa SD, Horwich A, Russell JM, Roberts JT, Cullen MH, Hodson NJ, et al. Optimal planning target volume for stage I testicular seminoma: a Medical Research Council randomised trial. Medical Research Council Testicular Tumor Working Group. *J Clin Oncol*1999;17:1146.
25 Moynihan C, Norman AR, Barbachano Y, Burchell L, Huddart R, Dearnaley DP, et al. Prospective study of factors predicting adherence to medical advice in men with testicular cancer. *J Clin Oncol*2009;27:2144-50.
26 International Germ Cell Cancer Collaborative Group. International germ cell consensus classification: a prognostic factor-based staging system for metastatic germ cell cancers. *J Clin Oncol*1997;15:594-603.
27 Mead GM, Cullen MH, Huddart R, Harper P, Rustin GJ, Cook PA, et al. A phase II trial of TIP (paclitaxel, ifosfamide and cisplatin) given as second-line (post-BEP) salvage chemotherapy for patients with

---

TIPS FOR NON-SPECIALISTS

- Refer patients with testicular lumps to a urologist under the two week suspected cancer referral pathway
- Patients may present with gynaecomastia owing to the production of human chorionic gonadotrophin, or with backache or chest symptoms from metastases
- Assessment of a germ cell cancer includes histological review; computed tomography of the thorax, abdomen, and pelvis; and monitoring of serum tumour markers
- Cure rates are more than 90% even in those with metastases, but treatment can be less intensive when disease is diagnosed at an earlier stage

---

ONGOING RESEARCH

- Germ cell cancers are more common in first degree relatives of affected men and genetic studies are trying to identify predisposing genes
- Because surveillance for stage I seminoma seems to be a safe and practicable option, an ongoing Medical Research Council (MRC) trial, TRISST, is investigating the optimal radiological techniques and schedule
- There is limited evidence that a single cycle of bleomycin, etoposide, and cisplatinum is sufficient in the adjuvant setting to prevent recurrence in stage I non-seminoma, and further supportive evidence will come from the current MRC prospective 111 trial
- The risks of cardiac events and second cancers were increased in patients given curative treatment before 1990, and we need to determine whether newer chemotherapy and radiotherapy regimens have reduced these risks. We also need a better understanding of the mechanisms underlying these toxicities

---

ADDITIONAL EDUCATIONAL RESOURCES

Resources for healthcare professionals

- European Association of Urology Guidelines. Testicular cancer. 2012 edition. www.uroweb.org/guidelines/online-guidelines/
- Beyer J, Albers P, Altena R, Aparicio J, Bokemeyer C, Busch J, et al. Maintaining success, reducing treatment burden, focusing on survivorship: highlights from the third European consensus conference on diagnosis and treatment of germ-cell cancer. *Ann Oncol* 2013;24:878-88
- Scottish Intercollegiate Guidelines Network. Management of adult testicular germ cell tumours. 2011. www.sign.ac.uk/pdf/sign124.pdf
- Laguna MP, Albers P, Bokemeyer C, Richie JP, eds. Cancer of the testis. Springer, 2010.
- Horwich A, Shipley J, Huddart R. Testicular germ-cell cancer. *Lancet* 2006;367:754-65. Useful review

Resources for patients

- The following websites all provide patient information resources:
- Cancer Research UK (www.cancerresearchuk.org/cancer-help/type/testicular-cancer/)
- Macmillan Cancer Support (www.macmillan.org.uk)
- Healthtalk online (www.healthtalkonline.org/cancer/testicular_cancer)
- Everyman (www.everyman-campaign.org/)

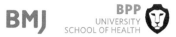

metastatic germ cell cancer: a medical research council trial. *Br J Cancer*2005;93:178-84.

28 International Prognostic Factors Study Group. Prognostic factors in patients with metastatic germ cell tumors who experienced treatment failure with cisplatin-based first-line chemotherapy. *J Clin Oncol*2010;28:4906-11.

29 Feldman DR, Sheinfeld J, Bajorin DF, Fischer P, Turkula S, Ishill N, et al. TI-CE high-dose chemotherapy for patients with previously treated germ cell tumors: results and prognostic factor analysis. *J Clin Oncol*2010;28:1706-13.

30 Oldenburg J, Martin JM, Fossa SD. Late relapses of germ cell malignancies: incidence, management and prognosis. *J Clin Oncol*2006;24:5503-11.

31 Herrstedt J, Roila F; ESMO Guidelines Working Group. Chemotherapy-induced nausea and vomiting: ESMO clinical recommendations for prophylaxis. *Ann Oncol*2009;20(suppl 4):ii154-8.

32 O'Sullivan JM, Huddart RA, Norman AR, Nicholls J, Dearnaley DP, Horwich A. Predicting the risk of bleomycin lung toxicity in patients with germ-cell tumours. *Ann Oncol* 2003;14:91-6.

33 Glendenning JL, Barbachano Y, Norman AR, Dearnaley DP, Horwich A, Huddart RA. Long-term neurologic and peripheral vascular toxicity after chemotherapy treatment of testicular cancer. *Cancer*2010;116:2322-31.

34 Lampe H, Horwich A, Norman A, Nicholls J, Dearnaley DP. Fertility after chemotherapy for testicular germ cell cancers. *J Clin Oncol*1997;15:239-45.

35 Singhera M, Lees K, Huddart R, Horwich A. Minimizing toxicity in early-stage testicular cancer treatment. *Expert Rev Anticancer Ther*2012;12:185-93.

36 De Wit R, Roberts JT, Wilkinson P, de Mulder PH, Mead GM, Fossa SD, et al. Equivalence of three or four cycles of bleomycin, etoposide, and cisplatin chemotherapy and of a 3- or 5-day schedule in good-prognosis germ cell cancer: a randomized study of the European Organization for Research and Treatment of Cancer Genitourinary Tract Cancer Cooperative Group and the Medical Research Council. *J Clin Oncol*2001;19:1629-40.

37 Christian JA, Huddart RA, Norman A, Mason M, Fossa S, Aass N, et al. Intensive induction chemotherapy with CBOP/BEP in patients with poor prognosis germ cell tumors. *J Clin Oncol*2003;21:871-7.

38 Kaye SB, Mead GM, Fossa S, Cullen M, deWit R, Bodrogi I, et al. Intensive induction-sequential chemotherapy with BOP/VIP-B compared with treatment with BEP/EP for poor-prognosis metastatic nonseminomatous germ cell tumor: a Randomized Medical Research Council/European Organization for Research and Treatment of Cancer study. *J Clin Oncol*1998;16:692-701.

39 Motzer RJ, Nichols CJ, Margolin KA, Bacik J, Richardson PG, Vogelzang NJ, et al. Phase III randomized trial of conventional-dose chemotherapy with or without high-dose chemotherapy and autologous hematopoietic stem-cell rescue as first-line treatment for patients with poor prognosis metastatic germ cell tumors. *J Clin Oncol*2007;25:247-56.

40 Huddart RA, Norman A, Moynihan C, Horwich A, Parker, Nicolls E, et al. Fertility, gonadal and sexual function in survivors of testicular cancer. *Br J Cancer*2005;93:200-7.

41 Greenfield DM, Walters SJ, Coleman RE, Hancock BW, Snowden JA, Shalet SM, et al. Quality of life, self-esteem, fatigue, and sexual function in young men after cancer: a controlled cross-sectional study. *Cancer*2010;116:1592-601.

42 Van den Belt-Dusebout AW, de Wit R, Gietema JA, Horenblas S, Lowman MW, Ribot JG, et al. Treatment-specific risks of second malignancies and cardiovascular disease in 5-year survivors of testicular cancer. *J Clin Oncol*2005;25:4370-8.

43 Robinson D, Moller H, Horwich A. Mortality and incidence of second cancers following treatment for testicular cancer. *Br J Cancer*2007;96:529-33.

44 Huddart RA, Norman A, Shahidi M, Horwich A, Coward D, Nicholls J, et al. Cardiovascular disease as a long-term complication of treatment for testicular cancer. *J Clin Oncol*2003;21:1513-23.

45 Travis LB, Beard CAJM, Dahl AA, Feldman DR, Oldenburg J, Daugaard G, et al. Testicular cancer survivorship: research strategies and recommendations. *J Natl Cancer Inst*2010;102:1130.

46 Haugnes H S, Bosl G J, Boer H, Gietema J A, Brydøy M, Oldenburg J, et al. Long-term and late effects of germ cell testicular cancer treatment and implications for follow-up. *J Clin Oncol* 2012;30:3752-63.

Related links

bmj.com/archive
- Managing cows' milk allergy in children (*BMJ* 2013;347:f5424)
- Personality disorder (*BMJ* 2013;347:f5276)
- Dyspepsia (*BMJ* 2013;347:f5059)
- Tourette's syndrome (*BMJ* 2013;347:f4964
- Developing role of HPV in cervical cancer prevention (*BMJ* 2013;347:f4781)

bmj.com
- Get Cleveland Clniic CME credits for ths article
- Oncology updates from BMJ

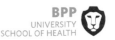
Identifying brain tumours in children and young adults

S H Wilne consultant paediatric oncologist[1], R A Dineen clinical associate professor[2], R M Dommett National Institute for Health Research clinical lecturer[3], T P C Chu research fellow in epidemiology[2], D A Walker professor of paediatric oncology[2]

[1]Department of Paediatric Oncology, Nottingham University Hospitals NHS Trust, Queens Medical Centre, Nottingham NG7 2UH, UK

[2]Faculty of Medicine and Health Sciences, University of Nottingham, Nottingham, UK

[3]School of Clinical Sciences, University of Bristol, Bristol, UK

Correspondence to: S H Wilne
sophie.wilne@nuh.nhs.uk

Cite this as: BMJ 2013;347:f5844

‹DOI› 10.1136/bmj.f5844
http://www.bmj.com/content/347/bmj.f5844

Healthcare professionals caring for children need to promptly identify the child or young person with a serious underlying condition from the majority who present with minor self limiting illness. Recognising when a child might have cancer can be particularly difficult. Despite the perception that cancer is rare in children, an average general practice will see a child or young person with a new cancer every six years, and a quarter of the tumours will be brain tumours (personal communication, Patricia O'Hare, 2013).[1] Early diagnosis can be crucial—evidence from cohort studies shows that it can improve short term and long term outcomes.[2][3][4][5] This review summarises current evidence on the presentation and recognition of brain tumours in children and young adults and provides an overview of the treatment and long term care strategies for this population.

What brain tumours occur in children?

The term "brain tumour" encompasses a large number of different tumour types that have different cells of origin and clinical course (table 1). The most common brain tumours in children and young people are pilocytic astrocytomas, medulloblastomas, ependymomas, high grade gliomas, and germ cell tumours.[6][7] Histologically, brain tumours are assigned a World Health Organization grade of 1-4 according to features suggesting malignancy, such as pleomorphic nuclei, high mitotic rate, and vascular invasion. Grades 1 and 2 are regarded as benign and 3 and 4 as malignant,[8] although the correlation between histological grade and patient outcome is poor. A low grade tumour that is not susceptible to treatment and is in a crucial area of the brain, such as the brain stem, is more likely to be fatal than

certain high grade tumours that are resectable and sensitive to chemoradiotherapy.[9][10]

What are the risk factors for brain tumours in children?

As is true for most childhood cancers, no cause or trigger can be identified for most brain tumours. Several genetic syndromes, however, are associated with an increased risk of brain tumours (table 2)[7]

The development of some childhood brain tumours is related to changes in the local tumour (brain) environment that are linked to age. Children with neurofibromatosis type 1 have a 10-20% risk of developing an intracranial pilocytic astrocytoma, particularly in the optic pathways, owing to loss of neurofibromin 1 (the product of the *NF1* gene), which is a negative regulator of cell growth through the mitogen activated protein kinases/extracellular signal regulated kinases pathway. Not every child with neurofibromatosis type 1 develops an optic pathway glioma, and almost all children with the condition who develop one are under the age of 7 years. Therefore there is an interaction between germline *NF1* mutations, the age of the child, and another unknown factor that results in the development of an optic pathway glioma in some but not all children with the condition.

Studies in mouse models of neurofibromatosis type 1 have shown that reduced cAMP production in the brain is needed for the development of tumours. Mouse and human tissue studies have shown that cAMP levels vary with polymorphisms in cAMP regulators,[11] and that cAMP levels in the optic pathway are lower in young children than in older ones. These findings explain why optic pathway gliomas occur in only some young children with neurofibromatosis type 1.

Intracranial germ cell tumours provide another less well understood example. With the exception of mature teratomas, intracranial germ cell tumours are very rare in young children but are much more common as adolescence proceeds, in parallel with the onset of puberty. Presumably, this is a result of the hormonal drive to gonadal development interacting with potential tumour cells within the brain.

Case-control and cohort studies have shown that exposure to ionising radiation is the only environmental factor associated with brain tumours.[7] Brain or central nervous system radiotherapy for a previous cancer is the most common cause of exposure to high doses of ionising radiation, and secondary high grade gliomas and meningiomas have been reported in these populations.[12] Children who undergo computed tomography (CT) also have a risk of radiation induced cancer. A recently published epidemiological study found 608 excess cancers (of which 147 were brain tumours) in 680 211 patients who had a CT scan between the ages of 0 and 19 years, with children less than 5 years being particularly at risk.[13]

SOURCES AND SELECTION CRITERIA

We searched Medline, Embase, and the Cochrane Library for review articles. Key words were brain tumour(s), brain tumor(s), and diagnosis. Articles were restricted to English language and all children. We also used personal reference libraries and consulted experts.

SUMMARY POINTS

- Each week in the United Kingdom, 10 children and young people are diagnosed with a brain tumour
- An average general practice sees a new childhood cancer every six years; a quarter of these will be brain tumours
- Earlier diagnosis of brain tumours in children and young adults improves long term outcomes
- Diagnosis requires recognition of the specific combinations of symptoms and signs seen with tumours in different areas of the brain and with raised intracranial pressure, followed by brain imaging
- The developmental stage of the child affects tumour presentation; young children may not be able to describe visual abnormalities and headache
- Include a focused history (looking for corroborative symptoms and risk factors) and assessment of vision, motor skills, growth, and puberty in children or young people who present with symptoms or signs suggestive of a brain tumour

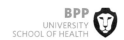

Table 1   Classification of brain tumours that occur in children and young people

Tumour group	Tumour	Location	WHO* grade	Approximate frequency (%)
Embryonal tumours: arise from transformation of undifferentiated and immature neuroepithelial cells	Medulloblastoma	Cerebellum	4	20
	Central primitive neuroectodermal tumour	Cerebral hemispheres	4	5
	Atypical teratoid or rhabdoid tumour	Throughout the brain	4	1
Glial tumours: arise from glial (supporting) cells	Astrocytoma	Throughout the brain	Pilocytic astrocytomas: 1; pilomyxoid astrocytomas: 2; anaplastic astrocytomas: 3; glioblastoma multiforme: 4	45
	Oligodendroglioma	Cerebral hemispheres	Oligodendroglioma: 2; anaplastic oligodendroglioma: 3	4
	Ependymoma	Throughout the ventricular system	Ependymoma: 2; anaplastic ependymoma: 3	10
	Choroid plexus tumours	Choroid plexus (within lateral ventricle)	Choroid plexus papilloma: 1; choroid plexus carcinoma: 3	2
Neuronal and glioneuronal tumours: arise from nerve cells	Ganglioglioma	Throughout the brain	1	3
	Dysembryoplastic neuroepithelial tumour	Cerebral hemispheres	1	2
Pineal parenchymal tumours: arise from melatonin secreting cells in the pineal glands (pineocytes)	Pineoblastoma	Pineal gland	2	1
	Pineocytoma	Pineal gland	4	1
Germ cell tumours: arise from germ cells that have become mislocated during embryonic development	Germinomas	Throughout the midline brain—for example, pituitary and pineal regions, hypothalamus, and third ventricle	Not included in WHO grading	4
	Teratomas			
	Embryonal carcinoma and yolk sac tumours			
Other developmental tumours	Craniopharyngioma	Epithelial tumour of sellar region (arises from Rathke's pouch epithelium)		
Meningiomas: arise from meningeal cells	Meningioma	Throughout the meninges	Meningioma: 1; atypical meningiomas: 2; anaplastic meningiomas: 3	2

*WHO=World Health Organization.

Table 2   Genetic syndromes associated with brain tumours in children and young people

Syndrome*	Prevalence (UK newborns)	Associated brain tumour	Clinical characteristics
Neurofibromatosis type 1	1/2500-3000	Astrocytomas; meningiomas; schwannomas	Skin: cafe au lait patches, axillary freckles, neurofibromas; bones: scoliosis, pseudarthrosis; learning and behavioural difficulties; peripheral nerve sheath tumours
Tuberous sclerosis	1/6000	Subependymal giant cell astrocytoma	Skin: hypomelanic nodules, angiofibromas, shagreen patch, ungula fibromas; heart: rhabdomyomas; Brain: cortical tubers, subependymal nodules, epilepsy; kidneys: angiomyolipomas; learning and behavioural difficulties
Neurofibromatosis 2	1/25 000	Schwannomas; meningiomas; ependymomas	Schwannomas (bilateral vestibular schwannomas); cataracts
Von Hippel-Lindau disease	1/36 000	Haemangioblastomas	Cerebellar and retinal haemangioblastoma, phaeochromocytoma, renal cysts, renal carcinoma, pancreatic cysts, pancreatic carcinoma, endolymphatic sac tumours
Li-Fraumeni syndrome	Unknown, rare	Astrocytomas; choroid plexus carcinoma	Early onset soft tissue sarcomas; leukaemia; osteosarcoma; melanoma; cancer of the breast, colon, pancreas, adrenal cortex, and brain
Turcot syndrome	Unknown, rare	Astrocytomas; medulloblastoma	Multiple adenomatous polyps, colorectal cancer and central nervous system tumours

How do brain tumours present in children and young people?

The symptoms and signs of brain tumours are varied and determined by the part of the brain affected, the developmental stage and ability of the child or young person, and whether or not intracranial pressure is raised. There is usually a clinical evolution in the time period between initial symptom onset and diagnosis. In a retrospective four centre cohort study of 139 children with a brain tumour, an average of one symptom or sign was reported at symptom onset, but this increased to six at the time of diagnosis.[14]

Figure 1 shows the combinations of symptoms and signs at diagnosis caused by tumours developing in different parts of the brain and the frequency with which they occur.[15] This information was obtained from a meta-analysis of the presenting symptoms and signs in 4171 children who were newly diagnosed with a brain tumour. Recognition of these specific combinations of symptoms and signs is an essential step towards diagnosis. Cerebellar tumours present with ataxia, nystagmus, head tilt, and poor coordination (www.youtube.com/watch?v=SwcQoTv_4Vw). At least 75% of cerebellar tumours obstruct the flow of cerebrospinal fluid through the aqueduct and into the fourth ventricle so also present with symptoms and signs of

Table 3   Brain tumour presentation according to age*

Pre-school (<5 years)	Primary school (5-11 years)	Secondary school (12-18 years)
Persistent or recurrent vomiting	Persistent or recurrent headache†	Persistent or recurrent headache†
Problems with balance, coordination, or walking	Persistent or recurrent vomiting	Persistent or recurrent vomiting
Abnormal eye movements	Problems with balance, coordination, or walking	Problems with balance, coordination, or walking
Behavioural change (particularly lethargy)	Abnormal eye movements	Abnormal eye movements
Fits or seizures (not with a fever)	Blurred or double vision†	Blurred or double vision†
Abnormal head position such as wry neck, head tilt, or persistent stiff neck	Behavioural change	Behavioural change
Progressively increasing head circumference†	Fits or seizures	Fits or seizures
	Abnormal head position such as wry neck, head tilt, or persistent stiff neck	Delayed or arrested puberty, slow growth†

*Based on a systematic review,[15] combined with clinical expertise and experience.
†Symptoms that differ according to age group.

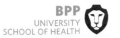

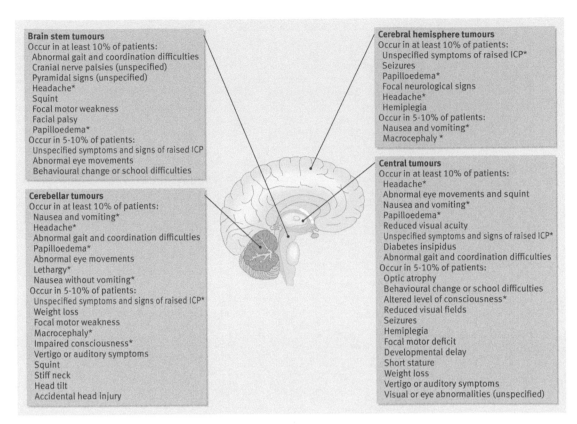

Brain stem tumours
Occur in at least 10% of patients:
  Abnormal gait and coordination difficulties
  Cranial nerve palsies (unspecified)
  Pyramidal signs (unspecified)
  Headache*
  Squint
  Focal motor weakness
  Facial palsy
  Papilloedema*
Occur in 5-10% of patients:
  Unspecified symptoms and signs of raised ICP
  Abnormal eye movements
  Behavioural change or school difficulties

Cerebellar tumours
Occur in at least 10% of patients:
  Nausea and vomiting*
  Headache*
  Abnormal gait and coordination difficulties
  Papilloedema*
  Abnormal eye movements
  Lethargy*
  Nausea without vomiting*
Occur in 5-10% of patients:
  Unspecified symptoms and signs of raised ICP*
  Weight loss
  Focal motor weakness
  Macrocephaly*
  Impaired consciousness*
  Vertigo or auditory symptoms
  Squint
  Stiff neck
  Head tilt
  Accidental head injury

Cerebral hemisphere tumours
Occur in at least 10% of patients:
  Unspecified symptoms of raised ICP*
  Seizures
  Papilloedema*
  Focal neurological signs
  Headache*
  Hemiplegia
Occur in 5-10% of patients:
  Nausea and vomiting*
  Macrocephaly *

Central tumours
Occur in at least 10% of patients:
  Headache*
  Abnormal eye movements and squint
  Nausea and vomiting*
  Papilloedema*
  Reduced visual acuity
  Unspecified symptoms and signs of raised ICP*
  Diabetes insipidus
  Abnormal gait and coordination difficulties
Occur in 5-10% of patients:
  Optic atrophy
  Behavioural change or school difficulties
  Altered level of consciousness*
  Reduced visual fields
  Seizures
  Hemiplegia
  Focal motor deficit
  Developmental delay
  Short stature
  Weight loss
  Vertigo or auditory symptoms
  Visual or eye abnormalities (unspecified)

Fig 1 Brain tumour presentation according to tumour location. *Symptom or sign caused by raised intracranial pressure (ICP)

raised intracranial pressure (headache, vomiting, lethargy, increasing head circumference, papilloedema, reduced level of consciousness).

Central brain tumours present with reduced visual acuity and fields, wandering or roving eye movements in young children (owing to loss of visual fixation), and damage to the hypothalamic-pituitary axis.

This last feature leads to abnormal pubertal progression (precocious, arrested, or delayed), growth failure, diabetes insipidus, and diencephalic syndrome in young children (emaciation despite normal energy intake). Central tumours may also obstruct the flow of cerebrospinal fluid, leading to symptoms and signs of raised intracranial pressure.

Brain stem tumours present with swallowing difficulties, facial asymmetry and squint (owing to lower cranial nerve damage), hemiplegia, poor coordination, and abnormal gait (owing to long tract involvement). Cerebral hemisphere tumours are least likely to cause neurological signs and often present with focal seizures; they can also cause hemiplegia or a more focal motor weakness.

The developmental stage and ability of the child can also alter the presentation of tumours. For example, at least 20% of midline tumours cause visual impairment owing to compression of the optic chiasm and optic tracts. Older children can recognise that visual loss is abnormal and have the language skills to express this. Younger children lack this ability and are good at navigating familiar environments, so they can develop marked loss before this is recognised. Similarly, raised intracranial pressure causes headache. Older children can describe this, but younger children are often not good at localising pain and don't have the language skills to describe headache; instead, they may appear unsettled, lethargic, or withdrawn. Table 3 shows the most common symptoms and signs of brain tumours in different age groups.

Red flag symptoms

Attempts to reduce delays in diagnosis of tumours have identified "red flag" symptoms and signs that trigger referral to a "fast track" investigation and diagnostic service in secondary care. A population based case-control study determined the predicative value of such symptoms and signs in identifying children with a subsequent diagnosis of cancer presenting to primary care.[16] The red flags were taken from National Institute for Health and Care Excellence (NICE) referral guidelines for suspected cancer.[17] Just over a quarter of patients diagnosed as having cancer had any red flag symptom recorded in the previous three months, and a third in the preceding year.

However, red flag symptoms also occurred in children and young people who did not have a tumour (1.4% in three months and 5.4% in 12 months). Occurrence of a red flag symptom or sign increased the likelihood of a cancer diagnosis from 0.35 to 5.5 in 10 000 children at three months and from 1.4 to 7.0 in 10 000 children over a year. Symptoms and signs with the highest predictive value for brain tumours were abnormal movement, visual symptoms, vomiting, headache, pain, and seizures.

Thus, red flag symptoms and signs do occur in brain tumours, but their lack of specificity limits their usefulness in identifying children and young people requiring rapid brain imaging to diagnose or exclude a brain tumour. Further evidence for this is provided by the routes to diagnosis study of all patients diagnosed as having cancer in England between 2006 and 2008, which found that only 2% of all childhood cancers were diagnosed through a "two week" wait referral.[18]

Cohort and case-control studies have shown an association between frequency of consultation and subsequent tumour diagnosis. The specificity of consultation frequency alone is low, but it is improved if combined with a red flag symptom. For example, of 10 000 children attending their GP with

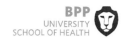

visual symptoms within a three month period, six would be diagnosed as having cancer, but if they had consulted on three or more occasions (for any reason), this number increases to 23.[19] Referral should therefore be carefully considered for children with repeated consultations and a red flag symptom.

What should I do if I suspect that a child has a brain tumour?

Include a brain tumour in the (often very wide) differential diagnosis of any child or young person presenting with the symptoms and signs shown in fig 1. Their presence should trigger a focused history (including family history and any predisposing genetic factors) and examination to look for corroborative findings (particularly the symptom and sign clusters associated with tumours in specific locations). Include motor and visual assessment, pubertal staging, and comparison of the child's height and weight with previous growth and age appropriate norms in the examination. It can be difficult to assess the visual function of pre-school children, so if necessary refer them to community optometry or ophthalmology. Children who present with symptoms of critical raised intracranial pressure (persistent headache and vomiting, confusion, drowsiness, reduced consciousness level) require urgent imaging of the central nervous system so, if in primary care, refer them the same day to local paediatric services.

The much harder management decision in both primary and secondary care is for children who appear reasonably well at assessment but who have a symptom or sign that could be caused by a brain tumour. In this situation, the clinician must decide whether no further action is needed and the family can be reassured; whether a period of watchful waiting and subsequent review is needed; or whether symptoms, signs, and additional examination findings are specific enough to merit referral for secondary care review or imaging.

A short period of watchful waiting can be helpful because symptoms and signs often evolve with time in children with brain tumours. Brain tumours however can progress rapidly, so review children who present with headache within four weeks and those with all other symptoms and signs within two weeks. Tell parents and carers to return sooner if their child deteriorates. Book a follow-up appointment for young people at their initial consultation because they tend to be less reliable at returning with persisting symptoms.

NHS evidence endorsed clinical guidelines advising on assessment and indications for referral and imaging of children and young people who may have a brain tumour have been published.[20] The guidelines and other information sources are available on the HeadSmart website (www.headsmart.org.uk), which also advises on specific clinical situations where reassurance, review, or referral is an appropriate action.

How is a brain tumour confirmed?

Imaging of the central nervous system is needed to confirm or refute the diagnosis of a brain tumour. Imaging is used to confirm the presence of an intracranial mass lesion and to identify complications that require urgent intervention, such as the presence of a large mass effect or hydrocephalus. Both CT and magnetic resonance imaging (MRI) are suitable for this purpose. The widespread availability, ease of access, and speed of CT mean that this modality is widely used as first line imaging in children with suspected brain tumours. CT is particularly useful for emergency scanning of children who present in extremis, where time does not allow MRI, or for young children who would otherwise require general anaesthesia to undergo MRI in centres where access to general anaesthesia is limited.

However, in centres with good access to paediatric MRI services, MRI is used in preference to CT for children with suspected brain tumours. A brief protocol consisting of axial T2 weighted imaging can be used to effectively exclude a large intracranial mass lesion and takes around five minutes to perform. Full tumour MRI protocols may take more than an hour but provide both accurate anatomical localisation (including neuroaxis dissemination) and additional biological information, such as chemical composition, cellularity, and vascularity.

How are brain tumours treated in children and young people?

Brain tumours require multidisciplinary management, and the care of children and young people with brain tumours should be coordinated by their regional paediatric neurosurgery and neuro-oncology service. Treatment will be determined by the tumour type and location as well as the age of the child; it may involve surgery, chemotherapy, and radiotherapy. Research in paediatric neuro-oncology requires international collaboration, and patients are offered participation in clinical trials when available; our experience is that most families and young people welcome this opportunity.

Sequential clinical trials have led to great improvements in survival for many children and young people with brain tumours (fig 2).[21] [22] However, survival varies greatly between

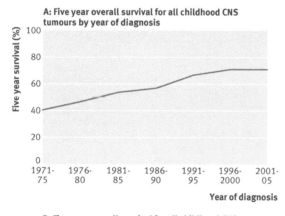

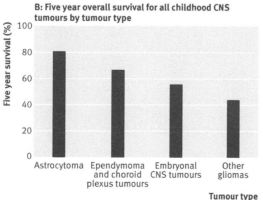

Fig 2 Five year overall survival for childhood (age 0-15 years) brain tumours by year of diagnosis (A) and tumour type (B). Data from the national registry of childhood tumours and the Office for National Statistics[21] [22]

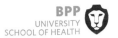

different tumour types and locations. Recent progress in biotechnology has enabled identification of novel pathway aberrations in multiple tumour types and led to the search for novel anti-tumour agents that can act on these pathways.[23] [24] [25] Treatment of young children is particularly challenging because brain directed treatment can have a serious impact on the child's subsequent development. Current clinical strategies used to minimise the side effects of treatment include the use of intraventricular chemotherapy and proton radiotherapy.[26] [27] [28]

Rehabilitation and support for reintegration into education and society are essential. Children and young people should be assessed by neuropsychology, physiotherapy, occupational therapy, and speech and language services at diagnosis and ongoing care provided if needed. Return to education can be particularly challenging, and early communication with the child or young person's education provider to obtain advice on what support is likely to be needed facilitates this process. Children and young people treated with chemoradiotherapy for brain tumours often develop cognitive difficulties, particularly with the speed of processing, and it is important that this is recognised and supportive strategies implemented.[29] [30] Children often require lifelong additional care, so early engagement with primary care is essential.

Contributors: SHW drafted the initial version. RAD, TPCC, and RMD provided advice on specific sections. All authors reviewed and contributed to subsequent versions. SHW is guarantor.

Funding: The authors received no funding to write this article.

Competing interests: We have read and understood the BMJ Group policy on declaration of interests and declare the following interests: RMD, RAD, TPCC have none. DAW is an expert witness in the field of clinical practice in childhood brain tumours, codirector of a university research centre related to children's brain tumour research and principal investigator for the "HeadSmart Be Brain Tumour Aware" campaign, which is a Health Foundation funded collaborative national project. SHW is one of the coinvestigators for the "HeadSmart Be Brain Tumour Aware" campaign.

Provenance and peer review: Not commissioned; externally peer reviewed.

1 Cancer Research UK. Cancer incidence by age. www.cancerresearchuk.org/cancer-info/cancerstats/incidence/age/.

2 Batchelder P, Foreman N, MaddenJ, Wilkinson C, Handler M. Catastrophic presentations in pediatric brain tumors [abstract]. *Neuro oncology*2010;12:ii76.

3 Reimers T, Ehrenfels S, Mortensen E, Schmiegelow M, Sonderkaer S, Carstensen H, et al. Cognitive deficits in long-term survivors of childhood brain tumours: identification of predictive factors. *Med Pediatr Oncol*2003;40:26-34.

4 Yule S, Hide T, Cranney M, Simpson E, Barrett A. Low grade astrocytomas in the west of Scotland 1987-96: treatment, outcome and cognitive function. *Arch Dis Childhood*2001;84:61-4.

5 Chou S, Digre K. Neuro-ophthalmic complications of raised intracranial pressure, hydrocephalus and shunt malfunction. *Neurosurg Clin N Am*1999;10:587-608.

6 Stiller C, Allen M, Eatock E. Childhood cancer in Britain: the national registry of chidhood tumours and incidence rates 1978-1987. *Eur J Cancer*1995;31:2028-34.

7 Stiller C, Bleyer W. Epidemiology. In: Taylor R, Walker D, Perilongo G, Punt J, eds. Brain and spinal tumours of childhood. Arnold, 2004:35-49.

8 Louis D, Ohgaki H, Wiestler O, Cavenee W, Burger P, Jouvet A, et al. The 2007 WHO classification of tumours of the central nervous system. *Acta Neuropathol* 2007;114:97-109.

9 Korones D, Fisher P, Kretschmar C, Zhou T, Chen Z, Kepner J, et al. Treatment of children with diffuse intrinsic brian stem glioma with radiotherapy, vincristine and oral VP-16: a children's oncology group phase II study. *Pediatr Blood Cancer*2008;50:227-30.

10 Packer R, Gajjar A, Vezina G, Rorke-Adams L, Burger P, Robertson P, et al. Phase III study of craniospinal radiation therapy followed by adjuvant chemotherapy for newly diagnosed average-risk medulloblastoma. *J Clin Oncol*2006;25:4202-8.

11 Warrington N, Woerner M, Daginakatte G, Dasgupta B, Perry A, Gutmann DH, et al. Spatiotemporal differences in CXCL 12 expression and cyclic AMP underlie the unique pattern of optic pathway glioma growth in neurofibromatosis type 1. *Cancer Res*2007;67:8588-95.

12 Banerjee J, Paakko E, Harila M, Herva R, Tuominen J, Koivula A, et al. Radiation-induces meningiomas: a shadow in the sucess story of childhood leukaemia. *Neurooncology*2009;11:543-9.

13 Matthews JD, Forsythe AV, Brady Z, Butler MW, Georgen SK, Byrnes GB, et al. Cancer risk in 680 000 people exposed to computer tomography scans in childhood or adolescence: data linkage study of 11 million Australians. *BMJ*2013;346:f2360.

14 Wilne S, Collier J, Kennedy C, Jenkins A, Grout J, Mackie S, et al. Progression from first symptoms to diagnosis in childhood brain tumours. *Eur J Pediatr*2011;71:87-93.

15 Wilne S, Collier J, Kennedy C, Grundy R, Wlaker D. Presentation of childhood CNS tumours: a systematic review and meta-analysis. *Lancet Oncol*2007;8:685-95.

16 Dommett R, Redaniel M, Stevens M, Hamilton W, Martin RM. Features of childhood cancer in primary care: a population-based case-control study. *Br J Cancer*2012;106:982-7.

17 National Institute for Health and Care Excellence. Referral for suspected cancer. CG27. 2005. www.nice.org.uk/CG27.

18 Ellis-Brookes L, McPhail S, Ives A, Greenslade M, Shelton J, Hiorn S, et al. Routes to diagnosis for cancer—determining the patient journey using multiple routine data sets. *Br J Cancer*2012;107:1220-6.

19 Dommett R, Redaniel T, Stevens M, Martin R, Hamilton W. Risk of childhood cancer with symptoms in primary care: a population-based case control study. *Br J Gen Pract*2013;63:22-9.

20 Wilne S, Koller K, Collier J, Kennedy C, Grundy R, Walker D. The diagnosis of brain tumours in children: a guideline to assist healthcare professionals in the assessment of children who may have a brain tumour. *Arch Dis Child*2010;95:534-9.

21 Childhood Cancer Research Group. Survival from childhood cancer, Great Britain, 1971-2005. 2010. www.ccrg.ox.ac.uk/datasets/survivalrates.shtml.

22 Cancer Research UK. Childhood cancer survival statistics. www.cancerresearchuk.org/cancer-info/cancerstats/childhoodcancer/survival/ .

23 Franz D, Belousova E, Sparagana S, Bebin M, Frost M, Kuperman R, et al. Efficacy and safety of everolimus for subependymal giant cell astrocytomas associated with tuberous sclerosis complex (EXIST-1): a multicentre, randomised, placebo-controlled phase 3 trial. *Lancet*2013;381:125-32.

24 Picard D, Miller S, Hawkins C, Bouffet E, Rogers HA, Chan TS, et al. Markers of survival and metastatic potential in childhood CNS primitive neuro-ectodermal brain tumours: an integrative genomic analysis. *Lancet Oncol*2012;13:838-48.

25 Low J, Sauvage F. Clinical experience with hedgehog pathway inhibitors. *J Clin Oncol*2010;28:5321-26.

26 Von Bueren A, von Hoff K, Pietsch T, Gerber N, Warmuth-Metz M, Deinlein F, et al. Treatment of young children with localised medulloblastoma by chemotherapy alone: results of the multicentretrial HIT 2000 confirming the porgnostic impact of radiotherapy. *Neurooncology*2011;13:669-79.

ADDITIONAL EDUCATIONAL RESOURCES

Resources for healthcare professionals

- HeadSmart (www.headsmart.org.uk)—Guidance on the identification and management of children and young people presenting with signs or symptoms that could be caused by a brain tumour

- Royal College of General Practitioners (http://elearning.rcgp.org.uk/course/info.php?id=99)—Education module using case illustrations to educate healthcare professionals about the presentation of childhood brain tumours

- BMJ Learning (http://learning.bmj.com/learning/module-intro/sarcomas-brain-tumours-children.html?moduleId=10042893&locale=en_GB)—Education module using case illustrations to educate healthcare professionals about the presentation of childhood brain and bone tumours

- National Institute for Health and Care Excellence. Referral for suspected cancer. CG27. www.nice.org.uk/cg027

- Neuro Foundation (www.nfauk.org/)—Information about neurofibromatosis, including advice on managing children and young people with the condition

- Tuberous Sclerosis Association (www.tuberous-sclerosis.org/)—Clinical guidelines for the management of people with tuberous sclerosis

Resources for patients and families

- HeadSmart (www.headsmart.org.uk)—Information on how brain tumours present and what to do if you are concerned that you or your child could have a brain tumour

- Neuro Foundation (www.nfauk.org/)—Information about neurofibromatosis including cause, potential complications, and management; also a source of advice and support

- Tuberous Sclerosis Association (www.tuberous-sclerosis.org/)—Information about tuberous sclerosis including cause, potential complications, and management; also a source of advice and support

- Brain Tumour Charity (www.thebraintumourcharity.org/)—The largest UK brain tumour charity. Provides information about brain tumours, including diagnosis and treatment options, plus support and a helpline

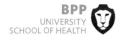

27 Merchant T, Hua C, Shukla H, Ying X, Nill S, Oelfke U. Proton versus photon radiotherapy for common pedaitric brain tumors: comparison of models of dose characteristics and their relationships to cognitive function. *Pediatr Blood Cancer*2008;51:110-17.

28 Brodin N, Vogelius I, Maraldo M, Munck A, Rosenschold P, Aznar M, et al. Life years lost—comparing potentially fatal late complications after radiotherapy for pediatric medulloblsatoma on a common scale. *Cancer*2012;118:5432 40.

29 Pruitt D, Ayyanger R, Craig K, White A, Neufeld J. Pediatric brain tumor rehabilitation. *J Pediatr Rehabil Med*2011;4:59-70.

30 Nazemi K, Butler R. Neuropsychological rehabilitation for survivors of childhood and adolescent brain tumors: a view of the past and a vision for a promising future. *J Pediatr Rehabil Med*2011;4:37-46.

Related links

bmj.com
- Get Cleveland Clinic CME creditrs for this article

bmj.com/archive
- Gout (*BMJ* 2013;347:f5648)
- Testicular germ cell tumours (*BMJ* 2013;347:f5526)
- Managing cows' milk allergy in children (*BMJ* 2013;347:f5424)
- Personality disorder (*BMJ* 2013;347:f5276)
- Dyspepsia (*BMJ* 2013;347:f5059)

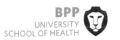

Head and neck cancer—Part 1: Epidemiology, presentation, and prevention

H Mehanna director and honorary associate professor[1], V Paleri consultant surgeon and honorary clinical senior lecturer[2], C M L West professor of radiation biology[3], C Nutting director[4]

[1]Institute of Head and Neck Studies and Education, University Hospitals Coventry, Coventry CV2 2DX

[2]Otolaryngology-Head and Neck Surgery, Newcastle upon Tyne Hospitals NHS Trust, Newcastle upon Tyne

[3]University of Manchester, Manchester

[4]Head and Neck Unit, Royal Marsden NHS Foundation Trust, London

Correspondence to: H Mehanna hishammehanna@aol.com

Cite this as: BMJ 2010;341:c4684

‹DOI› 10.1136/bmj.c4684
http://www.bmj.com/content/341/bmj.c4684

Head and neck cancers include cancers of the upper aerodigestive tract (including the oral cavity, nasopharynx, oropharynx, hypopharynx, and larynx), the paranasal sinuses, and the salivary glands. Cancers at different sites have different courses and variable histopathological types, although squamous cell carcinoma is by far the most common. The anatomical sites affected are important for functions such as speech, swallowing, taste, and smell, so the cancers and their treatments may have considerable functional sequelae with subsequent impairment of quality of life. Decisions about treatment are usually complex, and they must balance efficacy of treatment and likelihood of survival, with potential functional and quality of life outcomes. Patients and their carers need considerable support during and after treatment.

In this first part of a two article series, we review the common presentations of head and neck cancer. We also discuss common investigations and new diagnostic techniques, as well as briefly touching on screening and prevention. In this review, we have used evidence from national guidelines, randomised trials, and level II-III studies. We have limited our discussions to squamous cell carcinoma of the head and neck, which constitutes more than 85% of head and neck cancers.

How common is head and neck cancer and who gets it?

Cancer of the mouth and oropharynx is the 10th most common cancer worldwide, but it is the seventh most common cause of cancer induced mortality.[1]

In 2002, the World Health Organization estimated that there were 600 000 new cases of head and neck cancer and 300 000 deaths each year worldwide, with the most common sites being the oral cavity (389 000 cases a year), the larynx (160 000), and the pharynx (65 000).[2] The male to female ratio reported by large scale epidemiological studies and national cancer registries varies from 2:1 to 15:1 depending on the site of disease.[w1] The incidence of cancers of the head and neck increases with age. In Europe, 98% and 50% of patients diagnosed are over 40 and 60 years of age, respectively.[w2]

What regions have the highest incidence?

A high incidence of head and neck cancer is seen in the Indian subcontinent, Australia, France, Brazil, and Southern Africa (table). Nasopharyngeal cancer is largely restricted to southern China. The incidence of oral, laryngeal, and other smoking related cancers is declining in North America and western Europe, primarily because of decreased exposure to carcinogens, especially tobacco.[2] In contrast, because of the 40 year temporal gap between changes in population tobacco use and its epidemiological effects, the worst of the tobacco epidemic has yet to materialise in developing countries. WHO projections estimate worldwide mortality figures from mouth and oropharyngeal cancer in 2008 to be 371 000. This is projected to rise to 595 000 in 2030 because of a predicted rise in mortality in South East Asia (182 000 in 2008 to 324 000 in 2030). Modest rises are predicted in Africa, the Americas, and the Middle East, whereas mortality in Europe is expected to remain stable.[3]

Several retrospective analyses of samples collected from patients recruited in randomised trials, as well as retrospective patient series, have shown recent changes in epidemiology and pathogenesis of head and neck cancers related to the human papillomavirus (HPV), especially oropharyngeal carcinoma. A rapid rise in HPV related oropharyngeal cancers in particular has been shown in epidemiological studies from the developed world.[4] For example, the United Kingdom has seen a doubling in the incidence of oropharyngeal cancer (from 1/100 000 population to 2.3/100 000) in just over a decade.[5] A recent retrospective study showed a progressive proportional increase in the detection of HPV in oropharyngeal squamous cell carcinomas in Stockholm over the past three decades: 23% in the 1970s, 29% in 1980s, 57% in 1990s, 68% between 2000 and 2002, 77% between 2003 and 2005, and 93% between 2006 and 2007.[6] Other prospective studies, such as ones from the United States, have also reported proportional increases.

What are the risk factors for head and neck cancer?

Tobacco and alcohol

The major risk factors are tobacco (smoking and smokeless products such as betel quid) and alcohol. They account for about 75% of cases, and their effects are multiplicative when combined.[7] [w3] Smoking is more strongly associated with laryngeal cancer and alcohol consumption with cancers of the pharynx and oral cavity.[w4] Pooled analyses of 15 case-control studies showed that non-smokers who have

---

SOURCES AND SELECTION CRITERIA

We used the terms "head and neck", "larynx", "oral", and "oropharynx"—with each limited by "cancer", "diagnosis", and "treatment" separately—to search the Medline, Embase, PubMed, Cochrane, CINAHL, and AMED databases. We also used them to cross check national guidelines, reference lists, textbooks, and personal reference lists. We assessed over 1000 identified abstracts for relevance.

SUMMARY POINTS

- The incidence of head and neck cancer is relatively low in developed countries and highest in South East Asia
- The main risk factors are smoking and heavy alcohol consumption
- Incidence of human papillomavirus related oropharyngeal carcinoma is rising rapidly in developed countries and is easily missed. It has a different presentation and better prognosis than other head and neck cancers
- Patients with head neck cancer often present with hoarseness, throat pain, tongue ulcers, or a painless neck lump, and symptoms for longer than three weeks' duration should prompt urgent referral
- No strong evidence supports visual examination or other screening methods in the general population

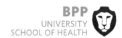

Data for head and neck cancers in 2004 in WHO regions*						
	Africa	The Americas†	Eastern Mediterranean	Europe	South East Asia	Western Pacific
Population	737 536	874 380	519 688	883 311	1 671 904	1 738 457
Incidence	30	38	29	72	195	74
Mortality	22	25	22	51	158	56

*Numbers should be multiplied by 1000.
†North America, South America, and Canada.

three or more alcoholic drinks (beer or spirits) a day have double the risk of developing the disease compared with non-drinkers (odds ratio 2.04, 95% confidence interval 1.29 to 3.21).[8 9]

Genetic factors

Most people who smoke and drink do not develop head and neck cancer, however, and a genetic predisposition has been shown to be important. The International Head And Neck Cancer Epidemiology Consortium (INHANCE) carried out pooled analyses of epidemiological studies that examined risks associated with the disease.[7] This work confirmed the role of genetic predisposition that had been suggested by small studies. A family history of head and neck cancer in a first degree relative is associated with a 1.7-fold (1.2 to 2.3) increased risk of developing the disease.[7] Genetic polymorphisms in genes encoding enzymes involved in the metabolism of tobacco and alcohol have been linked with an increased risk of the disease. For example, a meta-analysis of 30 studies showed that a polymorphism in $GSTM1$, which encodes a protein involved in the metabolism of xenobiotics (glutathione S transferase), was associated with a 1.23 (1.06 to 1.42) increased risk of developing head and neck cancer.[w5]

Viral infection

Viral infection is a recognised risk factor for cancer of the head and neck. The association between Epstein-Barr virus infection and the development of nasopharyngeal cancer was first recognised in 1966.[w6] More recently, HPV has attracted attention.[4] Recent observational studies have found that this virus is a strong risk factor for the development of head and neck cancer, especially oropharyngeal cancer (63, 14 to 480), and they suggest that HPV infection—especially infection with HPV subtype 16 (HPV-16)—is an aetiological factor.[10 w7] The disease is thought to be sexually transmitted. A pooled analysis of eight multinational observational studies that compared 5642 cases of head and neck cancer with 6069 controls found that the risk of developing oropharyngeal carcinoma was associated with a history of six or more lifetime sexual partners (1.25, 1.01 to 1.54), four or more lifetime oral sex partners (3.36, 1.32 to 8.53), and—for men—an earlier age at first sexual intercourse (2.36, 1.37 to 5.05).[11]

HPV related oropharyngeal carcinoma is a distinct disease entity. Patients are younger (usually 40-50 years old), often do not report the usual risk factors of smoking or high alcohol intake, and often present with a small primary tumour and large neck nodes. This may lead to delayed diagnosis.

Other risk factors

Other risk factors identified from pooled analyses of case-control studies include sex (men are more likely to have head and neck cancer than women),[7] a long duration of passive smoking (odds ratio for >15 years at home: 1.60, 1.12 to 2.28),[7] low body mass index (odds ratio for body mass index 18: 2.13, 1.75 to 2.58),[w8] and sexual behaviour (for example, odds ratio for cancer of the base of tongue in men with a history of same sex sexual contact: 8.89, 2.14 to 36.8).[11] Some evidence points to a role of occupational exposure, poor dental hygiene, and dietary factors, such as low fruit and vegetable intake.[w9]

How does head and neck cancer present?

Patients with head and neck cancers present with a variety of symptoms, depending on the function of the site where they originate. Laryngeal cancers commonly present with hoarseness, whereas pharyngeal cancers often present late with dysphagia or sore throat. Many often present with a painless neck node. Patients with head and neck cancer can present with non-specific symptoms or symptoms commonly associated with benign conditions, however, such as sore throat or ear pain.[w10] Box 1 lists "red flag symptoms" that practice guidelines consider to warrant urgent referral and consultation with a specialist head and neck clinician. UK guidelines specify that urgent referral should mean that patients are seen within two weeks.[12] Head and neck centres often run a dedicated clinic—a neck lump clinic—to diagnose such patients. Box 2 describes unusual clinical scenarios in which clinicians may miss a diagnosis of cancer.

BOX 1 "RED FLAG" SYMPTOMS AND SIGNS OF HEAD AND NECK CANCER[12]

Any of the following lasting for more than three weeks.

Symptoms
- Sore throat
- Hoarseness
- Stridor
- Difficulty in swallowing
- Lump in neck
- Unilateral ear pain

Signs
- Red or white patch in the mouth
- Oral ulceration, swelling, or loose tooth
- Lateral neck mass
- Rapidly growing thyroid mass
- Cranial nerve palsy
- Orbital mass
- Unilateral ear effusion

How are suspicious lesions investigated?

A recent *BMJ* clinical review discussed the investigation of oral lesions in detail.[13] Examination of any lesion of the head or neck should include palpation of the entire neck for lymph nodes, and examination of the scalp and the whole oral cavity, including tongue, floor of mouth, buccal mucosa, and tonsils. Dentures should be removed before examination. The nose and ears should also be examined, especially if no other abnormalities are found. Flexible nasolaryngoscopy allows proper examination of the nasal cavities, postnasal space, base of the tongue, larynx, and hypopharynx. Box 3 summarises the investigations that are performed in specialist care.

Diagnosis of the cancer is confirmed on histology of the biopsy from the primary site. The new technique of

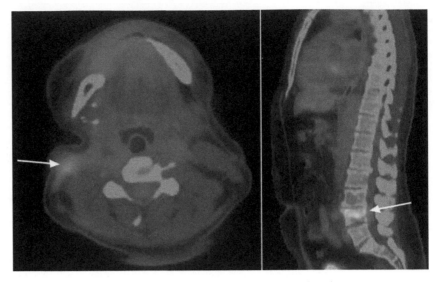

Positron emission tomography-computed tomography scans showing: left, recurrence in neck (arrow) in a patient who had previously undergone a neck dissection and chemoradiotherapy; and right, 53 year old man with adenoid cystic carcinoma of the parotid gland showing spinal metastases in the fourth lumbar vertebra

---

BOX 2 PRESENTATIONS WHERE CANCER MIGHT EASILY BE MISSED

Persistently enlarged neck nodes in younger patients (30-50 years)
These are often human papillomavirus related tumours. Patients often do not have the usual risk factors for head and neck cancer—they are often non-smokers and do not drink alcohol heavily. Tumours are often small or occult within normal looking tonsils. Because of patient's young age, absence of risk factors, and unusual presentation, the problem might be confused with benign reactive nodal enlargement and the diagnosis delayed.

Persistent unilateral otalgia with no signs of ear infection in patients over 30
Patients with this problem should also be considered for early referral to a head and neck surgeon who can do a full examination of the upper aerodigestive tract with a flexible nasolaryngoscope to exclude pharyngeal and postnasal space tumours.

Recent onset wheeze in a patient over 40, usually a heavy smoker
The "wheeze" is in fact a mild biphasic stridor mistaken for wheeze and the patient, who may also have breathlessness, may be misdiagnosed as having sequelae of chronic obstructive airway disease or late onset asthma and may be treated as such. This presentation, however, may be that of a slow growing laryngeal carcinoma. Clinicians should consider this diagnosis in patients with late onset wheeze or asthma that does not respond to drugs in patients who smoke or give a history of heavy alcohol intake.

BOX 3 INVESTIGATIONS USED FOR HEAD AND NECK CANCER

Imaging
- Computed tomography scanning from the skull base to the diaphragm is the first line investigation to assess nodal metastasis and identify the primary tumour site and tumour size

Magnetic resonance imaging is indicated for:
- Oral cavity and oropharyngeal tumours; it provides better information than because of the absence of interference from dental amalgam and the better delineation of soft tissue extension
- Cases where extension through the laryngeal cartilage is suspected but cannot be conclusively determined on computed tomography
- Ultrasound guided fine needle aspiration performed by experienced practitioners is highly accurate and used by some centres to diagnose nodal metastasis and determine its distribution[14]
- Positron emission tomography-computed tomography scanning is used to investigate occult primary and distant metastases in some cases
- Sentinel node biopsy is used to detect nodal metastases in cases with a high risk of occult metastasis. A radioactive tracer with blue dye is injected into the lesion, often a mouth cancer, and under general anaesthesia a Geiger counter locates the node with highest radioactivity, which is removed. If the node contains tumour, the patient undergoes neck dissection

Histological confirmation of diagnosis
- Examination under anaesthetic and biopsy allows assessment of the size and extent of the primary tumour
- Fine needle aspiration or core biopsy, often under ultrasound guidance, can provide cytological evidence of nodal metastasis[14]

---

fusion positron emission tomography-computerised tomography has become one of the most important diagnostic tools for head and neck cancers. It combines normal computed tomography scanning with functional imaging using 18F-fluorodeoxyglucose (18F-FDG), which is taken up preferentially by cells with high metabolic activity, especially cancer cells (fig). This technique can therefore help identify occult primary tumours, which are relatively common and not detected by examination and conventional imaging. The technique may also have a role in the assessment of persistent nodal disease after treatment, and in the monitoring and follow-up of patients with head and neck cancer in the longer term, but sufficient evidence to support this is not yet available.[15]

To prove that a tumour is caused by HPV, virus specific DNA must be identified within the tumour and it must be shown that it has undergone transcription. HPV DNA can be demonstrated by polymerase chain reaction or in situ

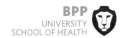

HPV related oropharygeal cancer may theoretically be prevented by vaccination against HPV-16, although no strong evidence is available to support this. Currently, most national HPV vaccination programmes include only girls, because several health economics assessments did not support the cost effectiveness of including boys.[21] However the rapid increase in HPV related oropharygeal cancer has led some health professionals to call for a reassessment of the cost effectiveness of including boys in such programmes.[4]

Thanks to Olu Adesanya, University Hospitals Coventry and Warwickshire, for supplying the figures, and to Mr and Mrs Culling for supplying the resources for patients and carers

Contributors: HM originated the idea. All authors helped plan, conduct, and report the review. All authors are guarantors.

Competing interests: All authors have completed the Unified Competing Interest form at www.icmje.org/coi_disclosure.pdf (available on request from the corresponding author) and declare that they had no financial support for the submitted work; HM is the director of an institute that does contract work for GSK, which has interests in head and neck cancers; he has also received grants from NCC-Health Technology Assessment Unit, Cancer Research UK, and Macmillan Research Fund. CN has received three clinical trial grants from Cancer Research UK and is principal investigator on a drug trial sponsored by Bayer; all authors have no other relationships or activities that could appear to have influenced the submitted work.

Provenance and peer review: Commissioned; externally peer reviewed.

hybridisation. Transcription can be demonstrated by using immunohistochemistry to identify expression of p16, a downstream product of HPV DNA transcription.[16]

Can we screen for head and neck cancer?

Data are available for oral cancer screening only. It is unclear whether treating premalignant lesions can prevent the occurrence of invasive cancer.[W11] A Cochrane review of randomised controlled trials of screening for oral cancer or precursor oral lesions found no strong evidence to support visual examination or other methods of screening for oral cancer in the general population.[17] The sensitivity of visual examination of the mouth for detecting oral precancerous and cancerous lesions varies from 58% to 94% and the specificity from 76% to 98%. These figures may be even lower for areas affected by HPV related oropharyngeal cancer, such as the tonsil and base of tongue, which are less accessible. Randomised studies in areas of high incidence have suggested that opportunistic visual screening of high risk groups may reduce mortality.[18] In special groups such as patients with Fanconi's anaemia, who have a higher lifetime risk of developing head and neck cancer, it is recommended that everyone over the age of 10 is screened every four months.[19]

Can head and neck cancer be prevented?

Prevention of head and neck cancer is closely linked to the success of tobacco control programmes. After pooling more than 50000 sets of individual level data from case-control studies, INHANCE estimated that quitting tobacco smoking for one to four years reduces the risk of developing head and neck cancer (0.70, 0.61 to 0.81 compared with current smoking), with further risk reduction at 20 years or more (0.23, 0.18 to 0.31), at which time risk is similar to that of never smokers.[5] For alcohol use, a beneficial effect was seen only after 20 years or more of quitting (0.60, 0.40 to 0.89 compared with current drinking).[20]

1 WHO. The global burden of disease: 2004 update. 2008. www.who.int/evidence/bod.
2 Boyle P, Levin B, eds. World cancer report. International Agency for Research on Cancer, 2008.
3 Mathers CD, Loncar D. Projections of global mortality and burden of disease from 2002 to 2030. PLoS Med2006;3:e442.
4 Mehanna H, Jones TM, Gregoire V, Ang KK. Oropharyngeal carcinoma related to human papillomavirus. BMJ2010;340:c1439.
5 Oxford Cancer Intelligence Unit. Profile of head and neck cancers in England. 2010. http://library.ncin.org.uk/docs/100504-OCIU-Head_and_Neck_Profiles.pdf.
6 Nasman A, Attner P, Hammarstedt L, Du J, Eriksson M, Giraud G, et al. Incidence of human papillomavirus (HPV) positive tonsillar carcinoma in Stockholm, Sweden: an epidemic of viral-induced carcinoma? Int J Cancer2009;125:362-6.
7 Conway DI, Hashibe M, Boffetta P, Wunsch-Filho V, Muscat J, La Vecchia C, et al. Enhancing epidemiologic research on head and neck cancer: INHANCE—the International Head and Neck Cancer Epidemiology Consortium. Oral Oncol2009;45:743-6.
8 Purdue MP, Hashibe M, Berthiller J, La Vecchia C, Dal Maso L, Herrero R, et al. Type of alcoholic beverage and risk of head and neck cancer—a pooled analysis within the INHANCE Consortium. Am J Epidemiol2009;169:132-42.
9 Hashibe M, Brennan P, Benhamou S, Castellsague X, Chen C, Curado MP, et al. Alcohol drinking in never users of tobacco, cigarette smoking in never drinkers, and the risk of head and neck cancer: pooled analysis in the International Head and Neck Cancer Epidemiology Consortium. J Natl Cancer Inst2007;99:777-89.
10 WHO. IARC monographs on the evaluation of carcinogenic risks to humans. Vol 90—human papillomaviruses. International Agency for Research on Cancer, 2007. http://monographs.iarc.fr/ENG/Monographs/vol90/index.php.
11 Heck JE, Berthiller J, Vaccarella S, Winn DM, Smith EM, Shan'gina O, et al. Sexual behaviours and the risk of head and neck cancers: a pooled analysis in the International Head and Neck Cancer Epidemiology (INHANCE) Consortium. Int J Epidemiol2010;39:166-81.
12 National Institute for Health and Clinical Excellence. Improving outcomes in head and neck cancers—the manual. 2004. http://guidance.nice.org.uk/csghn/guidance/pdf/English .

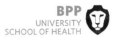

13   Paleri V, Staines K, Sloan P, Douglas A, Wilson J. Evaluation of oral ulceration in primary care. *BMJ* 2010;340:c2639.

14   Van den Brekel MW, Castelijns JA, Stel HV, Golding RP, Meyer CJ, Snow GB. Modern imaging techniques and ultrasound-guided aspiration cytology for the assessment of neck node metastases: a prospective comparative study. *Eur Arch Otorhinolaryngol* 1993;250:11-7.

15   Isles MG, McConkey C, Mehanna HM. A systematic review and meta-analysis of the role of positron emission tomography in the follow up of head and neck squamous cell carcinoma following radiotherapy or chemoradiotherapy. *Clin Otolaryngol* 2008;33:210-22.

16   Singhi AD, Westra WH. Comparison of human papillomavirus in situ hybridization and p16 immunohistochemistry in the detection of human papillomavirus-associated head and neck cancer based on a prospective clinical experience. *Cancer* 2010;116:2166-73.

17   Kujan O, Glenny AM, Oliver RJ, Thakker N, Sloan P. Screening programmes for the early detection and prevention of oral cancer. *Cochrane Database Syst Rev* 2006;3:CD004150.

18   Sankaranarayanan R, Ramadas K, Thomas G, Muwonge R, Thara S, Mathew B, et al; for the Trivandrum Oral Cancer Screening Study Group. Effect of screening on oral cancer mortality in Kerala, India: a cluster-randomised controlled trial. *Lancet* 2005;365:1927-33.

19   Fanconi Anaemia Clinical Network. Clinical standards of care in the UK. www.fanconi.org.uk/clinical-network/standards-of-care/.

20   Marron M, Boffetta P, Zhang ZF, Zaridze D, Wünsch-Filho V, Winn DM, et al. Cessation of alcohol drinking, tobacco smoking and the reversal of head and neck cancer risk. *Int J Epidemiol* 2010;39:182-96.

21   Kim JJ, Goldie SJ. Cost effectiveness analysis of including boys in a human papillomavirus vaccination programme in the United States. *BMJ* 2009;339:b3884.

BMJ   BPP
UNIVERSITY
SCHOOL OF HEALTH

Head and neck cancer—Part 2: Treatment and prognostic factors

H Mehanna director and honorary associate professor[1], C M L West professor of radiation biology[2], C Nutting director[3], V Paleri consultant surgeon and honorary clinical senior lecturer[4]

[1]Institute of Head and Neck Studies and Education, University Hospitals Coventry, Coventry CV2 2DX

[2]University of Manchester, Manchester

[3]Head and Neck Unit, Royal Marsden NHS Foundation Trust, London

[4]Otolaryngology-Head and Neck Surgery, Newcastle upon Tyne Hospitals NHS Trust, Newcastle upon Tyne

Correspondence to: H Mehanna
hishammehanna@aol.com

Cite this as: BMJ 2010;341:c4690

‹DOI› 10.1136/bmj.c4690
http://www.bmj.com/content/341/bmj.c4690

In this second of a two part series, we discuss recent advances in the management of cancers of the head and neck. We also discuss the important prognostic factors, including the importance of human papillomavirus (HPV) positivity in the newly discovered HPV related cancers of the head and neck. As before, we have used evidence from national guidelines, randomised trials, and level II-III studies. We have also limited our discussions to squamous cell carcinoma of the head and neck, which constitutes more than 85% of head and neck cancers.

What determines prognosis in head and neck cancer?

Site and TNM stage

The most important prognostic factors are site and TNM (tumour, node, metastasis) stage. The table details the survival rates of patients diagnosed with head and neck cancer at different sites. Patients with tumours that are larger and have spread to nodes and other tissues have poorer survival. Guidelines for head and neck carcinomas from the Royal College of Pathologists state that other accepted features related to clinical outcome are grade, pattern of invasion, proximity of carcinoma to resection margins, and the presence of extranodal spread. A large meta-analysis showed that extranodal spread more than halved the chances of surviving for five years (odds ratio 2.7, 95% confidence interval 2.1 to 3.7).[1] [w1]

Comorbid illness

The results of large meta-analyses of clinical trial data show that poor performance status (poor fitness and presence of comorbidities) is associated with an adverse prognosis.[2] [3] A systematic review of the effect of comorbidity on survival from head and neck cancer found that for laryngeal cancer, for example, the risk of death is significantly related to comorbidity (hazard ratio 1.5-13.5, depending on the comorbidity).[4] A systematic quantitative review of the association of anaemia and survival in patients with cancer showed that anaemia increased the relative risk of death in patients with head and neck cancer by 47%.[w2] Meta-analyses of clinical trial data show that advancing age is associated with a decreased probability of survival.[2] [3] [w3]

Molecular markers

Molecular markers of prognosis have been studied but none has yet entered routine clinical reporting. A systematic review and meta-analysis found no conclusive value for p53 as a prognostic factor because of heterogeneity across studies.[w4] Another meta-analysis of tumour expression of the angiogenic vascular endothelial growth factor in 1002 patients found that patients who were positive for this growth factor had nearly double the risk of death (relative risk 1.88, 1.43 to 2.45) at two years.[w5] A large body of evidence associates tumour hypoxia with adverse prognosis, and hypoxia associated markers have shown promising results, in particular hypoxia inducible factor 1α and carbonic anhydrase 9.[5] High tumour expression of the epidermal growth factor receptor was linked with a poor prognosis in several studies, and also predicted benefit from accelerated radiotherapy.[w6] [w7]

How to treat cancers of the head and neck?

Management is increasingly being delivered by specialists, whose main interest is cancers of the head and neck. Multidisciplinary care has now become the standard of care, often encouraged by national guidelines and protocols.[6] The complexities of combined surgery and radiotherapy, as well as rehabilitation, mean that a team of health professionals is needed to deliver high quality care to patients treated for head and neck cancer. An ideal team usually includes head and neck surgeons from different disciplines, clinical and medical oncologists, clinical nurse specialists, speech and language therapists, dietitians, psychologists, restorative dentists, prosthodontists, and social workers. Although we have no data to prove that multidisciplinary treatment has improved care, intuitively and anecdotally that seems to be the case.

Radiotherapy and surgery are the two most common treatments for cancers of the head and neck. The choice of treatment modality depends on individual factors related to the site of the tumour and stage, but also patient preference.

Early stage tumours

Case series, often retrospective and from single centres, have shown that for early stage tumours in many sites surgical excision or radiotherapy have similar cure rates but a different side effect profile.[7] [w8] Radiotherapy may offer better organ preservation, and for some cancers where function is important it is the treatment of choice.

SUMMARY POINTS

- The main prognostic factors are stage, site of disease, and comorbidities
- Treatment decisions should involve a multidisciplinary team of health professionals and the patient, and must balance efficacy and survival with potential functional and quality of life outcomes
- Early stage cancers are usually treated by either surgery or radiotherapy
- More advanced tumours usually require both surgery and chemoradiotherapy
- The disease and its treatments can cause substantial functional impairment and reduced quality of life
- Patients and their carers need considerable support during and after treatment

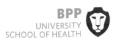

Five year survival rates for patients diagnosed with head and neck cancer in 1996-9 in England and Wales[23]	
Site	5 year survival rate (%)
Lip	93
Larynx	65
Oral cavity	51
Tongue	49
Oropharynx	44
Hypopharynx	19

For example, radiotherapy allows preservation of natural speech and swallowing in carcinomas of the tongue base. A recent advance in surgical treatment, transoral carbon dioxide laser (fig 1), reduces morbidity with improved organ preservation compared with open surgery. Prospective and retrospective case series have shown good outcomes for organ preservation in certain cancers, such as early glottic cancers and tonsillar cancers, because this technique causes less tissue damage than open surgery.[w9 w10] However, there have been no randomised comparisons of radiotherapy and carbon dioxide laser surgery. For some sites (such as the oral cavity), mainly retrospective single centre case series have shown that surgical excision alone may be curative,[7] and that it is associated with a highly satisfactory functional outcome.[w11]

Advanced tumours

For advanced squamous cell carcinoma of the head and neck, single modality treatment (surgery or radiotherapy) is associated with poorer outcomes,[8] and randomised studies have shown that combined use of surgery and postoperative radiotherapy, or combined chemotherapy and radiotherapy, offer the highest chance of achieving a cure.[8 9]

Primary reconstruction, using microvascular free flaps, of large defects after surgical resection of oral tumours especially, and laryngopharyngectomy (removal of the larynx and pharynx), is now a standard treatment that improves functional abilities and quality of life.[w12 w13]

Patients with HPV related cancer

Retrospective analyses of samples from patients recruited in large randomised trials and retrospective case series show that patients with HPV related oropharyngeal carcinoma seem to respond better to a variety of treatments, including chemoradiotherapy or surgery and radiotherapy,[10 11 12] than those with non-HPV related head and neck tumours. Because these patients are generally younger, they may survive for several decades with substantial side effects and functional impairment as a consequence of the treatment they receive, and this may have implications for carers, the health system, and social care.

Recent advances in surgery

Transoral surgery using the carbon dioxide laser under microscope guidance is now a widely accepted technique that can help in organ preservation, mainly in early disease.[w10] More recently, robotic surgery (fig 2) has been used and evaluated, especially for transoral resection of cancers of the base of the tongue and the tonsils. The high definition stereoscopic view, with three dimensional input, and the manoeuvrability of the robotic grasper provide improved access and visualisation. This technique allows resection of more extensive tumours located in difficult to reach areas than is possible using traditional transoral resection with microscopic guidance.[w14] Reports of early outcomes using robotic surgery, usually in combination with postoperative radiotherapy, show functional outcomes comparable to other treatment modalities.[w14] A recent prospective feasibility study of 45 patients reported no involved margins, but 56% and 17.8% patients needed postoperative chemoradiotherapy or radiotherapy respectively.[w14] No data on long term outcomes are available yet.

Reconstruction of large defects using microvascular free flaps comes at a considerable economic cost through substantial investment in microvascular expertise and postoperative care, as well as rehabilitation and support services. Newer techniques that result in less donor site morbidity and may have better functional outcomes, such as anterolateral thigh free flaps, circumflex iliac flaps, and scapular flaps, are increasingly used in preference to other more established flaps.

Patients undergoing bony reconstruction may now have osseo-integrated implants placed at the same time to allow dental and prosthetic rehabilitation after treatment has been completed. This has improved functional and aesthetic outcomes and increased patient satisfaction in retrospective and prospective case series.[w15]

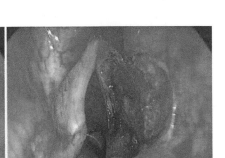

Fig 1 Cancer of the left vocal cord before resection (left) and immediately after resection with a carbon dioxide laser (right)

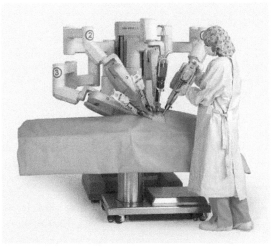

Fig 2 Surgical robot. Intuitive Surgical, with permission

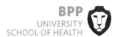

Recent advances in radiotherapy

In recent years radiotherapy has benefited from advances in cancer imaging, high speed computer software that optimises treatment planning (intelligently selecting the most appropriate beam direction and shape), and developments in radiation delivery technology. It is now one of the most technology driven branches of medicine. A tightly fitted moulded perspex mask, which is custom made for the patient, is used to immobilise the patient in the same specific orientation and position on the table during the delivery of the daily radiotherapy on an outpatient basis. Radiation treatment is delivered by computer driven linear accelerators with sub-millimetre accuracy, so that radiation is focused on the tumour bearing tissues and radiation of normal tissue structures is minimised.

A recent UK randomised trial of 88 patients found that intensity modulated radiotherapy, a new form of radiotherapy that allows better control of radiation dose delivery to the head and neck, reduced radiation induced xerostomia (the main long term side effect of standard radiotherapy) from 75% to 39% (P=0.004) at 12 months after treatment (fig 3).[13] A similar improvement in side effects was seen in a randomised controlled study for patients with nasopharyngeal cancer.[14]

Large randomised controlled studies have shown improvements in local tumour control with accelerated radiotherapy (radiation delivered over a shorter time period) or hyperfractionated radiotherapy (delivery of a higher dose of radiation in two to three low dose fractions a day).[15] These treatments have not shown consistent improvements in overall survival, but have resulted in increased short term mucosal toxicity; they have therefore not been adopted widely outside of North America.

Newer developments using particle therapy, such as proton therapy or stereotactic radiotherapy, may spare particularly radiosensitive organs close to tumours (such as the brain and spinal cord). However, these new technologies, especially proton therapy, are not yet widely available, their benefits have not been proved, and they cost considerably more than standard radiotherapy techniques.

Recent advances in chemotherapy

In a large meta-analysis of 93 trials and more than 17 000 patients, concomitant chemotherapy (given during radiotherapy) was shown to improve locoregional

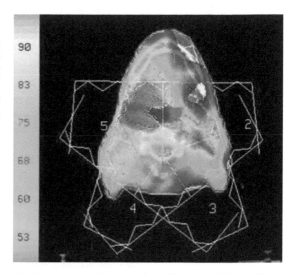

Fig 3 Dosimetry planning for a patient being treated with intensity modulated radiotherapy. The diagram shows the doses of radiotherapy delivered to each organ. Through use of sophisticated planning and delivery methods, this technique enables the one parotid gland (arrow) to be spared high doses of radiotherapy

control rates and was associated with a 6.5% increase in survival (P<0.0001). The benefits were largely confined to chemotherapy given during radiotherapy rather than in the adjuvant or neoadjuvant setting. In addition, combining chemotherapy with radiation improves the rates of organ conservation. Cisplatin chemotherapy schedules were the most effective.[16 w16 w17]

Two randomised controlled trials have shown that concomitant use of cisplatin and radiotherapy after surgery increases tumour control and overall survival in high risk patients with positive resection margins or extracapsular lymph node spread.[17 18]

Recently, the concurrent administration of cetuximab, an antiepidermal growth factor receptor antibody, with radiotherapy, was shown to increase overall survival and locoregional control in patients with squamous cell carcinoma of the head and neck in a large randomised controlled trial.[19 w18] This was the first time that a biologically targeted treatment was shown to be effective in the treatment of head and neck cancer.

Although concomitant chemotherapy has been shown to improve outcomes for head and neck cancer, the role of neoadjuvant chemotherapy (chemotherapy given before start of radiotherapy) remains controversial. Two recent phase II and phase III randomised studies suggested that the addition of docetaxel to cisplatin and fluorouracil given before definitive radiotherapy improved survival. However, the use of non-standard radiotherapy and chemoradiation schedules in these trials has led to uncertainty about the benefits of this approach when standard chemoradiotherapy is prescribed.[20 21]

What are the complications of treatment?

Surgical complications

Surgical procedure times vary from one to 12 hours, and patients often have a high burden of concurrent medical illness. These patients are prone to complications arising from prolonged anaesthesia, such as pulmonary consolidation and deep venous thrombosis. Depending on the nature of the procedure, patients may also be at increased risk of postoperative aspiration and its consequences. Although it is not a complication, the end stoma resulting from

---

A PATIENT'S PERSPECTIVE

When I first saw the ulcer under my tongue, I thought that I just hadn't noticed it before. At that time I was smoking around 35-40 cigarettes a day. My busy life meant that it was three months before I visited my general practitioner and was referred to the specialist. The penny dropped, and I realised that this could be cancer.

After investigations, I had an operation to remove the cancerous ulcer. The tumour had spread to my lymph glands and had attached itself to a nerve that worked my tongue, which had to be cut to remove the tumour. This troubled me because I knew it would affect my speech and possibly, in the long term, my career. I coped well after the operation and was allowed home after a week. Unknowingly, this had been a stroll in the park compared with what was to come.

I started chemoradiotherapy and was offered the option to participate in clinical trials for a new drug. For the next six weeks, every weekday I made a 50 mile round trip to the hospital for treatment. At first I went on my own as I thought that I coped better this way. However, 15 days into the treatment, I had to be driven. I had by now become unable to eat or even drink and had a tube inserted in my stomach. I felt very down, for the first time in many years. I would come home from the treatment and go straight to bed after a five minute battle with the stairs. This period was the lowest part of my life. I said to myself, could this have been avoided?

When I look back on this journey, I tend to forget the bad things and think of the positive ones; the people who helped me, my family, my friends, and my partner who was my rock throughout my treatment. I now enjoy good health and have my life back on track.Tony, *Newcastle upon Tyne*

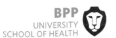

laryngectomy may affect patients' activities of daily living because of problems with body image and the need for daily tracheo-oesophageal valve care to maintain speech through the valve.

Because most surgical procedures are of the clean-contaminated variety, where the oral or pharyngeal lumen is opened at some point in the procedure, case series report postoperative surgical site infection rates of 20-40%.[w19 w20]

Other early complications include haemorrhage from major vessels and wound breakdown, the last of which is especially common in patients who have had radiation before surgery. In a prospective study of the outcome of surgical salvage of failed chemoradiotherapy for laryngeal cancer in patients from a randomised controlled trial, a third of patients developed a salivary fistula into the neck.[22] Rarely, injury to the lymphatic duct on the left side of the neck can lead to a lymph leak that can take up to a few weeks to settle.

Surgery can injure or require sacrifice of important neuromuscular structures to ensure tumour clearance. Injury to the spinal accessory nerve, which leads to shoulder dysfunction, and removal of the sternocleidomastoid muscle, which causes loss of contour to the neck, may also occur. Other cranial nerves (VII, X, and XII) and the sympathetic chain are also prone to injury depending on the extent of the tumour. Although microvascular free flap reconstructions have a consistently high success rate (>95%), failure of a flap can have considerable complications that can lead to prolonged hospital stay and a delay in any planned postoperative radiotherapy.

In the longer term, patients present with functional problems such as impaired swallowing and speech and voice problems, or weak shoulder. They may have to care for an end stoma. These sequelae will require input from various health professionals to achieve rehabilitation.

Complications of chemoradiotherapy

Acute complications of radiotherapy to the head and neck region include radiation dermatitis, xerostomia, excessive mucus production, and painful mucositis. Consequently, patients often reduce their intake of food and liquids and some may require nasogastric feeding or percutaneous gastrostomy to maintain adequate nutrition. The addition of concomitant chemotherapy may exacerbate the severity and duration of these acute effects. The acute effects of radiation typically settle four to six weeks after treatment is completed.

Serious late radiation toxicity is seen in as many as 82% of patients at five years,[23] and it may include xerostomia, fibrosis of soft tissues, dysphagia, and osteo-radionecrosis of the mandible.[23] These complications are important because they are usually permanent. Some, like xerostomia, improve over time,[13] but others, such as pharyngeal stenosis, are occasionally progressive and sometimes resistant to treatment. Minimising the volume of the tissues receiving radiotherapy (for example, by sparing salivary glands or bone) can reduce the rate of these complications, as shown in the PARSPORT trial.[13]

What quality of life do treated patients have?

Studies exploring quality of life outcomes in patients with head and neck cancer have shown greater impairment of quality of life for combined than for single modality treatments.[w21] Several large prospective cohorts studies have shown that patients' quality of life is greatly reduced during treatment but starts to improve about three months after treatment ends and continues to improve for one to two years, with little further improvement thereafter.[w21] More recently, data suggest a possible deterioration in quality of life in the long term (10 years) in survivors of head and neck cancer, but it is not clear whether this is the result of late sequelae of treatment or the development of other related or unrelated comorbidities.[24] Clearly, however, late effects of treatment, especially dry mouth and swallowing problems, are important determinants of long term quality of life.[25]

Interestingly, quality of life outcomes do not seem to differ significantly between the different treatment modalities, at least in the short to medium term, because several small retrospective and prospective cohort studies have reported similar outcomes for both radiotherapy and transoral laser conservation surgery for early laryngeal tumours.[w22] Similar quality of life outcomes have been reported for patients who have had laryngectomy (removal of the larynx) compared with those who have had organ sparing chemoradiotherapy for the treatment of advanced laryngeal cancer.[w23] Of note, qualitative studies have shown that a cure is the primary concern of patients with head and neck cancer, followed by prolongation of survival and then quality of life.[26] This is by no means consistent, however, and patients differ in their priorities,[26] which highlights the importance of involving patients fully in the decision making and treatment process.

How can recurrent or metastatic cancer be treated?

In patients with metastatic or locally recurrent head and neck cancer, treatment is usually palliative. If the recurrence occurs in previously untreated tissues of the head and neck then surgery and chemoradiation may be used as local salvage treatments. If not, chemotherapy with cisplatin and fluorouracil may be used to reduce symptoms. A recent randomised controlled trial found that the addition of an epidermal growth factor receptor inhibitor (cetuximab) to the above schedule produced a modest prolongation of overall survival.[27]

TIPS FOR NON-SPECIALISTS

- When following up patients with head and neck cancer who have been treated, watch out for:
- Recurrence of pretreatment symptoms, such as hoarseness
- New pain in head and neck
- Persistent cough or haemoptysis
- New ulcers, bleeding, or neck lumps
- Hypothyroidism after radiotherapy

ONGOING RESEARCH QUESTIONS

- To understand the epidemiology, prognosis, and optimum treatment of patients with human papillomavirus induced head and neck cancer
- To understand the optimum schedules for combination of radiotherapy, growth factor receptor inhibition, and chemotherapy
- To delineate the role of robotic surgery in transoral resection of oropharyngeal and laryngeal tumours and other head and neck surgical procedures, such as minimally invasive thyroidectomy
- To individualise the treatment and management of head and neck cancers on the basis of tumour cell biomarkers

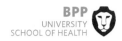

ADDITIONAL EDUCATIONAL RESOURCES

Resources for healthcare professionals

- WHO. The global burden of disease: 2004 update. 2008. www.who.int/evidence/bod
- National Cancer Comprehensive Network (www.nccn.org/index.asp)—Guidelines on treatment of cancers including head and neck in US
- Scottish Intercollegiate Guidelines Network. Diagnosis and management of head and neck cancer guidelines. Guideline no 90. 2006. www.sign.ac.uk/guidelines/fulltext/90/index.html
- National Institute for Health and Clinical Excellence. Improving outcomes in head and neck cancers—the manual. 2004. http://guidance.nice.org.uk/csghn/guidance/pdf/English
- Fanconi Anaemia Clinical Network. Clinical standards of care in the UK. www.fanconi.org.uk/clinical-network/standards-of-care/

Resources for patients and carers

- Cancer Research UK (www.cancerresearchuk.org)—National site that covers all cancers; very easy to navigate with lots of information
- Macmillan (www.macmillan.org.uk)—National site that covers all cancers; easy to navigate; need to type larynx into the search engine
- Merseyside Head and Neck Cancer Centre (www.headandneckcancer.co.uk)—Suitable for patients and carers in any part of the country, easy to navigate, very clear language and format
- Get A-Head (http://www.getahead.org.uk)—Easy to navigate, suitable for patients and carers in any part of the country, very informative; click on "patient info" then "helpful information"
- National Association of Laryngectomee Clubs (www.laryngectomy.org.uk)—Patient organised site with a wide selection of information for patients and professionals; hard copies are free on request
- Guidelines and Audit Implementation Network (http://www.gain-ni.org)—Informal learning course of six modules

Contributors: HM originated the idea. All authors helped plan, conduct, and report the review. All authors are guarantors.

Competing interests: All authors have completed the Unified Competing Interest form at www.icmje.org/coi_disclosure.pdf (available on request from the corresponding author) and declare that they had no financial support for the submitted work; HM is the director of an institute that does contract work for GSK, which has interests in head and neck cancers; he has also received grants from NCC-Health Technology Assessment Unit, Cancer Research UK, and Macmillan Fund. CN has received three clinical trial grants from Cancer Research UK and is principal investigator on a drug trial sponsored by Bayer; all authors have no other relationships or activities that could appear to have influenced the submitted work.

Provenance and peer review: Commissioned; externally peer reviewed.

Patient consent obtained.

1 Royal College of Pathologists. Standards and datasets for reporting cancers: datasets for histopathology reports on head and neck carcinomas and salivary neoplasms. 2nd ed. 2005. www.rcpath.org/resources/pdf/HeadNeckDatasetJun05.pdf .

2 Bourhis J, Overgaard J, Audry H, Ang KK, Saunders M, Bernier J, et al. Hyperfractionated or accelerated radiotherapy in head and neck cancer: a meta-analysis. Lancet2006;368:843-54.

3 Pignon JP, le Maitre A, Maillard E, Bourhis J. Meta-analysis of chemotherapy in head and neck cancer (MACH-NC): an update on 93 randomised trials and 17 346 patients. Radiother Oncol2009;92:4-14.

4 Paleri V, Wight RG, Silver CE, Haigentz M Jr, Takes RP, Bradley PJ, et al. Comorbidity in head and neck cancer: a critical appraisal and recommendations for practice. Head Neck2010 [forthcoming].

5 Silva P, Homer JJ, Slevin NJ, Musgrove BT, Sloan P, Price P, et al. Clinical and biological factors affecting response to radiotherapy in patients with head and neck cancer: a review. Clin Otolaryngol2007;32:337-45.

6 National Institute for Health and Clinical Excellence. Improving outcomes in head and neck cancers—the manual. 2004. http://guidance.nice.org.uk/csghn/guidance/pdf/English

7 Scottish Intercollegiate Guidelines Network. Head and neck cancers management, 2006, www.sign.ac.uk/guidelines/fulltext/90/index.html.

8 Bhalavat RI, Fakih AR, Mistry RC, Mahantshetty U. Radical radiation vs surgery plus post-operative radiation in advanced (resectable) supraglottic larynx and pyriform sinus cancers: a prospective randomized study. Eur J Surg Oncol2003;29:750-6.

9 Department of Veterans Affairs Laryngeal Cancer Study Group. Induction chemotherapy plus radiation compared with surgery plus radiation in patients with advanced laryngeal cancer. N Engl J Med1991;324:1685-90.

10 Fakhry C, Westra WH, Li S, Cmelak A, Ridge JA, Pinto H, et al. Improved survival of patients with human papillomavirus-positive head and neck squamous cell carcinoma in a prospective clinical trial. J Natl Cancer Inst2008;100:261-9.

11 Licitra L, Perrone F, Bossi P, Suardi S, Mariani L, Artusi, et al. High-risk human papillomavirus affects prognosis in patients with surgically treated oropharyngeal squamous cell carcinoma. J Clin Oncol2006;24:5630-6.

12 Ang KK, Harris J, Wheeler R, Weber R, Rosenthal DI, Nguyen-Tân PF, et al. Human papillomavirus and survival of patients with oropharyngeal cancer. N Engl J Med2010;363:24-35.

13 Nutting C, A'Hern R, Rogers MS, Sydenham MA, Adab F, Harrington K, et al. First results of a phase III multicenter randomized controlled trial of intensity modulated (IMRT) versus conventional radiotherapy (RT) in head and neck cancer (PARSPORT: ISRCTN48243537; CRUK/03/005)[abstract]. J Clin Oncol2009;27(suppl):18S.

14 Kam MK, Leung SF, Zee B, Chau RM, Suen JJ, Mo F, et al. Prospective randomized study of intensity-modulated radiotherapy on salivary gland function in early-stage nasopharyngeal carcinoma patients. J Clin Oncol2007;25:4873-9.

15 Fu KK, Pajak TF, Trotti A, Jones CU, Spencer SA, Phillips TL, et al. A Radiation Therapy Oncology Group (RTOG) phase III randomized study to compare hyperfractionation and two variants of accelerated fractionation to standard fractionation radiotherapy for head and neck squamous cell carcinomas: first report of RTOG 9003. Int J Radiat Oncol Biol Phys2000;48:7-16.

16 Pignon JP, Bourhis J, Domenge C, Designe L. Chemotherapy added to locoregional treatment for head and neck squamous-cell carcinoma: three meta-analyses of updated individual data. MACH-NC Collaborative Group. Meta-analysis of chemotherapy on head and neck cancer. Lancet2000;355:949-55.

17 Bernier J, Domenge C, Ozsahin M, Matuszewska K, Lefebvre JL, Greiner RH, et al. Postoperative irradiation with or without concomitant chemotherapy for locally advanced head and neck cancer. N Engl J Med2004;350:1945-52.

18 Cooper JS, Pajak TF, Forastiere AA, Jacobs J, Campbell BH, Saxman SB, et al. Radiation Therapy Oncology Group 9501/Intergroup. Postoperative concurrent radiotherapy and chemotherapy for high-risk squamous-cell carcinoma of the head and neck. N Engl J Med2004;350:1937-44.

19 Bonner JA, Harari PM, Giralt J, Azarnia N, Shin DM, Cohen RB, et al. Radiotherapy plus cetuximab for squamous-cell carcinoma of the head and neck. N Engl J Med2006;354:567-78.

20 Posner MR, Hershock DM, Blajman CR, Mickiewicz E, Winquist E, Gorbounova V, et al. Cisplatin and fluorouracil alone or with docetaxel in head and neck cancer. N Engl J Med2007;357:1705-15.

21 Vermorken JB, Remenar E, van Herpen C, Gorlia T, Mesia R, Degardin M, et al. Cisplatin, fluorouracil, and docetaxel in unresectable head and neck cancer. N Engl J Med2007;357:1695-704.

22 Weber RS, Berkey BA, Forastiere A, Cooper J, Maor M, Goepfert H, et al. Outcome of salvage total laryngectomy following organ preservation therapy: the Radiation Therapy Oncology Group trial 91-11. Arch Otolaryngol Head Neck Surg2003;129:44-9.

23 Denis F, Garaud P, Bardet E, Alfonsi M, Sire C, Germain T, et al. Late toxicity results of the GORTEC 94-01 randomized trial comparing radiotherapy with concomitant radiochemotherapy for advanced-stage oropharynx carcinoma: comparison of LENT/SOMA, RTOG/EORTC, and NCI-CTC scoring systems. Int J Radiat Oncol Biol Phys2003;55:93-8.

24 Mehanna HM, Morton RP. Deterioration in quality-of-life of late (10-year) survivors of head and neck cancer. Clin Otolaryngol2006;31:204-11.

25 Langendijk JA, Doornaert P, Verdonck-de Leeuw IM, Leemans CR, Aaronson NK, Slotman BJ. Impact of late treatment-related toxicity on quality of life among patients with head and neck cancer treated with radiotherapy. J Clin Oncol2008;26:3770-6.

26 List MA, Stracks J, Colangelo L, Butler P, Ganzenko N, Lundy D, et al. How do head and neck cancer patients prioritize treatment outcomes before initiating treatment? J Clin Oncol2000;18:877-84.

27 Rivera F, García-Castaño A, Vega N, Vega-Villegas ME, Gutiérrez-Sanz L. Cetuximab in metastatic or recurrent head and neck cancer: the EXTREME trial. Expert Rev Anticancer Ther2009;9:1421-8.

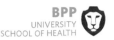

Low risk papillary thyroid cancer

Juan P Brito, assistant professor, endocrine fellow, and healthcare delivery scholar[1][2], Ian D Hay, professor of medicine and thyroidologist[1], John C Morris, professor of medicine, thyroidologist[1]

[1]Division of Endocrinology, Diabetes, Metabolism, and Nutrition, Mayo Clinic, Rochester, MN, USA

[2]Knowledge and Evaluation Research Unit, Mayo Clinic, Rochester, MN 55905, USA

Correspondence to: J C Morris Morris. John@mayo.edu

Cite this as: *BMJ* 2014;348:g3045

‹DOI› 10.1136/bmj.g3045
http://www.bmj.com/content/348/bmj.g3045

Thyroid cancer is one of the fastest growing diagnoses; more cases of thyroid cancer are found every year than all leukemias and cancers of the liver, pancreas, and stomach. Most of these incident cases are papillary in origin and are both small and localized. Patients with these small localized papillary thyroid cancers have a 99% survival rate at 20 years. In view of the excellent prognosis of these tumors, they have been denoted as low risk. The incidence of these low risk thyroid cancers is growing, probably because of the use of imaging technologies capable of exposing a large reservoir of subclinical disease. Despite their excellent prognosis, these subclinical low risk cancers are often treated aggressively. Although surgery is traditionally viewed as the cornerstone treatment for these tumors, there is less agreement about the extent of surgery (lobectomy v near total thyroidectomy) and whether prophylactic central neck dissection for removal of lymph nodes is needed. Many of these tumors are treated with radioactive iodine ablation and thyrotropin suppressive therapy, which—although effective for more aggressive forms of thyroid cancer—have not been shown to be of benefit in the management of these lesions. This review offers an evidence based approach to managing low risk papillary thyroid cancer. It also looks at the future of promising alternative surgical techniques, non-surgical minimally localized invasive therapies (ethanol ablation and laser ablation), and active surveillance, all of which form part of a more individualized treatment approach for low risk papillary thyroid tumors.

Introduction

Thyroid nodules are common. Depending on the population studied and the method of detection used, the prevalence of thyroid nodules varies from 5% by palpation to 30-67% by ultrasound evaluation.[1][2][3] Although most of these thyroid nodules are benign, 5-20% are malignant.[4] Therefore, thyroid cancer could be common in the population. This notion is supported by cadaveric studies from Finland, where a third of patients who died from non-thyroid related conditions were found to have thyroid cancer.[5]

The large reservoir of subclinical thyroid cancer has become more evident with the use of imaging technology. Thyroid cancer is now one of the fastest growing diagnoses; more cases of thyroid cancer are found every year in United States than all leukemias and cancers of the liver, pancreas, and stomach.[6] Despite its high prevalence, thyroid cancer

is an uncommon cause of death. Most patients with these lesions have an excellent prognosis and, because these tumors follow a highly indolent course they have been denoted as "low risk thyroid cancer."[7]

Several organizations and experts have provided guidance on these low risk tumors for both clinicians and patients.[8][9][10][11] Owing to uncertainty about the definition, epidemiology, and management of these cancers, many patients receive similar care to that for more aggressive thyroid cancers. New evidence has led to a better understanding of this condition and may herald a revolution in its management. Here, we review the available evidence and current challenges, and we provide a future perspective on the diagnosis and management of low risk thyroid cancer.

Definition

The most important predictor of prognosis for thyroid cancer is the histology of the primary tumor. Papillary and follicular thyroid cancers are differentiated thyroid cancers derived from follicular cells and represent 90% of all thyroid cancers.[8] Papillary thyroid cancer has a favorable prognosis, with a mortality of 1-2% at 20 years.[12] By contrast, follicular thyroid cancer is associated with a mortality of 10-20% at 20 years.[8] Other thyroid cancers—medullary, anaplastic, and poorly differentiated thyroid cancer—have an even worse prognosis. Patients with medullary thyroid cancer have a 25-50% mortality at 10 years,[8] and most patients with poorly differentiated and anaplastic thyroid cancer die within a few years (five year mortality of 90%).[13] Therefore, by definition, low risk thyroid cancer refers to papillary thyroid cancer only.

Low risk papillary thyroid cancers are generally not associated with well recognized predictors of mortality, such as higher grade and aggressive phenotype, local invasion, or distant metastatic disease.[14][15] Several classification systems have been developed that include these features and are used to stratify patients into risk categories.[16]

Classification systems

Figure 1 shows the features that denote low risk papillary thyroid cancer for each of the classification systems. These prognostic scoring and staging systems require the final histological interpretation and, in the case of MACIS, the assessment of residual disease after primary surgical resection.[12] Using these systems, 80-85% of papillary cancers are classified as low risk.[12][8][16] Although these scores consistently report an excellent prognosis for those classified as low risk (99% at 20 years), they are not designed to predict tumor recurrence.

In its clinical practice guidelines for differentiated thyroid carcinoma, the American Thyroid Association (ATA) suggested a three level classification scheme for predicting recurrence, which requires a dynamic assessment of the risk of recurrence and death over the clinical course of the thyroid cancer.[8] The ATA panel characterized low risk thyroid cancers as:

SOURCES AND SELECTION CRITERIA

We conducted a comprehensive search of Medline, Embase, the Cochrane Central Register of Controlled Trials, the Cochrane Database of Systematic Reviews, and Scopus from each database's inception to January 2014. The search strategy was designed and conducted by one of the study investigators (JPB). We used controlled vocabulary supplemented with keywords to search for "low risk thyroid cancer "and "low risk papillary thyroid cancer". We included observational and randomized studies published in English that included patients with low risk thyroid cancer as well as reviews, meta-analyses, and clinical guidelines for the treatment and management of thyroid cancer. The reference lists from primary studies and narrative reviews were searched, and we consulted with experts in the field to obtain any additional references of importance.

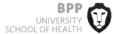
	AGES[13]	AMES[18]	MACIS[12]	TNM[19]
Prognostic factors	Age, Grade, Extent (invasion and distant metastasis), and Size	Age, Metastasis, extrathyroid Extension, tumor Size, and sex	Metastasis, Age, Completeness of resection, Invasion, and tumor Size	Tumor size, invasiveness, Nodal spread, distal Metastasis
Low risk	Score <4: 0.05 x age (if age ≥40) +1 (if grade 2) +1(if extrathyroid) +3 (if distant spread) +0.2 x tumor size in cm	Criteria: Men ≤40 or women ≤50 OR Older patients (without extrathyroid extension) Primary cancers <5 cm No distant metastasis	Score <6: 3.1 (if aged ≤39 years) or 0.08 x age (if aged ≥40 years), +0.3 x tumor size (cm), +1 (if incompletely resected), +1 (if locally invasive), +3 (if distant metastasis present)	Criteria: Stage I or II Younger than 45 years without distant metastasis or older than 45 years with tumor less than 4 cm and without regional or distant metastasis
Disease specific survival	99% at 20 years	99% at 20 years	99% at 20 years	100% at 5 years

Fig 1 Definition of low risk thyroid cancer according to different staging systems

- Lesions with no regional or distant metastasis or extra-thyroidal tumor invasion
- Absence of histology that is associated with aggressive papillary thyroid cancers, such as tall cell, insular, or columnar cell carcinoma
- Resection of all macroscopic tumor (assessed from surgical report or, if conducted, from whole body radioactive iodine scan).

The guidelines also suggested that, if radioactive iodine is given, low risk thyroid cancer should have no uptake of iodine-131 outside the thyroid bed on the first whole body radioactive iodine scan after treatment.

Similar recurrence stratification systems have been proposed by other thyroid societies, such as the Latin American Thyroid Society.[20]

Delayed risk stratification

Finally, many have argued that the low risk categorization should also consider the effect of initial treatment and require patients to be re-stratified according to the results of the first medical visit (8-12 months). This strategy, called delayed risk stratification, aims to classify patients who are falsely staged intermediate or high risk more accurately. A retrospective analysis that evaluated the predictive value of this approach found that about 50% of intermediate-high risk patients were re categorised as low risk after the first visit.[21]

This approach was further validated by a recent retrospective analysis, where delayed risk stratification predicted recurrence in a cohort of patients in whom the presence of antibodies against thyroglobulin could interfere with accurate assessment of this important tumor marker. This is an important finding, because 25% of patients with well differentiated thyroid cancer have anti-thyroglobulin antibodies.[22] Although these staging strategies are useful for clinicians and patients to decide postoperative management (adjunctive therapy, frequency, and intensity of follow-up) they are based on conventional clinicopathologic criteria. Ideally, low risk thyroid cancer should be identified before moving to treatment options, particularly before definitive surgery.

Molecular markers

Molecular based markers have the potential to improve the diagnosis of thyroid nodules and the risk stratification of thyroid cancers. Two intracellular pathways have been identified that play a role in thyroid cancer—the MAPK (mitogen activated protein kinase) and PI3K-AKT-MTOR (phosphatidylinositide 3-kinase-protein kinase B-mammalian target of rapamycin) pathways. Aberrant activation of the MAPK pathway results in tumor promotion, whereas mutations in the PI3K-AKT-MTOR pathway decrease expression of tumor suppressor genes.[23]

One mutation, the T1799A *BRAF* mutation in the MAPK pathway, has been studied as a prognostic molecular marker for aggressive clinicopathological outcomes. A recent meta-analysis of 2470 patients with papillary thyroid cancer found that this mutation was associated with an increased risk of tumor recurrence (relative risk 1.93, 95% confidence interval 1.61 to 2.32), lymph node metastasis (1.32, 1.20 to 1.45), extrathyroidal extension (1.71, 1.50 to 1.94), and advanced stage thyroid cancer (1.70, 1.45 to 1.99).[24] The meta-analysis also found a null effect on distant metastasis (0.95, 0.63 to 1.44).[24]

In a large retrospective multicenter study of 1890 patients,[25] the *BRAF* mutation was associated with a significantly increased cancer related mortality (5.3%, 3.9% to 7.1% in *BRAF* positive patients v 1.1%, 0.5% to 2.0% in *BRAF* negative patients (P<0.01), with a median follow-up of 33 months (interquartile range 13-67).

However, the association was no longer significant after adjusting for clinical and histopathological features, and the tumors in most patients with *BRAF* mutations still behaved in a low risk manner—only 95% of patients with a *BRAF* mutation had a death that was related to papillary thyroid cancer.[25] Similarly, recent large retrospective cohorts comprising 429 and 766 patients with papillary thyroid cancer found no association between a *BRAF* mutation and tumor multicentricity, lymphovascular invasion, extranodal extension, central neck involvement, advanced stage (III-IV), distant metastasis, or cause specific survival.[26] [27]

These results raise the question of whether the presence of this mutation provides any prognostic value over the existing clinical staging systems for low risk thyroid cancer.[28] Other markers are being explored. For example, mutations in the gene encoding the telomerase promoter (*TERT*), which can lead to persistent telomere lengthening, are indicators of clinically aggressive thyroid tumors and correlate with worse disease specific mortality. In a retrospective study of 647 patients with thyroid tumors,[29] *TERT* mutations were associated with a high risk of disease specific mortality in patients with papillary thyroid cancer (hazard ratio 23.8, 1.3 to 415) compared with those without the mutation. No *TERT* mutations were found in tumors less than 1 cm. Although this and other promising tumors markers (such as micro-RNA markers and epigenetic changes in tumor genes) could potentially be translated into practice to help define and differentiate low risk from high risk thyroid cancer, clinicopathological features are currently the best way to predict mortality and recurrence.

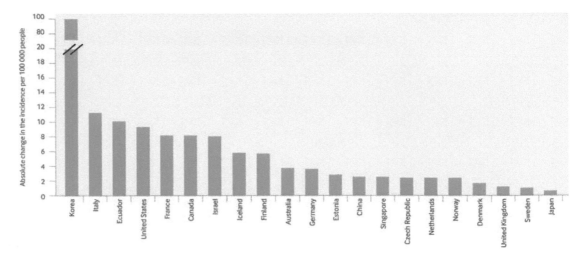

Fig 2 Absolute change in the incidence of thyroid cancer per 100000 per year calculated from the first date and last date of data insertion from each country[30]

Epidemiology

Thyroid cancer is the most common endocrine cancer and accounts for about 2% of all cancers in women and men.[30] Over the past three decades, the incidence of thyroid cancer has risen worldwide (fig 2).[31] The surge of new cases is growing more rapidly in countries where healthcare expenditure is driven by the private rather than the public sector, which have a low proportion of public health expenditure and a high proportion of private health financing.[32] For example, in the US the incidence of well differentiated thyroid cancer increased from 4.9 per 100000 to 14.3 per 100000 between 1975 and 2009.[33] Similarly, in South Korea, a country that relies heavily on patients' direct payment supplemented by private insurance,[28 32] the incidence of thyroid cancer increased from 10.6 per 100000 per year in 1996 to 111.3 per 100000 per year in 2010 in women, making thyroid cancer the most common cause of cancer among South Korean women.[34]

Geographic variation

The rate of increase in the incidence of thyroid cancers varies across countries. In Europe, for instance, the incidence of thyroid cancer in France resembles that seen in the US (3.4/100000 per year in 1983 to 11.7/100000 per year in 2002), the incidence in Sweden has not changed as dramatically (2.4/100000 per year in 1958 to 3.5/100000 per year in 2002).[35]

Geographic variation is also seen within countries. A recent report from Belgium showed that, between 2004 and 2006, the incidence of thyroid cancer was lower in the northern than in the southern part of the country (4.1/100000 v 8.3/100000).[36] Interestingly, the worldwide rise in the incidence of thyroid cancer has not been accompanied by an increase in mortality from this cancer, suggesting that these increasingly common incident cases represent a mild form of the disease that rarely causes death.

Increased detection

In countries where further analysis based on subtype and size of the tumor has been conducted, low risk thyroid cancer accounts for 90% of incident cases.[37] It has been suggested that the explosion of new cases of thyroid cancer, especially low risk papillary thyroid cancer, is due to the development and use of imaging technologies capable of exposing a large reservoir of subclinical disease.[38] In support of this hypothesis, many autopsy studies have shown that

thyroid cancer is common among people who die from non-thyroid related causes. Two studies, one in Spain and one in Finland,[5] analyzed the entire gland histologically.[5 39] They concluded that the frequency of thyroid cancer was 24% and 36%, respectively, suggesting the presence of a large reservoir of undiagnosed, and arguably clinically unimportant, disease.

Although it is not clear whether this pool of subclinical disease has changed over time, our capacity to detect it has changed. Increased availability of sensitive imaging technology may have increased the diagnosis of "occult" thyroid cancers. A recent retrospective study found that, among incident cases of thyroid cancer, 39% were detected through the use of imaging (mainly neck sonography and computer tomography), 15% were detected by pathological studies, and the remaining 46% were detected by palpation.[40] At least half of cases detected incidentally through imaging could have been labeled as low risk cancers. This is supported by a recent analysis of the US Surveillance, Epidemiology, and End Results Program (SEER) database,[41] which showed that the incidence of thyroid cancer was positively associated with markers of access to these technologies, such as college education, white collar employment, and higher family income. Incidence was negatively correlated with being uninsured, in poverty, unemployed, of non-white ethnicity, non-English speaking, and lacking high school education.

Risk factors

It has been suggested that the increased frequency of thyroid cancer might also reflect a new risk factor, not yet identified, that is causing the surge of incidence without affecting mortality. Candidates for these risk factors are increased exposure to low dose ionizing radiation from radiographic imaging as well as hormonal or nutritional factors.[42 43 44] The association of these risk factors with low risk thyroid cancer is weak and inconsistent, and no causal pathways have been described to link them to the increased incidence of thyroid cancer. Although other novel risk factors may play a role in the surge of new thyroid cancer cases, it is unlikely that they can explain the magnitude and geographic distribution of this surge worldwide.

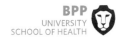

Treatment options for low risk thyroid cancer

Traditionally, the management of low risk papillary thyroid cancer involved removal of the primary tumor. Patients undergo preoperative assessment including neck ultrasound to map neck lymph nodes and fine needle aspiration biopsy of suspicious nodes. In those patients identified as having localized disease by this preoperative assessment, the most common treatment is surgical thyroidectomy. This permits removal of the primary tumor, facilitates postoperative treatment, and enables accurate staging and follow-up.[8] Although it is generally agreed that surgery is fundamental to the management of these tumors, there is less agreement about the extent of the surgery (lobectomy v near total thyroidectomy) and whether prophylactic central neck dissection for removal of lymph nodes is needed.

Thyroidectomy

No randomized trials have investigated the advantages of total thyroidectomy over lobectomy for patients with low risk papillary thyroid cancer. Thyroidectomy may remove the entire thyroid (total thyroidectomy) or may consist of ipsilateral total lobectomy and contralateral subtotal lobectomy, with only a small amount of thyroid tissue left to safeguard parathyroid function (near total thyroidectomy).

The rationale for thyroidectomy in these patients is that there are fewer recurrences with this intervention than with lobectomy. This argument is supported by a population based study from the National Cancer Data Base.[45] The study population comprised 52 173 patients undergoing thyroid surgery for papillary thyroid cancer. For tumors 1 cm or more, lobectomy resulted in a higher risk of recurrence (hazard ratio 1.15, 1.02 to 1.3) and non-disease specific mortality (1.31, 1.07 to 1.6). In view of this study and other benefits of thyroidectomy (possible future treatment with radioactive iodine and facilitation of follow-up with thyroglobulin), the ATA recommended that for patients with tumors greater than 1 cm, the initial surgical procedure should be a near total or total thyroidectomy unless there are contraindications to this surgery.[8] Other thyroid guidelines provide similar recommendations.[8 9 10 11]

Prophylactic central node dissection

The inclusion of prophylactic central node dissection (PCND)—resection of level VI, central compartment cervical lymph nodes in a patient with no evidence of lymph node involvement on physical examination, preoperative imaging, or intraoperative imaging[8]—during initial surgery is controversial.[46] This approach differs from the standard practice of performing central compartment dissection for visually or palpable lymph nodes seen at surgery, or seen preoperatively on preoperative ultrasound.

The argument supporting PCND is that nodal metastasis, which may be invisible on preoperative imaging (such as neck ultrasound), may be correlated with the persistence and recurrence of papillary thyroid cancer and that tumors often metastasize to cervical lymph nodes.[47] Retrospective studies of patients with tumors less than 1 cm who underwent node dissection showed the presence of microscopic nodal disease in 12-60% of patients.[48 49 50] In addition, proponents of PCND argue that this surgical intervention may also facilitate proper staging and postoperative tumor marker follow-up because it improves the assessment and removal of occult metastases.[51]

The argument against PCND is based on the uncertainty about its benefits for recurrence and mortality. A meta-analysis of retrospective studies,[52] comprising 1264 patients undergoing thyroidectomy or PCND, showed no difference in the risk of recurrence of thyroid cancer 1.05 (0.48 to 2.31) between the two groups. These results conflict with the results of a more recent meta-analysis of retrospective studies comprising 3331 patients.[53] In this systematic review, PCND was associated with a lower risk of short term (less than five years) locoregional recurrence than thyroidectomy alone (4.7% v 8.6%; pooled incidence rate ratio 0.65, 0.48 to 0.86). However, these results are confounded by the patients in the PCND group being 2.6 times more likely to receive radioactive iodine than those in the thyroidectomy group.

In addition, a retrospective study with a longer follow-up period evaluated disease specific survival for patients who underwent PCND for low risk thyroid cancer against historical cohorts without PCND. It showed that in 13 years of follow-up the rate of disease specific mortality was similar for both groups at 1.9%.[54] These findings are supported by a similar retrospective Norwegian study and a prospective Korean study.[55 56] This evidence suggests that PCND might not change the incidence of recurrence or disease specific mortality for patients with low risk papillary thyroid cancer.

The most salient argument against routine application of PCND is that its performance may increase the risk of complications of thyroidectomy, such as recurrent laryngeal nerve injury and hypoparathyroidism, especially if the surgeon is relatively inexperienced in the procedure.[46]

Lobectomy

The role of surgery for thyroid cancer is to clear the neck of disease. Some argue that this goal is achievable by a more conservative procedure—lobectomy. This intervention differs from a bilateral lobar resection (near total or total thyroidectomy) in that a hemi-thyroidectomy is performed, which removes only the lobe of the thyroid containing the nodule that harbors the malignant cells (determined by fine needle aspiration biopsy before surgery).

A recent large observational study based on the SEER database, analyzed 22 724 patients who had undergone surgery for papillary thyroid cancer between 1988 and 2001.[57] Controlling for tumor size, no survival benefit was seen with more aggressive surgical treatment for those patients with low risk tumors (total thyroidectomy v lobectomy). The lack of difference in survival between these two interventions is backed up by an earlier institutional retrospective study of 1038 patients and a database analysis of 53 856 patients in the National Cancer Data Base from 1985 to 1995.[58 59] The ATA recommends that thyroid lobectomy alone may be sufficient treatment for small (<1 cm), low risk, unifocal, intrathyroidal thyroid cancers in the absence of previous head and neck irradiation or radiologically or clinically involved cervical nodal metastasis.[8]

Trade-off

There is much uncertainty about the benefits of these surgical procedures for low risk papillary thyroid cancer. Total thyroidectomy and PCND could facilitate follow-up and staging of low risk tumors and might decrease the need for further intervention and the inherent anxiety associated with such procedures. However, patients with low risk tumors who undergo more invasive surgical procedures do not live longer than those who undergo lobectomy. It is likely that, because of the indolent course of low risk thyroid cancer, these two procedures are equivalent—it is

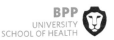

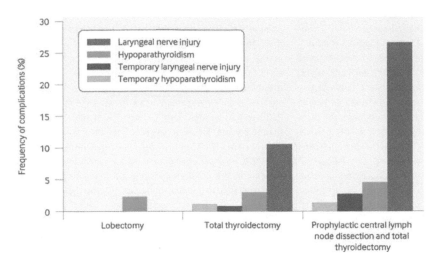

Fig 3 Frequency of complications of different surgical procedures for low risk papillary thyroid cancer calculated from relevant comparative cohorts[51 56 61 62 63]

difficult to show benefit of any intervention when the risk of mortality is close to 1-2% after 20 years of follow-up. However, all patients who have thyroidectomy need thyroid replacement (with its own burden of treatment and follow-up), compared with only half of patients who have lobectomy.[60] Finally, the morbidity associated with surgical intervention is directly and inversely correlated with the extent of surgical intervention and the surgeon's experience (fig 3).

Adjuvant therapies
Postoperative radioiodine remnant ablation
Radioiodine remnant ablation (RRA) aims to destroy the residual normal thyroid tissue seen after thyroidectomy. It differs from radioiodine "treatment," which is meant to destroy known residual thyroid cancer. However, it is often considered adjuvant therapy in cases where the risk of recurrence and mortality is a concern.[8]

Although radioactive iodine was first used to treat metastatic thyroid cancer in 1940,[64] it was not until 1960 that it was used to ablate postoperative remnant tissue.[65] By the 1990s, administration of RRA had become the standard of care for patients with thyroid cancer. The goals of RRA were, initially, to destroy microscopic residual disease and, more recently, to allow accurate surveillance with tumor markers (serum thyroglobulin measurements).

Nevertheless, over the past two decades evidence has emerged of a lack of any significant benefit of RRA for low risk papillary thyroid cancer. One of the first studies to suggest this lack of benefit was a large retrospective cohort of 1163 patients with a MACIS score less than 6 (low risk papillary thyroid cancer). These patients were treated between 1970 and 2000 and underwent near total or total thyroidectomy performed by a small group of specialized surgeons. After a follow-up of 20 years, in both the 527 node positive and the 636 node negative cases, cause specific mortality and tumor recurrence were the same in those who had surgery without postoperative RRA and in those who received postoperative RRA.[66 67] Furthermore, two systematic reviews investigating the effectiveness of radioactive iodine for treatment of patients with thyroid cancer found unclear benefits of RRA for low risk patients with papillary cancer and no statistically valid improvement in mortality or disease specific survival.[68 69]

Finally, RRA in low risk papillary thyroid cancer did not reduce recurrence in multifocal node positive disease.[70] In

addition, a recent large prospective multicenter study with a follow-up of 10.3 years found similar overall survival (95.8% v 94.6%) and disease-free survival (hazard ratio 0.73, 0.43 to 1.25) in patients with low risk thyroid cancer who received RRA after surgery versus those who had surgery alone.[71]

Despite this lack of benefit for RRA in patients with low risk thyroid cancer, its use has increased. In the US, the use of this technique in these patients increased from four in 100 patients to 38 in 100 patients between 1973 and 2007.[72] This finding is supported by a time trend analysis of 89 219 patients with well differentiated thyroid cancer treated at 981 hospitals associated with the US National Cancer Data Base between 1990 and 2008.[73] In this analysis the increased use of RRA for low risk thyroid cancer varied between hospitals, and this was attributed to unexplained hospital characteristics, suggesting considerable variation in practice for these patients. This use of RRA for low risk patients was perhaps driven by the belief that this treatment improves the specificity of postoperative thyroglobulin assays, which may detect persistent or recurrent disease.

Enthusiasm for the use of RRA to facilitate follow-up was tempered by a recent retrospective study of 290 consecutive patients with low risk thyroid cancer treated with thyroidectomy alone who underwent yearly follow-up with serum thyroglobulin assays.[74] It found that after about five years, thyroglobulin was undetectable in 95% of patients not treated with RRA compared with 99% in a matched cohort of patients treated with RRA. Only one patient who was not treated with RRA had a recurrence, as detected by an increase in thyroglobulin. This indicates that thyroglobulin continues to be a reliable marker of follow-up for patients with low risk thyroid cancer who did not receive RRA.

The administration of radioactive iodine is not risk free—it is associated with short term side effects (dry eyes, altered taste, and inflammation of salivary glands) and perhaps an increase in salivary gland cancers and leukemia.[72] In view of this evidence, recent guidelines do not recommend the use of RRA in patients with low risk thyroid cancer with lesions less than 1 cm who do not have high risk features (such as aggressive variants and vascular invasion). They recommend that it is used only in those with documented lymph node metastasis or other high risk features.[8 10]

Thyrotropin suppressive therapy
Similar to normal follicular cells, thyroid cancer cells express thyrotropin receptors and respond to this hormone by increasing cell growth.[75] Therefore, postoperative thyrotropin suppressive therapy has played a major role in the treatment of well differentiated thyroid cancer since the first report of regression of papillary thyroid cancer in two patients given thyroid extracts in 1937.[76]

In support of this practice, a meta-analysis of 4174 patients with well differentiated thyroid cancer showed that thyrotropin suppressive therapy reduced the risk of disease progression or recurrence and death (relative risk 0.73, 0.6 to 0.88).[77] Although it is generally agreed that patients with high risk thyroid cancers should receive suppressive therapy to maintain thyrotropin concentrations below 0.1 mU/L,[78 79] such treatment did not improve the rate of recurrence or disease specific survival in patients with low risk papillary thyroid cancer.[80]

Therefore, the goal of thyroid hormone treatment should be different for patients with low risk papillary thyroid cancer than for those with indeterminate or high risk disease. For low risk patients, post-thyroidectomy thyrotropin

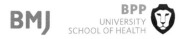

suppressive therapy should provide adequate replacement to avoid symptoms of hypothyroidism and thyrotoxicosis. Older patients, who are more likely to develop cardiovascular disease (atrial fibrillation and arrhythmia) and bone loss as a result of subclinical thyrotoxicosis, should be managed with less tight goals (thyrotropin 1-2.5 mU/L) than younger patients (thyrotropin 0.5-1 mU/L), who are less sensitive to the adverse effects of treatment.[81 82] The European and ATA guidelines for patients with low risk thyroid cancer recommend a thyrotropin concentration of 0.5-1 mU/L.[8 10]

Emerging treatments

After thyroid surgery, postoperative treatments (RRA and thyrotropin suppressive therapy) have not shown significant clinical benefit for patients with low risk thyroid cancer. However, for some patients, depending on the context and their preferences, even conventional surgery might not be desirable. Over the past decade, other management options have been studied for patients with low risk thyroid cancer.

Alternative surgical techniques

Although open surgery with a residual neck scar is the traditional technique for thyroidectomy, recent studies have reported that endoscopic thyroidectomy is also feasible for patients who wish to avoid a cervical incision. Endoscopic surgery, using extracervical access (for example, axillary, anterior chest, or breast), is an approach to the thyroid gland that uses video-endoscopic equipment through small and hidden incisions. One form of this endoscopic technique is robotic thyroidectomy, where the surgeon is assisted by an advanced robotic system that may allow better visualization and dexterity.

A meta-analysis of randomized clinical trials that compared video assisted interventions with conventional thyroidectomy in thyroid nodules and low risk papillary thyroid cancer found no significant difference in the risk of transient laryngeal nerve palsy or hypoparathyroidism.[83] In addition, video assisted techniques reduced postoperative pain at six hours and improved cosmetic results, although operative times were longer. Of note, the robotic technique has not received US Food and Drug Administration approval for thyroidectomy because of concerns regarding unreported adverse effects.[84]

Minimally invasive therapy for patients with low risk thyroid cancer

When surgery is neither indicated nor desired, non-surgical minimally invasive therapies are available. These treatments are based on the principle that focused and accurate destruction of tumor tissue will induce small vessel thrombosis and coagulative necrosis within the tumor, and they have been proposed by some as excellent options for primary treatment of low risk papillary thyroid cancer.

Ultrasound guided percutaneous ethanol ablation involves the direct intratumoral injection of 95% ethanol under careful ultrasound guidance and local anesthesia. Although this technique is effective and safe (small risk of temporary hoarseness) for benign cystic thyroid nodules and nodal metastasis in papillary thyroid cancer,[85 86] limited evidence is available on its efficacy in low risk thyroid cancer. A case series described three patients, with five intrathyroid foci of papillary microcarcinoma, whose biopsy confirmed papillary thyroid cancer lesions were treated by ethanol ablation within the intact thyroid.[87] In all cases, the lesions became avascular and smaller and one disappeared.

These promising results are limited by a lack of a comparator group and selection bias.

Others, however, have raised concerns that this treatment can cause random distribution of ethanol within the thyroid gland, with possible seepage into surrounding cervical tissues and local side effects.[88 89] They propose that thermal ablation with lasers may be a better alternative treatment for thyroid cancer owing to its predictable and well defined area of necrosis.[90] A recent study evaluated the efficacy of laser ablation of low risk papillary thyroid cancer as primary treatment in three patients.[91] All patients underwent percutaneous laser treatment of thyroid cancer lesions in the operating room immediately before surgical removal of the thyroid. Subsequent pathological and immunohistochemical analyses of the extirpated thyroid glands showed destruction of the malignant cells.

Radiofrequency ablation is another possible non-invasive treatment for primary low risk papillary thyroid cancer. This technique has been used successfully to ablate tumors in the liver, lung, and kidney.[92] A recent systematic review of prospective studies found that it is safe and effective in the treatment for symptomatic benign thyroid nodules and is effective in treating locoregional recurrence of thyroid cancers.[92 93] However, no studies have yet been reported for primary treatment of low risk thyroid cancer.

Active surveillance

Two large Japanese observational studies of 1465 patients with thyroid cancer were conducted on the basis of the hypothesis that most low risk papillary thyroid cancers do not need immediate or eventual thyroid surgery.[94 95] Patients were offered the option of active surveillance or thyroidectomy. Those who chose active surveillance were followed closely with neck ultrasound at six months and then annually for an average of five years (range 1-19). By the end of the follow-up only a minority of patients had lymph node metastasis (<2%) or experienced asymptomatic lesion growth (5%). No cases of disease specific mortality were seen in the observed patients. None of the other traditional risk factors for lymph node metastasis (multicentricity or size at diagnosis) were linked to any adverse outcomes.

Following the example of these Japanese studies, the Memorial Sloan-Kettering Cancer Center in New York City has begun an active surveillance program for patients with low risk papillary thyroid cancer who do not wish to proceed with surgery.[96] The table presents the most important characteristics and finding of these cohorts.

Active surveillance protocols have also been developed for recurrent localized disease after thyroidectomy. In a retrospective study of 166 patients with low risk thyroid cancer with at least one abnormal lymph node after thyroidectomy, the median size of lymph nodes at the start of the observation period was 1.3 cm (range 0.5-2.7).[97] After a median follow-up of 3.5 years, growth of at least 3 mm and 5 mm was seen in 33 (20%) and 15 (9%), respectively, whereas the nodules disappeared in 23 (14%). No local complications or disease related mortality were seen. A similar study from the same research group concluded that, when observed over a period of more than five years, only 10% of recurrent thyroid bed nodules from patients with low risk thyroid cancer increased substantially in size.[98] These two studies support the hypothesis that most low risk thyroid cancer lesions follow an indolent course and that many can be monitored safely without active intervention.

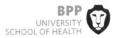

Studies on patients with low risk thyroid cancer undergoing active surveillance

Study	Definition of low risk	Patients (n)	Female (n (%))	Mean age (years (range))	Mean follow-up (years (range))	Growth >3 mm (n (%))	Lymph node metastasis (n (%))	Surgery at any follow up point (n (%))	Disease specific mortality
Sugitani (2010)[95]	<1 cm, no lymph node metastasis or extrathyroid invasion	230 (300 lesions)*	204 (89)	54 (23-84)	5 (1-17)	22 (7)	3 (1)	16 (5)	0
Ito (2013)[94]	<1 cm, no lymph node metastasis, extrathyroid invasion, or cytological findings suggesting high grade cancer; not close to trachea/dorsal thyroid surface	1235	1111 (90)	Unknown	5 (1-19)	58 (5)	19 (2)	191 (16)	0
Pace (2013)[96]	<1.5cm, no lymph node metastasis or extrathyroid invasion	71	50 (70)	52 (22-86)	1.3	0	0	3 (4)	0
All studies		1536	1365 (89)	NA	NA	80 (5)	22 (1.4)	210 (14)	0

*Analyzed by lesion.
NA=not applicable.

Patient centered and evidence based approaches

Despite their excellent prognosis patients with low risk papillary thyroid cancer still receive similar treatment to patients with aggressive disease and a worse prognosis. Perhaps the continued use of unnecessary treatments reflects uncertainty in the definition of "low risk thyroid cancer," which focuses on the lesions and not the patients.

Ideally, low risk papillary thyroid cancer should be managed in a way that achieves the lowest risk of mortality and morbidity with the lowest burden of treatment. For instance many argue that RRA facilitates disease related surveillance, but it clearly does not improve mortality and probably increases treatment related morbidity. Thus, this treatment might not be appropriate for a patient with low risk thyroid cancer.

Often, however, the balance between benefits (mortality and morbidity) and burden of treatment is not as clear as it is for surgical interventions (thyroidectomy v lobectomy). In such scenarios it is important to understand what the patient wants and needs, and what is most appropriate in the individual context.

Some patients might even opt for active surveillance because for them a surgical intervention brings more burden than benefit; fig 4 shows a decision tool to help clinicians review these management options with their patients. Many others may, in the future, decide for minimally invasive treatments (such as ultrasound guided percutaneous ethanol ablation or laser ablation) as these therapies become better understood and are more widely practiced.

To help patients make better decisions we should combine efforts to bring them the best comparative evidence about the efficacy and potential harm caused by each intervention. In low risk cancers with a low rate of events, a thyroid cancer network that helps create large databases for observational studies and samples for randomized clinical trials would be useful. Perhaps such a network might follow the example of pediatric cancer research, where a network sponsored by the US National Cancer Institute supports the enrollment of children diagnosed as having cancer to research registries. These networks facilitate the understanding and translation of evidence that might yield improvements in practice.[99]

Finally, we should explore the possible causes of this increase in the incidence of low risk papillary thyroid cancer. We have suggested that it probably reflects the increased use of imaging technologies. If this is the case, more research is needed to recognize which imaging techniques are more likely to find incidental small papillary thyroid cancers and investigate the appropriateness and usefulness of these tests.

Factors to take into account	Thyroid surgery		Active surveillance
	Partial thyroidectomy	**Total thyroidectomy**	
Need for lifelong thyroid replacement	Half of patients	All patients	No patients
Cost	$16 000-35 000 plus follow-up*		Cost of follow-up only
Follow-up	Yearly with blood test and thyroid ultrasound		Thyroid ultrasound every 6 months during the first year and every year thereafter†
Complications (LNI and HPT)/100 patients† — Temporary	1	5-25‡	Silent cancer growth of >3 mm in 5/100 patients and lymph node metastasis in 1/100 patients
Complications (LNI and HPT)/100 patients† — Permanent	No risk	2-5‡	
Mortality	1/1000 patients		95% CI 0/1000 to 3/1000 patients§

*Values estimated from several sources including patients forums. $16 000=£9500; €11 500.
†Suggested follow-up in observational trials to assess rate of growth and lymph node involvement.
‡High values for thyroidectomy plus prophylactic neck dissection.
§Estimated from observational trails of low risk thyroid cancer at 5 years.
LNI=laryngeal nerve injury; HPT=hypoparathyroidism.

Fig 4 Treatment options for patients with low risk papillary thyroid cancer

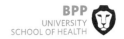

Conclusion

The diagnosis of thyroid cancer is rapidly increasing. This increase is occurring worldwide, but important geographic variations exist. Most of the new cases are small and localized papillary thyroid cancers that, because of their indolent course, are considered low risk. The main reason for this increase in the incidence of low risk papillary thyroid cancer is still unclear, but it probably reflects the discovery of a large reservoir of subclinical disease through the increased use of imaging.

Although clinicians are encountering patients with low risk thyroid cancer more often, guidelines and experts have not reached a consensus on the precise definition of this condition. This uncertainty in diagnosis is aggravated by the lack of high quality evidence from randomized clinical trials to elucidate the extent of the benefits and harms of currently available treatments. This lack of clarity has led many patients to receive treatments that are more appropriate for aggressive cancers. Many of these treatments can lead to adverse effects that might be perceived as unnecessarily harmful owing to the favorable prognosis of these lesions.

The challenges surrounding the diagnosis and management of low risk thyroid cancer should be seen as an opportunity to start collaborative networks around the globe that provide patients with faster and more reliable evidence about traditional and novel treatments. The outcomes of the trials should incorporate factors that help clinicians assess the burden of disease and also help them understand the burden of treatment and the outcomes that matter to patients. The era of a "one size fits all" management program for papillary thyroid cancer should end. Each patient is different and deserves a more individualized treatment approach.

Contributors: All authors contributed to the concepts and structure of this manuscript. JCM is guarantor.

Competing interests: We have read and understood BMJ policy on declaration of interests and declare the following interests: None.

Provenance and peer review: Commissioned; externally peer reviewed.

1 Tan GH, Gharib H. Thyroid incidentalomas: management approaches to nonpalpable nodules discovered incidentally on thyroid imaging. *Ann Intern Med*1997;126:226-31.
2 Reiners C, Wegscheider K, Schicha H, Theissen P, Vaupel R, Wrbitzky R, et al. Prevalence of thyroid disorders in the working population of Germany: ultrasonography screening in 96,278 unselected employees. *Thyroid*2004;14:926-32.
3 Braunstein G, Sacks W. Thyroid nodules. In: Braunstein GD, ed. Thyroid cancer. Springer US, 2012:45-61.
4 Brito JP, Yarur AJ, Prokop LJ, McIver B, Murad MH, Montori VM. Prevalence of thyroid cancer in multinodular goiter versus single nodule: a systematic review and meta-analysis. *Thyroid*2013;23:449-55.
5 Harach HR, Franssila KO, Wasenius VM. Occult papillary carcinoma of the thyroid. A "normal" finding in Finland. A systematic autopsy study. *Cancer*1985;56:531-8.
6 American Cancer Society. Cancer facts and figures 2012. www.cancer.org/acs/groups/content/@epidemiologysurveilance/documents/document/acspc-031941.pdf.

7 Roti E, degli Uberti EC, Bondanelli M, Braverman LE. Thyroid papillary microcarcinoma: a descriptive and meta-analysis study. *Eur J Endocrinol*2008;159:659-73.
8 Cooper DS, Doherty GM, Haugen BR, Kloos RT, Lee SL, Mandel SJ, et al. Revised American Thyroid Association management guidelines for patients with thyroid nodules and differentiated thyroid cancer. *Thyroid*2009;19:1167-214.
9 Pitoia F, Ward L, Wohllk N, Figuglietti C, Tomimori E, Gauna A, et al. Recommendations of the Latin American Thyroid Society on diagnosis and management of differentiated thyroid cancer. *Arq Bras Endocrinol Metabol*2009;53:884-7.
10 Pacini F, Schlumberger M, Dralle H, Elisei R, Smit JW, Wiersinga W. European consensus for the management of patients with differentiated thyroid carcinoma of the follicular epithelium. *Eur J Endocrinol*2006;154:787-803.
11 Harris PE. The management of thyroid cancer in adults: a review of new guidelines. *Clin Med*2002;2:144-6.
12 Hay ID, Bergstralh EJ, Goellner JR, Ebersold JR, Grant CS. Predicting outcome in papillary thyroid carcinoma: development of a reliable prognostic scoring system in a cohort of 1779 patients surgically treated at one institution during 1940 through 1989. *Surgery*1993;114:1050-7; discussion 57-8.
13 McIver B, Hay ID, Giuffrida DF, Dvorak CE, Grant CS, Thompson GB, et al. Anaplastic thyroid carcinoma: a 50-year experience at a single institution. *Surgery*2001;130:1028-34.
14 Toubeau M, Touzery C, Arveux P, Chaplain G, Vaillant G, Berriolo A, et al. Predictive value for disease progression of serum thyroglobulin levels measured in the postoperative period and after (131)I ablation therapy in patients with differentiated thyroid cancer. *J Nucl Med*2004;45:988-94.
15 Rouxel A, Hejblum G, Bernier MO, Boelle PY, Menegaux F, Mansour G, et al. Prognostic factors associated with the survival of patients developing loco-regional recurrences of differentiated thyroid carcinomas. *J Clin Endocrinol Metab*2004;89:5362-8.
16 Dean DS, Hay ID. Prognostic indicators in differentiated thyroid carcinoma. *Cancer Control*2000;7:229-39.
17 Hay ID, Grant CS, Taylor WF, McConahey WM. Ipsilateral lobectomy versus bilateral lobar resection in papillary thyroid carcinoma: a retrospective analysis of surgical outcome using a novel prognostic scoring system. *Surgery*1987;102:1088-95.
18 Cady B, Rossi R. An expanded view of risk-group definition in differentiated thyroid carcinoma. *Surgery*1988;104:947-53.
19 American Joint Committee on Cancer. Thyroid. In: Edge SB, Byrd DR, Compton CC, Fritz AG, Greene FL, Trotti A, eds. AJCC cancer staging manual. 7th ed. Springer, 2010:87-96.
20 Pitoia F, Bueno F, Urciuoli C, Abelleira E, Cross G, Tuttle RM. Outcome of patients with differentiated thyroid cancer risk stratified according to the American Thyroid Association and Latin-American Thyroid Society risk of recurrence classification systems. *Thyroid*2013;23:1401-7.
21 Castagna MG, Maino F, Cipri C, Belardini V, Theodoropoulou A, Cevenini G, et al. Delayed risk stratification, to include the response to initial treatment (surgery and radioiodine ablation), has better outcome predictivity in differentiated thyroid cancer patients. *Eur J Endocrinol*2011;165:441-6.
22 Jeon MJ, Kim WG, Park WR, Han JM, Kim TY, Song DE, et al. Modified dynamic risk stratification for predicting recurrence using the response to initial therapy in patients with differentiated thyroid carcinoma. *Eur J endocrinol*2014;170:23-30.
23 Xing M, Haugen BR, Schlumberger M. Progress in molecular-based management of differentiated thyroid cancer. *Lancet*2013;381:1058-69.
24 Tufano RP, Teixeira GV, Bishop J, Carson KA, Xing M. BRAF mutation in papillary thyroid cancer and its value in tailoring initial treatment: a systematic review and meta-analysis. *Medicine (Baltimore)*2012;91:274-86.
25 Xing M, Alzahrani AS, Carson KA, Viola D, Elisei R, Bendlova B, et al. Association between BRAF V600E mutation and mortality in patients with papillary thyroid cancer. *JAMA*2013;309:1493-501.
26 Gouveia C, Can NT, Bostrom A, Grenert JP, van Zante A, Orloff LA. Lack of association of BRAF mutation with negative prognostic indicators in papillary thyroid carcinoma: the University of California, San Francisco, experience. *JAMA Otolaryngol Head Neck Surg*2013;139:1164-70.
27 Ito Y, Yoshida H, Kihara M, Kobayashi K, Miya A, Miyauchi A. BRAF(V600E) mutation analysis in papillary thyroid carcinoma: is it useful for all patients? *World J Surg*2014;38:679-87.
28 Cappola AR, Mandel SJ. Molecular testing in thyroid cancer: BRAF mutation status and mortality. *JAMA*2013;309:1529-30.
29 Melo M, Rocha AG, Vinagre J, Batista R, Peixoto J, Tavares C, et al. TERT promoter mutations are a major indicator of poor outcome in differentiated thyroid carcinomas. *J Clin Endocrinol Metab*2014;99:E754-65.
30 Curado MP, Edwards B, Shin HR, Storm H, Ferlay J, Heanue M, et al. Cancer incidence in five continents. Vol IX. IARC Scientific Publications No. 160. International Agency for Research on Cancer, 2007. www.iarc.fr/en/publications/pdfs-online/epi/sp160/.
31 Kilfoy BA, Zheng T, Holford TR, Han X, Ward MH, Sjodin A, et al. International patterns and trends in thyroid cancer incidence, 1973-2002. *Cancer Causes Control*2009;20:525-31.
32 Lee TJ, Kim S, Cho HJ, Lee JH. The incidence of thyroid cancer is affected by the characteristics of a healthcare system. *J Korean Med Sci*2012;27:1491-8.

FUTURE RESEARCH QUESTIONS

- What is the contribution of imaging tests to the increased incidence of low risk thyroid cancer?
- Does any other risk factor explain the increased incidence of low risk thyroid cancer?
- What is the role of promising molecular markers in predicting recurrence and mortality in patients with low risk thyroid cancer?
- What are patients' values and preferences regarding the treatment decision for low risk thyroid cancer?
- What is the comparative effectiveness of active surveillance versus traditional management versus minimally invasive treatments for patients with low risk thyroid cancer?
- What is the role of shared decision making for patients with low risk thyroid cancer?

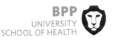

33 Davies L, Welch H. Current thyroid cancer trends in the united states. *JAMA Otolaryngol Head Neck Surg*2014;140:317-22.

34 Kweon SS, Shin MH, Chung IJ, Kim YJ, Choi JS. Thyroid cancer is the most common cancer in women, based on the data from population-based cancer registries, South Korea. *Jpn J Clin Oncol*2013;43:1039-46.

35 Ferlay J, Parkin DM, Curado MP, Bray F, Edwards B, Shin HR, et al. Cancer incidence in five continents. Vol I-IX: IARC CancerBase No. 9. International Agency for Research on Cancer, 2010. http://ci5.iarc.fr.

36 Van den Bruel A, Francart J, Dubois C, Adam M, Vlayen J, De Schutter H, et al. Regional variation in thyroid cancer incidence in Belgium is associated with variation in thyroid imaging and thyroid disease management. *J Clin Endocrinol Metab*2013;98:4063-71.

37 Davies L, Welch HG. Increasing incidence of thyroid cancer in the United States, 1973-2002. *JAMA*2006;295:2164-7.

38 Brito JP, Morris JC, Montori VM. Thyroid cancer: zealous imaging has increased detection and treatment of low risk tumours. *BMJ*2013;347:f4706.

39 Martinez-Tello FJ, Martinez-Cabruja R, Fernandez-Martin J, Lasso-Oria C, Ballestin-Carcavilla C. Occult carcinoma of the thyroid. A systematic autopsy study from Spain of two series performed with two different methods. *Cancer*1993;71:4022-9.

40 Malone MK, Zagzag J, Ogilvie JB, Patel KN, Heller KS. Thyroid cancers detected by imaging are not necessarily small or early stage. *Thyroid*2014;24:314-8.

41 Morris LG, Sikora AG, Tosteson TD, Davies L. The increasing incidence of thyroid cancer: the influence of access to care. *Thyroid*2013;23:885-91.

42 Hall EJ, Brenner DJ. Cancer risks from diagnostic radiology. *Br J Radiol*2008;81:362-78.

43 Negri E, Ron E, Franceschi S, Dal Maso L, Mark SD, Preston-Martin S, et al. A pooled analysis of case-control studies of thyroid cancer. I. Methods. *Cancer Causes Control*1999;10:131-42.

44 Dal Maso L, Bosetti C, La Vecchia C, Franceschi S. Risk factors for thyroid cancer: an epidemiological review focused on nutritional factors. *Cancer Causes Control*2009;20:75-86.

45 Bilimoria KY, Bentrem DJ, Ko CY, Stewart AK, Winchester DP, Talamonti MS, et al. Extent of surgery affects survival for papillary thyroid cancer. *Ann Surg*2007;246:375-81; discussion 81-4.

46 Carling T, Carty SE, Ciarleglio MM, Cooper DS, Doherty GM, Kim LT, et al. American Thyroid Association design and feasibility of a prospective randomized controlled trial of prophylactic central lymph node dissection for papillary thyroid carcinoma. *Thyroid*2012;22:237-44.

47 Machens A, Hinze R, Thomusch O, Dralle H. Pattern of nodal metastasis for primary and reoperative thyroid cancer. *World J Surg*2002;26:22-8.

48 Wada N, Duh QY, Sugino K, Iwasaki H, Kameyama K, Mimura T, et al. Lymph node metastasis from 259 papillary thyroid microcarcinomas: frequency, pattern of occurrence and recurrence, and optimal strategy for neck dissection. *Ann Surg*2003;237:399-407.

49 Gulben K, Berberoglu U, Celen O, Mersin HH. Incidental papillary microcarcinoma of the thyroid--factors affecting lymph node metastasis. *Langenbecks Arch Surg*2008;393:25-9.

50 Hughes DT, White ML, Miller BS, Gauger PG, Burney RE, Doherty GM. Influence of prophylactic central lymph node dissection on postoperative thyroglobulin levels and radioiodine treatment in papillary thyroid cancer. *Surgery*2010;148:1100-6; discussion 006-7.

51 Sywak M, Cornford L, Roach P, Stalberg P, Sidhu S, Delbridge L. Routine ipsilateral level VI lymphadenectomy reduces postoperative thyroglobulin levels in papillary thyroid cancer. *Surgery*2006;140:1000-5; discussion 1005-7.

52 Zetoune T, Keutgen X, Buitrago D, Aldailami H, Shao H, Mazumdar M, et al. Prophylactic central neck dissection and local recurrence in papillary thyroid cancer: a meta-analysis. *Ann Surg Oncol*2010;17:3287-93.

53 Lang BH, Ng SH, Lau LL, Cowling BJ, Wong KP, Wan KY. A systematic review and meta-analysis of prophylactic central neck dissection on short-term locoregional recurrence in papillary thyroid carcinoma after total thyroidectomy. *Thyroid*2013;23:1087-98.

54 Tisell LE, Nilsson B, Molne J, Hansson G, Fjalling M, Jansson S, et al. Improved survival of patients with papillary thyroid cancer after surgical microdissection. *World J Surg*1996;20:854-9.

55 Salvesen H, Njolstad PR, Akslen LA, Albrektsen G, Viste A, Soreide O, et al. Thyroid carcinoma: results from surgical treatment in 211 consecutive patients. *Eur J Surg*1991;157:521-6.

56 Roh JL, Park JY, Park CI. Total thyroidectomy plus neck dissection in differentiated papillary thyroid carcinoma patients: pattern of nodal metastasis, morbidity, recurrence, and postoperative levels of serum parathyroid hormone. *Ann Surg*2007;245:604-10.

57 Mendelsohn AH, Elashoff DA, Abemayor E, St John MA. Surgery for papillary thyroid carcinoma: is lobectomy enough? *Arch Otolaryngol Head Neck Surg*2010;136:1055-61.

58 Shaha AR, Shah JP, Loree TR. Low-risk differentiated thyroid cancer: the need for selective treatment. *Ann Surg Oncol*1997;4:328-33.

59 Hundahl SA, Fleming ID, Fremgen AM, Menck HR. A National Cancer Data Base report on 53856 cases of thyroid carcinoma treated in the US, 1985-1995. *Cancer*1998;83:2638-48.

60 Farkas EA, King TA, Bolton JS, Fuhrman GM. A comparison of total thyroidectomy and lobectomy in the treatment of dominant thyroid nodules. *Am Surg*2002;68:678-82; discussion 82-3.

61 Henry JF, Gramatica L, Denizot A, Kvachenyuk A, Puccini M, Defechereux T. Morbidity of prophylactic lymph node dissection in

the central neck area in patients with papillary thyroid carcinoma. *Langenbecks Arch Surg*1998;383:167-9.

62 Palestini N, Borasi A, Cestino L, Freddi M, Odasso C, Robecchi A. Is central neck dissection a safe procedure in the treatment of papillary thyroid cancer? Our experience. *Langenbecks Arch Surg*2008;393:693-8.

63 Roh JL, Park JY, Park CI. Prevention of postoperative hypocalcemia with routine oral calcium and vitamin D supplements in patients with differentiated papillary thyroid carcinoma undergoing total thyroidectomy plus central neck dissection. *Cancer*2009;115:251-8.

64 Keston AS, Ball RP, Frantz VK, Palmer WW. Storage of radioactive iodine in a metastasis from thyroid carcinoma. *Science*1942;95:362-3.

65 Blahd WH, Nordyke RA, Bauer FK. Radioactive iodine (I 131) in the postoperative treatment of thyroid cancer. *Cancer*1960;13:745-56.

66 Hay ID, Thompson GB, Grant CS, Bergstralh EJ, Dvorak CE, Gorman CA, et al. Papillary thyroid carcinoma managed at the Mayo Clinic during six decades (1940-1999): temporal trends in initial therapy and long-term outcome in 2444 consecutively treated patients. *World J Surg*2002;26:879-85.

67 Hay ID. Selective use of radioactive iodine in the postoperative management of patients with papillary and follicular thyroid carcinoma. *J Surg Oncol*2006;94:692-700.

68 Sawka AM, Thephamongkhol K, Brouwers M, Thabane L, Browman G, Gerstein HC. Clinical review 170: a systematic review and metaanalysis of the effectiveness of radioactive iodine remnant ablation for well-differentiated thyroid cancer. *J Clin Endocrinol Metab*2004;89:3668-76.

69 Sacks W, Fung CH, Chang JT, Waxman A, Braunstein GD. The effectiveness of radioactive iodine for treatment of low-risk thyroid cancer: a systematic analysis of the peer-reviewed literature from 1966 to April 2008. *Thyroid*2010;20:1235-45.

70 Hay ID, Hutchinson ME, Gonzalez-Losada T, McIver B, Reinalda ME, Grant CS, et al. Papillary thyroid microcarcinoma: a study of 900 cases observed in a 60-year period. *Surgery*2008;144:980-7; discussion 87-8.

71 Schvartz C, Bonnetain F, Dabakuyo S, Gauthier M, Cueff A, Fieffe S, et al. Impact on overall survival of radioactive iodine in low-risk differentiated thyroid cancer patients. *J Clin Endocrinol Metab*2012;97:1526-35.

72 Iyer NG, Morris LG, Tuttle RM, Shaha AR, Ganly I. Rising incidence of second cancers in patients with low-risk (T1No) thyroid cancer who receive radioactive iodine therapy. *Cancer*2011;117:4439-46.

73 Haymart MR, Banerjee M, Stewart AK, Koenig RJ, Birkmeyer JD, Griggs JJ. Use of radioactive iodine for thyroid cancer. *JAMA*2011;306:721-8.

74 Durante C, Montesano T, Attard M, Torlontano M, Monzani F, Costante G, et al. Long-term surveillance of papillary thyroid cancer patients who do not undergo postoperative radioiodine remnant ablation: is there a role for serum thyroglobulin measurement? *J Clin Endocrinol Metab*2012;97:2748-53.

75 Brabant G. Thyrotropin suppressive therapy in thyroid carcinoma: what are the targets? *J Clin Endocrinol Metab*2008;93:1167-9.

76 Dunhill TP. Surgery of the thyroid gland. *BMJ*1937;1:460-61. www.bmj.com/content/1/3975/568.

77 McGriff NJ, Csako G, Gourgiotis L, Lori CG, Pucino F, Sarlis NJ. Effects of thyroid hormone suppression therapy on adverse clinical outcomes in thyroid cancer. *Ann Med*2002;34:554-64.

78 Cooper DS, Specker B, Ho M, Sperling M, Ladenson PW, Ross DS, et al. Thyrotropin suppression and disease progression in patients with differentiated thyroid cancer: results from the national thyroid cancer treatment cooperative registry. *Thyroid*1998;8:737-44.

79 Pujol P, Daures JP, Nsakala N, Baldet L, Bringer J, Jaffiol C. Degree of thyrotropin suppression as a prognostic determinant in differentiated thyroid cancer. *J Clin Endocrinol Metab*1996;81:4318-23.

80 Jonklaas J, Sarlis NJ, Litofsky D, Ain KB, Bigos ST, Brierley JD, et al. Outcomes of patients with differentiated thyroid carcinoma following initial therapy. *Thyroid*2006;16:1229-42.

81 Bauer DC, Rodondi N, Stone KL, Hillier TA. Thyroid hormone use, hyperthyroidism and mortality in older women. *Am J Med*2007;120:343-9.

82 Kung AW, Yeung SS. Prevention of bone loss induced by thyroxine suppressive therapy in postmenopausal women: the effect of calcium and calcitonin. *J Clin Endocrinol Metab*1996;81:1232-6.

83 Sgourakis G, Sotiropoulos GC, Neuhauser M, Musholt TJ, Karaliotas C, Lang H. Comparison between minimally invasive video-assisted thyroidectomy and conventional thyroidectomy: is there any evidence-based information? *Thyroid*2008;18:721-7.

84 FDA. Form FDA-483. 2013. www.fda.gov/downloads/AboutFDA/CentersOffices/OfficeofGlobalRegulatoryOperationsandPolicy/ORA/ORAElectronicReadingRoom/UCM358468.pdf.

85 Lewis BD, Hay ID, Charboneau JW, McIver B, Reading CC, Goellner JR. Percutaneous ethanol injection for treatment of cervical lymph node metastases in patients with papillary thyroid carcinoma. *AJR Am J Roentgenol*2002;178:699-704.

86 Hay ID, Lee RA, Davidge-Pitts C, Reading CC, Charboneau JW. Long-term outcome of ultrasound-guided percutaneous ethanol ablation of selected "recurrent" neck nodal metastases in 25 patients with TNM stages III or IVA papillary thyroid carcinoma previously treated by surgery and (131)I therapy. *Surgery*2013;154:1448-55.

87 Hay ID, Lee RA. Ultrasound-guided percutaneous ethanol ablation represents a promising minimally invasive alternative to observation in papillary thyroid microcarcinoma. Abstracts of the 83rd Annual Meeting of the American Thyroid Association Meeting. October 16-20, 2013. San Juan, Puerto Rico. *Thyroid*2013;23(suppl 1):A-58:129.

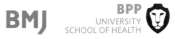

88 Guglielmi R, Pacella CM, Bianchini A, Bizzarri G, Rinaldi R, Graziano FM, et al. Percutaneous ethanol injection treatment in benign thyroid lesions: role and efficacy. *Thyroid*2004;14:125-31.

89 Papini E, Guglielmi R, Gharib H, Misischi I, Graziano F, Chianelli M, et al. Ultrasound-guided laser ablation of incidental papillary thyroid microcarcinoma: a potential therapeutic approach in patients at surgical risk. *Thyroid*2011;21:917-20.

90 Pacella CM, Bizzarri G, Guglielmi R, Anelli V, Bianchini A, Crescenzi A, et al. Thyroid tissue: US-guided percutaneous interstitial laser ablation-a feasibility study. *Radiology*2000;217:673-7.

91 Valcavi R, Piana S, Stecconi Bortolani G, Lai R, Barbieri V, Negro R. Ultrasound-guided percutaneous laser ablation of thyroid papillary microcarcinoma (PMC). a feasibility study on 3 cases with pathological and immunohistochemical evaluation. *Thyroid*2013;23:1578-82.

92 Fuller CW, Nguyen SA, Lohia S, Gillespie MB. Radiofrequency ablation for treatment of benign thyroid nodules: systematic review. *Laryngoscope*2014;124:346-53.

93 Shin JE, Baek JH, Lee JH. Radiofrequency and ethanol ablation for the treatment of recurrent thyroid cancers: current status and challenges. *Curr Opin Oncol*2013;25:14-9.

94 Ito Y, Miyauchi A, Kihara M, Higashiyama T, Kobayashi K, Miya A. Patient age is significantly related to the progression of papillary microcarcinoma of the thyroid under observation. *Thyroid*2014;24:27-34.

95 Sugitani I, Toda K, Yamada K, Yamamoto N, Ikenaga M, Fujimoto Y. Three distinctly different kinds of papillary thyroid microcarcinoma should be recognized: our treatment strategies and outcomes. *World J Surg*2010;34:1222-31.

96 Pace MD, Fagin JA, Bach A, Boucai L, Minkowltz G, Morris LG, et al. Properly selected patients with papillary thyroid cancer readily accept active surveillance when offered as a standard of care alternative to immediate surgery. Abstracts of the 83rd Annual Meeting of the American Thyroid Association Meeting. October 16-20, 2013. San Juan, Puerto Rico. *Thyroid*2013;23(suppl 1):A-116:8.

97 Robenshtok E, Fish S, Bach A, Dominguez JM, Shaha A, Tuttle RM. Suspicious cervical lymph nodes detected after thyroidectomy for papillary thyroid cancer usually remain stable over years in properly selected patients. *J Clin Endocrinol Metab*2012;97:2706-13.

98 Rondeau G, Fish S, Hann LE, Fagin JA, Tuttle RM. Ultrasonographically detected small thyroid bed nodules identified after total thyroidectomy for differentiated thyroid cancer seldom show clinically significant structural progression. *Thyroid*2011;21:845-53.

99 Ross JA SR, Pollock BH, Robison LL. Childhood cancer in the United States. A geographical analysis of cases from the Pediatric Cooperative Clinical Trials groups. *Cancer*1996;77:201-7.

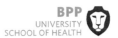

Oesophageal cancer

Jesper Lagergren professor and consultant of surgery[12], Pernilla Lagergren associate professor and senior lecturer in healthcare science[1]

[1]Upper Gastrointestinal Research, Department of Molecular Medicine and Surgery, Karolinska Institutet, Stockholm SE-171 76, Sweden

[2]Division of Cancer Studies, King's College London, UK

Correspondence to: J Lagergren
jesper.lagergren@ki.se

Cite this as: BMJ 2010;341:c6280

‹DOI› 10.1136/bmj.c6280
http://www.bmj.com/content/341/bmj.c6280

The incidence of oesophageal cancer is increasing. While the incidence of squamous cell carcinoma of the oesophagus has recently been stable or declined in Western societies, the incidence of oesophageal adenocarcinoma has risen more rapidly than that of any other cancer in many countries since the 1970s, particularly among white men.[1] The UK has the highest reported incidence worldwide, for reasons yet unknown.[2] Overall, the prognosis for patients diagnosed with oesophageal cancer is poor, but those whose tumours are detected at an early stage have a good chance of survival. We outline strategies for prevention and describe presenting features of oesophageal cancer to assist generalists in diagnosing and referring patients early. Treatment is often highly invasive and alters patients' quality of life. We review the evidence from large randomised clinical trials, meta-analyses, and large cohort and case-control studies (preferably those of population based design, since they carry a lower risk of selection bias).

Who gets oesophageal cancer?

The two main histological types of oesophageal cancer, adenocarcinoma and squamous cell carcinoma (fig 1), have different causes and patterns of incidence.[1] Although the incidence of adenocarcinoma has surpassed that of squamous cell carcinoma in many Western countries, squamous cell carcinoma still represents 90% of all oesophageal cancer cases in most Eastern countries. Register based cohort studies have found that the incidence of oesophageal cancer increases with age and the average age of onset is about 65 to 70 years. Generally, men are more affected than women: the striking 7:1 male predominance of oesophageal adenocarcinoma remains unexplained.[1]

The origins of oesophageal cancer are multifactorial, including interactions among environmental risk exposures and nucleotide polymorphisms of inflammatory and tumour growth promoting pathways. The two main risk factors for oesophageal adenocarcinoma are gastro-oesophageal reflux and obesity.[3] Some gene-environment interaction patterns differ between patients with and without reflux.[4] Polymorphisms of genes coding for the obesity linked insulin-like growth factor may also be markers of risk.[5]

The two main risk factors for squamous cell carcinoma of the oesophagus are tobacco smoking and high alcohol consumption, particularly in combination. The 3:1 male predominance is explained by differences in such exposures between the sexes. Infection with the bacterium *Helicobacter pylori*, which commonly occurs in the gastric mucosa, seems to reduce the risk of oesophageal adenocarcinoma by about half.[6] A possible mechanism is that the gastric atrophy that might follow such infection reduces the acidity and volume of the gastric juice, thereby lowering the risk of gastro-oesophageal reflux.[7]

Use of aspirin or non-steroidal anti-inflammatory drugs (NSAIDs) might decrease the risk of oesophageal cancer. A recent meta-analysis, mainly including case-control studies, showed a 35% decrease in the risk of oesophageal cancer among users of NSAIDs compared with non-users.[8] Factors affecting the choice of using NSAIDs, however, constitute a threat to the validity of observational studies, as highlighted in some investigations.[8] [9]

How does a patient with oesophageal cancer present?

The cardinal symptoms of oesophageal cancer are progressive dysphagia and weight loss. The dysphagia is typically linked with vomiting of undigested food. Earlier symptoms may include discomfort or occasionally pain when swallowing. If such symptoms persist they should prompt an upper endoscopy. However, elasticity of the oesophagus means that onset of symptoms may not occur until the tumour is at an advanced stage. Late symptoms include hoarseness, caused by tumour overgrowth of the left laryngeal nerve, severe cough linked with tumour fistula between the oesophagus and the respiratory tract, and signs of metastatic disease—for example, ascites or palpable lymph node metastases.

How is the diagnosis made?

Figure 2 shows a flowchart for diagnosis.

Referral

Patients presenting with symptoms indicative of oesophageal cancer should undergo urgent endoscopy, preferably within one week. Patients with typical symptoms together with macroscopic signs of tumour on endoscopy require immediate referral (without need for histological confirmation) to a unit with relevant experience, usually an upper gastrointestinal surgery unit.

SOURCES AND SELECTION CRITERIA

We searched PubMed to identify peer reviewed original articles, meta-analyses, and reviews. Search terms were oesophageal cancer, cancer of the oesophagus, oesophageal adenocarcinoma, oesophageal squamous cell carcinoma, neoplasm and oesophagus, and oesophageal neoplasm. Only papers written in English were considered. We mainly included studies published during the recent few years where we deemed the scientific validity to be adequate.

SUMMARY POINTS

- The incidence of oesophageal adenocarcinoma has increased during the past few decades, particularly among white men in the UK
- Oesophageal adenocarcinoma is associated with gastro-oesophageal reflux and obesity, whereas squamous cell carcinoma is associated with use of tobacco and alcohol
- Diagnosis is confirmed by endoscopy with biopsies, precise tumour stage is defined by more sophisticated radiological examinations
- A multidisciplinary approach is recommended in decision making and treatment
- Curatively intended treatment usually includes chemotherapy or radiochemotherapy followed by extensive surgery
- The overall prognosis for oesophageal cancer patients remains poor and several palliative options are available where cure is not possible

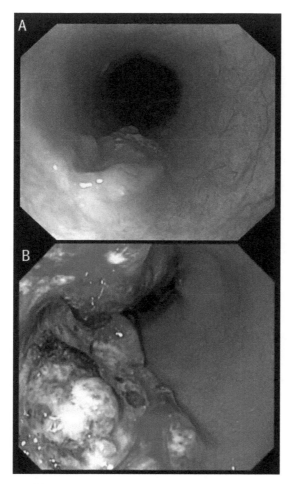

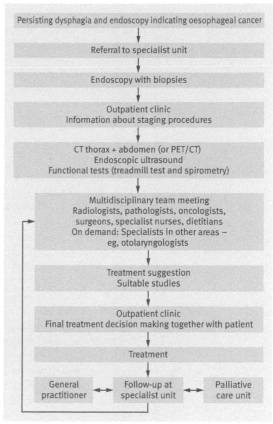

Fig 2 Diagnosis with multidisciplinary team for cancer of the oesophagus suitable for curatively intended surgery

Fig 1 (A) Small oesophageal squamous cell carcinoma seen on endoscopy. (B) Large necrotic and bleeding oesophageal adenocarcinoma seen on endoscopy. Used with permission from Dr Edgar Jaramillo

Primary tumour
The diagnosis is made by visualising a mass on endoscopy and by histological confirmation using biopsy samples collected from the mass and adjacent tissue. Figure 1 shows typical oesophageal cancer lesions as seen on endoscopy.

The importance of staging
Accurate staging allows for individually tailored treatment and the tumour needs to be staged before a treatment decision can be made. Recent advances in imaging techniques have contributed to more accurate staging. Cohort studies have shown that fluorodeoxyglucose combined positron emission tomography combined with computed tomography can be used to visualise early distant spread of tumours.[10] This tool has also shown promising results in the evaluation of the effects of preoperative oncological treatment.[11] Endoscopic ultrasonography can accurately measure the extent of local and regional tumour growth, which helps with staging.[12] More recently, endoscopic mucosal resection has become a useful staging technique for early intramucosal tumours. These tools have led to improved staging and less referral of patients with advanced or incurable disease for aggressive treatment.

Can oesophageal cancer be prevented?
Primary prevention
Avoidance of obesity, tobacco smoking, and alcohol intake decrease the risk of oesophageal cancer. Gastro-oesophageal reflux could also be reduced by controlling obesity and tobacco smoking, which are the two main established risk factors for reflux.

Secondary prevention
The hypothesis that antireflux medication and antireflux surgery reduce the incidence of oesophageal adenocarcinoma in people with reflux has been addressed mainly in uncontrolled studies. Robust data (from randomised trials, for example) supporting a preventive effect of antireflux medication against cancer are limited.[13] [14] A large population based cohort study found no reduction in the risk of oesophageal adenocarcinoma with time after antireflux surgery.[15] The potential preventive effect of NSAIDs needs to be evaluated in randomised trials.

Is there a role for endoscopic screening?
Endoscopic screening for early oesophageal cancer requires selection of an easily identifiable high risk group. One such group might be white men with severe reflux and obesity. However, the feasibility of screening has to be based on the individual's absolute risk, which takes the incidence of the cancer into account. The high prevalence of reflux and the low incidence of oesophageal adenocarcinoma make endoscopic screening programmes of people with reflux symptoms, with or without known risk factors, unfeasible.[3] Moreover, there are no data showing a reduction in deaths from oesophageal adenocarcinoma resulting from endoscopic screening.[16] A better defined and much smaller,

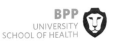

truly high risk group needs to be identified before any endoscopic screening can be considered. Measures other than endoscopy could be used for such screening in the future—for example, ingestible oesophageal sampling devices such as the Cytosponge.[17] The role of endoscopic surveillance of Barrett's oesophagus, a metaplasia associated with oesophageal adenocarcinoma, has been addressed in a recent review.[18]

What is the approach to making a decision about treatment?

Patients with invasive oesophageal cancer need to be thoroughly evaluated regarding fitness and tumour stage. Tumours with local overgrowth into adjacent tissues or organs (T4) or with distant metastases (M1) are usually not eligible for curatively intended treatment. Physical activity, biological age, and comorbidities are considered when patient fitness is evaluated, and treadmill tests and spirometry are used whenever needed to objectively assess fitness. The final treatment recommendation should be based on a multidisciplinary meeting, as shown in figure 2, in which experienced doctors representing surgery, oncology, radiology, and pathology should participate. A multidisciplinary review of the radiology examinations, pathology reports, and the objective and subjective fitness of the patient could improve the accuracy of the treatment decisions and facilitate inclusion into clinical trials.[19] [20] The final decision must thereafter be taken together with the patient. The doctor responsible for the patient must thoroughly explain the reasons for the recommendation of the meeting. If there are doubts about this recommendation, a second opinion from a multidisciplinary team in another hospital is valuable.

What is the best approach to organisation of care?

The optimal treatment of patients with oesophageal cancer requires the resources and skills of a well coordinated multidisciplinary team (fig 2). Increased centralisation of treatment for patients with cancer of the oesophagus puts additional strain on resources at large centres, and these patients have high needs for supportive care.[21] Such circumstances emphasise the need for good coordination and continuity of the complex care pathway. A randomised clinical trial has emphasised the important role of specialised contact nurses in maintaining and coordinating the care pathway.[22] These nurses ideally keep in close contact with each patient and take part in all appointments with them.

Treatment with intent to cure—what are the options?

Treatment with a curative intent is undertaken only in patients who are considered fit enough to undergo extensive surgery and who have a tumour without any signs of overgrowth or distant metastases. The most common tumour stages among resected oesophageal cancer patients are advanced primary cancer without invasion into surrounding tissue or organs (T2-T3) with local or regional lymph node metastases (N1).[23]

Surgical resection remains the main option for curative treatment. Whether to offer chemotherapy or chemoradiotherapy before surgery is controversial because underpowered trials have produced contradictory results. Although the majority of individual studies do not show any benefit from such a strategy, data from more recent and larger randomised clinical trials indicate that preoperative chemotherapy or chemoradiotherapy improve survival compared with surgery alone.[24] [25] Moreover, data from case series indicate a curative potential for chemoradiotherapy alone without surgery, particularly in older non-surgical candidate patients, but randomised trials are needed to support a nonsurgical strategy.[26] Nevertheless, chemoradiotherapy alone is used in many patients who are not fit enough for surgery or in those who choose not to undergo surgery. Currently, a typical treatment strategy in fit patients with the most commonly occurring tumour stages (II-III) is chemotherapy followed by surgery.[25]

Surgical resection

Which is the preferred surgical approach?

Oesophageal cancer surgery is an extensive procedure with substantial risk of postoperative complications and long term morbidity.[27] A recent review concluded that fit patients are possibly best treated by a transthoracic oesophagectomy with removal of local and regional lymph nodes and vessels along with the oesophageal specimen (extended en bloc, two field lymphadenectomy). However, for patients who are less fit or those with junctional tumours or tumours of the gastric cardia, a transhiatal approach with a partly blunt dissection in the chest (through an abdominal and neck incision, without opening the thoracic wall) with a neck anastomosis may be a better option.[28]

Where to have surgery?

Since the in-hospital mortality after oesophagectomy is lower when centres and surgeons are experienced in this procedure, centralisation to high volume units has taken place in recent years.[21] Much of the lower risk of mortality at centres dealing with high volumes of such cases seems to be explained by better handling of complications.[29] The risk of complications seems, however, to be more related to the skills of the individual surgeon than to volume alone.[30]

How to improve quality of life outcomes?

Large, population based cohort studies have shown that patients who undergo surgical resection of an oesophageal tumour have poor health related quality of life in the short and long term.[27] These findings highlight a need to improve the procedure—for example, by better tailoring of surgery, and through the development of less invasive techniques such as minimally invasive, robotic, and vagal nerve preserving oesophagectomy.[31] [32] [33] Such developments must, however, be based on results from large multicentre randomised clinical trials that are well designed rather than on case series. Generally, patients undergoing surgical resection should be enrolled in a randomised trial when possible.

Endoscopic treatments

Various endoscopic approaches are emerging as potential alternatives to surgical treatment in the highly selected group of patients with high grade dysplastic mucosa and early intramucosal oesophageal cancer.[34] [35] Such local procedures might be justified in view of the low likelihood of lymph node metastases in early tumours, but more research is needed before general clinical recommendations can be given. Endoscopic mucosal resection, photodynamic therapy, argon plasma coagulation, and radiofrequency ablation can all induce regression of dysplasia.[14] A large randomised trial found that radiofrequency ablation resulted in eradication rates of 94% in patients with dysplasia, compared with a sham treatment,[35] and it might become the endoscopic

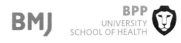

treatment of choice, combined with endoscopic mucosal resection for visible, focal lesions. Until longer term trials become available, however, radiofrequency ablation should only be used in expert centres with careful follow-up.[14] For the vast majority of patients with an invasive tumour, endoscopic therapy is, at least currently, not a treatment option.

Who will get palliative care and what will it involve?

Large population based cohort studies estimate that up to 75% of patients with oesophageal cancer are never treated with a curative intent, mainly because of advanced tumour stage or poor physical condition.[23] For incurable disease, patients need the support of expert palliative care professionals who are familiar with the pros and cons of the available palliative treatments. Several approaches can improve health related quality of life in patients who are ineligible for surgery (box), and the best approach involves treatment that is tailored to offer the best possible outcome for the patient. Patients with advanced oesophageal cancer have a short median survival and thus are no longer offered surgical resection for palliation only. A major challenge is to relieve dysphagia as effectively as possible. A recent Cochrane systematic review of interventions aimed at relieving dysphagia concluded that self expanding metallic stents and intraluminal brachytherapy (local radiotherapy) seem to offer the best palliation.[36] Chemotherapy and external beam radiotherapy can also palliate dysphagia. We stress that a well functioning care pathway is just as important for patients in whom the aim of therapy is palliation, as it is for those where curatively intended treatment is possible. Support from a palliative care team, including, for example, pain therapy, feeding, or general support, is valuable for these patients.

Is the prognosis for patients with oesophageal cancer improving?

Population based cohort studies have shown that the overall prognosis for patients with cancer of the oesophagus has improved slightly during the past 20 years.[37] However, despite efforts to improve surveillance, diagnostic procedures, and treatment, the overall five year survival in oesophageal adenocarcinoma remains lower than 15%.[37] Population based studies from Europe have shown the five year survival after curatively intended surgery for oesophageal adenocarcinoma to be 30-35%, a figure that has improved substantially during the past few years, whereas the population based five year survival for stage specific tumours has been reported to be 67%, 33%, and 8% in stages 0-I, II, and III, respectively.[23] Unfortunately, patients with tumour recurrence after surgery cannot usually be cured because of the lack of effective second line treatment.

Which might be the future directions?

Primary prevention by avoidance of preventable risk exposures might help to reduce the incidence of oesophageal cancer in the future. It should also be possible to identify true high risk patients for oesophageal cancer who might benefit from tailored surveillance strategies, possibly by combining risk factor information with future genetic markers that might predict a risk of progression.

Improvements in the treatment of oesophageal cancer, in regard to survival and to health related quality of life, are best achieved through large randomised clinical trials

to investigate new chemotherapeutic agents and new, less invasive, surgical approaches.

Contributors: JL and PL contributed to the concept and writing of this article.

Funding: JL and PL are funded by the Swedish Research Council and the Swedish Cancer Society.

Competing interests: Both authors have completed the Unified Competing Interest form and declare no support for the submitted work; no relationships that might have an interest in the submitted

---

PALLIATIVE THERAPY

- May include all or any of the following:
- Endoscopic stenting
- Brachytherapy
- Chemotherapy
- External radiotherapy
- Feeding through gastrostomy, jejunostomy, or intravenously
- Pain relief
- Best palliative supportive care

TIPS FOR NON-SPECIALISTS

- The cardinal symptoms of oesophageal cancer are progressive dysphagia and weight loss
- Any persisting dysphagia in adults should prompt an urgent endoscopy
- Typical symptoms in combination with an endoscopy indicating oesophageal cancer should be followed by referral to a unit with experience in the treatment of this tumour
- A majority of patients with oesophageal cancer need initial palliative therapy, usually provided at the referral hospital, and thereafter general palliative care

---

QUESTIONS FOR FUTURE RESEARCH

- Interaction between risk exposures and genetic factors might improve knowledge of the causes of oesophageal cancer
- Identification of preventive measures might decrease the incidence of oesophageal cancer
- Identification of true high risk groups for oesophageal cancer might provide possibilities for feasible future surveillance strategies
- Curative and palliative treatment of oesophageal cancer needs to be improved, and is best achieved through large randomised clinical trials

---

ADDITIONAL EDUCATIONAL RESOURCES

For healthcare professionals

- National Institute for Health and Clinical Excellence (www.nice.org.uk)—National body providing evidence based guidance on specific diseases and conditions
- Cancer Research UK (www.cancerresearchuk.org)—UK's leading cancer charity's website, containing information about the charity and about cancer

For patients

- Oesophageal Patients Association (www.opa.org.uk)—A large support group for patients with oesophageal cancer
- Patient UK (www.patient.co.uk)—Comprehensive source of health and disease information for patients
- Cancer Research UK (www.cancerresearchuk.org)
- British Society of Gastroenterology (www.bsg.org.uk/patients/patients/general/oesophageal-cancer.html)—Patient information from a large gastroenterology organisation

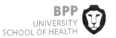

work; and no non-financial interests that may be relevant to the submitted work.

Provenance and peer review: Not commissioned; externally peer reviewed.

1   Cook MB, Chow WH, Devesa SS. Oesophageal cancer incidence in the United States by race, sex, and histologic type, 1977-2005. *Br J Cancer*2009;101:855-9.

2   Bollschweiler E, Wolfgarten E, Gutschow C, Holscher AH. Demographic variations in the rising incidence of esophageal adenocarcinoma in white males. *Cancer*2001;92:549-55.

3   Lagergren J, Ye W, Bergstrom R, Nyren O. Utility of endoscopic screening for upper gastrointestinal adenocarcinoma. *JAMA*2000;284:961-2.

4   Zhai R, Chen F, Liu G, Su L, Kulke MH, Asomaning K, et al. Interactions among genetic variants in apoptosis pathway genes, reflux symptoms, body mass index, and smoking indicate two distinct etiologic patterns of esophageal adenocarcinoma. *J Clin Oncol*2010;28:2445-51.

5   McElholm AR, McKnight AJ, Patterson CC, Johnston BT, Hardie LJ, Murray LJ. A population-based study of IGF axis polymorphisms and the esophageal inflammation, metaplasia, adenocarcinoma sequence. *Gastroenterology*2010;139:204-12.e3.

6   Rokkas T, Pistiolas D, Sechopoulos P, Robotis I, Margantinis G. Relationship between Helicobacter pylori infection and esophageal neoplasia: a meta-analysis. *Clin Gastroenterol Hepatol*2007;5:1413-7, 1417.e1-2.

7   Anderson LA, Murphy SJ, Johnston BT, Watson RG, Ferguson HR, Bamford KB, et al. Relationship between Helicobacter pylori infection and gastric atrophy and the stages of the oesophageal inflammation, metaplasia, adenocarcinoma sequence: results from the FINBAR case-control study. *Gut*2008;57:734-9.

8   Abnet CC, Freedman ND, Kamangar F, Leitzmann MF, Hollenbeck AR, Schatzkin A. Non-steroidal anti-inflammatory drugs and risk of gastric and oesophageal adenocarcinomas: results from a cohort study and a meta-analysis. *Br J Cancer*2009;100:551-7.

9   Heath EI, Canto MI, Piantadosi S, Montgomery E, Weinstein WM, Herman JG, et al. Secondary chemoprevention of Barrett's esophagus with celecoxib: results of a randomized trial. *J Natl Cancer Inst*2007;99:545-57.

10 Meyers BF, Downey RJ, Decker PA, Keenan RJ, Siegel BA, Cerfolio RJ, et al. The utility of positron emission tomography in staging of potentially operable carcinoma of the thoracic esophagus: results of the American College of Surgeons Oncology Group Z0060 trial. *J Thorac Cardiovasc Surg*2007;133:738-45.

11 Lordick F, Ott K, Krause BJ, Weber WA, Becker K, Stein HJ, et al. PET to assess early metabolic response and to guide treatment of adenocarcinoma of the oesophagogastric junction: the MUNICON phase II trial. *Lancet Oncol*2007;8:797-805.

12 Kelly S, Harris KM, Berry E, Hutton J, Roderick P, Cullingworth J, et al. A systematic review of the staging performance of endoscopic ultrasound in gastro-oesophageal carcinoma. *Gut*2001;49:534-9.

13 Nguyen DM, El-Serag HB, Henderson L, Stein D, Bhattacharyya A, Sampliner RE. Medication usage and the risk of neoplasia in patients with Barrett's esophagus. *Clin Gastroenterol Hepatol*2009;7:1299-304.

14 Rees JR, Lao-Sirieix P, Wong A, Fitzgerald RC. Treatment for Barrett's oesophagus. *Cochrane Database Syst Rev*2010;1:CD004060.

15 Lagergren J, Ye W, Lagergren P, Lu Y. The risk of esophageal adenocarcinoma after antireflux surgery. *Gastroenterology*2010;138:1297-301.

16 Rubenstein JH, Sonnenberg A, Davis J, McMahon L, Inadomi JM. Effect of a prior endoscopy on outcomes of esophageal adenocarcinoma among United States veterans. *Gastrointest Endosc*2008;68:849-55.

17 Kadri SR, Lao-Sirieix P, O'Donovan M, Debiram I, Das M, Blazeby JM, et al. Acceptability and accuracy of a non-endoscopic screening test for Barrett's oesophagus in primary care: cohort study. *BMJ*2010;341:c4372.

18 Jankowski J, Barr H, Wang K, Delaney B. Diagnosis and management of Barrett's oesophagus. *BMJ*2010;341:c4551.

19 Stephens MR, Lewis WG, Brewster AE, Lord I, Blackshaw GR, Hodzovic I, et al. Multidisciplinary team management is associated with improved outcomes after surgery for esophageal cancer. *Dis Esophagus*2006;19:164-71.

20 McNair AG, Choh CT, Metcalfe C, Littlejohns D, Barham CP, Hollowood A, et al. Maximising recruitment into randomised controlled trials: the role of multidisciplinary cancer teams. *Eur J Cancer*2008;44:2623-6.

21 Stitzenberg KB, Sigurdson ER, Egleston BL, Starkey RB, Meropol NJ. Centralization of cancer surgery: implications for patient access to optimal care. *J Clin Oncol*2009;27:4671-8.

22 Verschuur EM, Steyerberg EW, Tilanus HW, Polinder S, Essink-Bot ML, Tran KT, et al. Nurse-led follow-up of patients after oesophageal or gastric cardia cancer surgery: a randomised trial. *Br J Cancer*2009;100:70-6.

23 Rouvelas I, Zeng W, Lindblad M, Viklund P, Ye W, Lagergren J. Survival after surgery for oesophageal cancer: a population-based study. *Lancet Oncol*2005;6:864-70.

24 Medical Research Council Oesophageal Cancer Working Group. Surgical resection with or without preoperative chemotherapy in oesophageal cancer: a randomised controlled trial. *Lancet*2002;359:1727-33.

25 Gebski V, Burmeister B, Smithers BM, Foo K, Zalcberg J, Simes J. Survival benefits from neoadjuvant chemoradiotherapy or chemotherapy in oesophageal carcinoma: a meta-analysis. *Lancet Oncol*2007;8:226-34.

26 Morgan MA, Lewis WG, Casbard A, Roberts SA, Adams R, Clark GW, et al. Stage-for-stage comparison of definitive chemoradiotherapy, surgery alone and neoadjuvant chemotherapy for oesophageal carcinoma. *Br J Surg*2009;96:1300-7.

27 Djarv T, Lagergren J, Blazeby JM, Lagergren P. Long-term health-related quality of life following surgery for oesophageal cancer. *Br J Surg*2008;95:1121-6.

28 Lagarde SM, Vrouenraets BC, Stassen LP, van Lanschot JJ. Evidence-based surgical treatment of esophageal cancer: overview of high-quality studies. *Ann Thorac Surg*2010;89:1319-26.

29 Ghaferi AA, Birkmeyer JD, Dimick JB. Variation in hospital mortality associated with inpatient surgery. *N Engl J Med*2009;361:1368-75.

30 Rutegard M, Lagergren J, Rouvelas I, Lagergren P. Surgeon volume is a poor proxy for skill in esophageal cancer surgery. *Ann Surg*2009;249:256-61.

31 Gemmill EH, McCulloch P. Systematic review of minimally invasive resection for gastro-oesophageal cancer. *Br J Surg*2007;94:1461-7.

32 Galvani CA, Gorodner MV, Moser F, Jacobsen G, Chretien C, Espat NJ, et al. Robotically assisted laparoscopic transhiatal esophagectomy. *Surg Endosc*2008;22:188-95.

33 Pring C, Dexter S. A laparoscopic vagus-preserving Merendino procedure for early esophageal adenocarcinoma. *Surg Endosc*2010;24:1195-9.

34 Prasad GA, Wu TT, Wigle DA, Buttar NS, Wongkeesong LM, Dunagan KT, et al. Endoscopic and surgical treatment of mucosal (T1a) esophageal adenocarcinoma in Barrett's esophagus. *Gastroenterology*2009;137:815-23.

35 Shaheen NJ, Sharma P, Overholt BF, Wolfsen HC, Sampliner RE, Wang KK, et al. Radiofrequency ablation in Barrett's esophagus with dysplasia. *N Engl J Med*2009;360:2277-88.

36 Sreedharan A, Harris K, Crellin A, Forman D, Everett SM. Interventions for dysphagia in oesophageal cancer. *Cochrane Database Syst Rev*2009;4:CD005048.

37 Sundelof M, Ye W, Dickman PW, Lagergren J. Improved survival in both histologic types of oesophageal cancer in Sweden. *Int J Cancer*2002;99:751-4.

Related links

bmj.com/archive

- Managing frostbite (2010;341:c5864)
- Management of venous ulcer disease (2010;341:c6045)
- Translating genomics into improved healthcare (2010;341:c5945)
- Extracorporeal life support (2010;341:c5317)
- Managing diabetic retinopathy (2010;341:c5400)

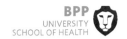

The diagnosis and management of gastric cancer

Sri G Thrumurthy honorary research fellow[1], M Asif Chaudryo esophagogastric surgeon[2], Daniel Hochhauser Kathleen Ferrier professor of medical oncology[3], Muntzer Mughal honorary clinical professor and head [1]

[1]Department of Upper Gastrointestinal Surgery, University College London Hospital, London NW1 2BU, UK

[2]Department of Upper Gastrointestinal Surgery, St Thomas' Hospital, London, UK

[3]UCL Cancer Institute, University College London, London, UK

Correspondence to: M Mughal muntzer.mughal@uclh.nhs.uk

Cite this as: BMJ 2013;347:f6367

‹DOI› 10.1136/bmj.f6367
http://www.bmj.com/content/347/bmj.f6367

Age standardised mortality rates for gastric cancer are 14.3 per 100 000 in men and 6.9 per 100 000 in women worldwide.[1] Incidence shows clear regional and sex variations—rates are highest in eastern Asia, eastern Europe, and South America and lowest in northern and southern Africa.[1] Early diagnosis is crucial because of the possibility of early metastasis to the liver, pancreas, omentum, oesophagus, bile ducts, and regional and distant lymph nodes.[2] Using evidence from large randomised controlled trials, meta-analyses, cohort studies, and case-control studies this review aims to outline preventive strategies, highlight the presenting features of gastric cancer, and guide generalists in early diagnosis, referral, and treatment.

What is gastric cancer?

Gastric cancer refers to tumours of the stomach that arise from the gastric mucosa (adenocarcinoma), connective tissue of the gastric wall (gastrointestinal stromal tumours), neuroendocrine tissue (carcinoid tumours), or lymphoid tissue (lymphomas). This review will focus on gastric adenocarcinoma (›90% of all gastric cancers), which may be polypoid, ulcerating, or diffuse infiltrative (linitis plastica) in macroscopic form.

Who gets gastric cancer?

Epidemiological data from the American Cancer Society suggest that gastric cancer is the fourth most common cancer in men (after lung, prostate, and colorectal cancer) and the fifth most common cancer in women (after breast, cervical, colorectal, and lung cancer) globally.[3] Gastric

cancer accounts for 8% of the total number of cases of cancer and 10% of annual deaths from cancer worldwide. It has a significantly higher fatality to case ratio (70%) than prostate (30%) and breast (33%) cancer.[4]

Men are twice as likely as women to develop gastric cancer,[3] with an expected worldwide incidence of 640 000 cases in men and 350 000 cases in women in 2011[3] (fig 1) and peak age of incidence of 60-84 years.[5] [6] The global incidence of gastric cancer has decreased significantly over time—the age standardised incidence in the United Kingdom decreased from 44 per 100 000 in 1975-77 to 18 per 100 000 in 2006-08).[7] This is partly because of reductions in chronic *Helicobacter pylori* infection and smoking in the developed world and partly the result of increased use of refrigeration, availability of fresh fruit and vegetables, and decreased reliance on salted or preserved foods.[3] [8]

What are the risk factors for gastric cancer?

Helicobacter pylori

H pylori infection is widely regarded as the most important modifiable risk factor for gastric cancer. More than 2 billion people are infected worldwide, although fewer than 0.5% will develop gastric adenocarcinoma.[4] A meta-analysis of 34 cohort and case-control studies found that *H pylori* carried a relative risk of gastric cancer of 3.02 (95% confidence interval 1.92 to 4.74) in high risk settings (China, Japan, and Korea) and 2.56 (1.99 to 3.29) in low risk settings (western Europe, Australia, and United States).[10]

Cigarette smoking

A meta-analysis of 42 cohort, case-cohort, and nested case-control studies across Asia, Europe, and the US found a relative risk of 1.53 (1.42 to 1.65) of developing gastric cancer in people who smoked.[11] Results from a retrospective cohort study of 699 patients, of whom 59% were current or ex-smokers, showed that tobacco use was associated with a 43% increase in disease recurrence and death from gastric cancer (hazard ratio 1.43, 1.08 to1.91; P=0.01).[12] Smoking was also an independent and significant risk factor for other measures of recurrence and survival, including five year disease-free survival (1.46; P=0.007) and overall survival (1.48; P=0.003).[12]

In a Norwegian prospective cohort study with 69 962 participants, the absolute lifetime risk of gastric cancer was 0.776% in heavy smokers (›20 cigarettes/day), 1.511% in long term smokers (≥30 years), and 0.658% in those who had never smoked.[13]

Alcohol

A meta-analysis of 44 case-control and 15 cohort studies of 34 557 cases of gastric cancer found a slightly increased risk (relative risk 1.07, 1.01 to 1.13) in people with light to moderate alcohol consumption and a greater increase (1.20, 1.01 to 1.44) for heavy alcohol drinkers (≥4 drinks/day).[14] A

SOURCES AND SELECTION CRITERIA

We searched PubMed to identify peer reviewed original articles, meta-analyses, and reviews. Search terms were gastric cancer, cancer of the stomach, gastric adenocarcinoma, gastro-oesophageal cancer, gastric neoplasm, and neoplasm of the stomach. We considered only those papers that were written in English, published within the past 10 years, and which described studies that had adequate scientific validity.

SUMMARY POINTS

- The incidence of gastric cancer is highest in eastern Asia, eastern Europe, and South America, and it affects twice as many men as women
- Risk factors for gastric cancer include *Helicobacter pylori* infection, cigarette smoking, high alcohol intake, excess dietary salt, lack of refrigeration, inadequate fruit and vegetable consumption, and pernicious anaemia
- Patients present with weight loss and abdominal pain, although those with proximal or gastro-oesophageal junction tumours may present with dysphagia
- Upper gastrointestinal endoscopy with biopsy is used to confirm the diagnosis; precise tumour stage is defined by more sophisticated radiological investigations
- Multidisciplinary approach to treatment: early gastric cancer is treated with surgery alone, whereas advanced disease is usually managed with chemotherapy before and after surgery, or postoperative chemoradiation
- Metastatic disease is managed with chemotherapy or chemoradiation as well as supportive care measures

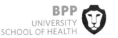

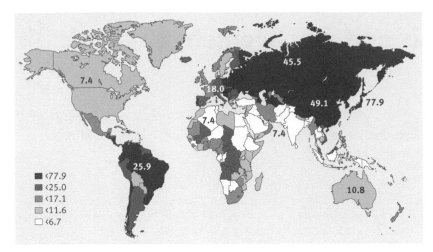

Fig 1 Worldwide annual incidence (per 100 000) of gastric cancer in men. Numbers on the map indicate regional average values. Adapted, with permission, from an article by the International Agency for Research on Cancer[9]

prospective European cohort study estimated that a high alcohol intake (>60 g/day) carried a relative risk of gastric cancer of 1.65 (1.06 to 2.58) and an absolute lifetime risk of 0.256%.[15]

Dietary salt and food preservation
A meta-analysis of cohort studies from the World Cancer Research Fund found that each gram of salt consumed each day increased the relative risk of gastric cancer by a factor of 1.08 (1.00 to 1.17).[16] A Japanese prospective cohort study with 2467 participants found an independent association between salt intake and incidence of gastric cancer. Compared with people who consumed less than 10 g of salt per day, those who consumed more than 16 g per day had a relative risk of 2.98 (1.53 to 5.82) of developing gastric cancer.[17] This correlation was stronger in the presence of H pylori infection and atrophic gastritis, suggesting that mucosal damage induced by salt intake increases the risk of persistent H pylori infection.[4]

The lack of refrigeration and use of salt based food preservatives have been associated with an increased risk of gastric cancer in socioeconomically deprived regions.[18] A cross sectional Korean study of multiple national statistics databases found a threefold decrease in age standardised mortality from gastric cancer between 1983 and 2007 (46.1/1 000 000 v 16.9/100 000), which was significantly and independently correlated with an increase in the number of refrigerators per household.[19]

Dietary fruit and vegetables
A Swedish cohort study of 82 002 participants and a total of 139 cases of gastric cancer found that an intake of two to five servings of fruit and vegetables a day decreased the risk of gastric cancer when compared with less than

one serving a day (hazard ratio 0.56, 0.34 to 0.93). This suggested a 44% reduction in the incidence of gastric cancer with increased fruit and vegetable intake.[20] A meta-analysis of cohort studies from the World Cancer Research Fund suggested a relative risk of 0.81 (0.58 to 1.14) per 100 g per day of non-starchy vegetables and fruit consumed.[16]

Pernicious anaemia
A recent meta-analysis of 27 cohort and case-control studies found an overall relative risk for gastric cancer in pernicious anaemia of 6.8 (2.6 to 18.1).[21] Although heterogeneity between the studies was not significant at the 5% level, the quality of the studies was variable, so further high quality studies are needed to confirm this higher risk before instigating surveillance for these patients.

Genetic syndromes
Hereditary diffuse gastric cancer is a syndrome caused by a germline mutation in the CDH1 gene, which encodes E-cadherin, a calcium dependent cell adhesion protein involved in cell-cell interaction and cell polarity. The condition is characterised by early onset (age <40 years) of diffuse gastric adenocarcinoma, an autosomal dominant inheritance pattern, and increased risk of lobular breast cancer and signet ring cell colon cancer.[22] Prospective analysis of a genetic database showed that this mutation carries a cumulative risk of gastric cancer of 67% in men and 83% in women.[23]

Lynch syndrome, an autosomal dominant syndrome involving defective DNA mismatch repair and an increased risk of colorectal and other visceral cancers, is also associated with a higher incidence of gastric cancer.[24] A Dutch prospective cohort study of 2014 people found an increased lifetime risk of gastric cancer in both men (8%) and women (5.3%),[25] prompting consideration of surveillance gastroscopy for patients with this syndrome who carry an MLH1 or MSH2 mutation.

How do patients with gastric cancer present?
Because patients with gastric cancer often present with vague and non-specific symptoms, the diagnosis is challenging. Data from the US National Cancer Institute suggest that patients are typically male smokers aged 60-84 years,[5] who exhibit the cardinal symptoms of upper abdominal pain and weight loss.[26] Less common symptoms are nausea, dysphagia (in proximal and gastro-oesophageal junction tumours), and evidence of melaena. Typical textbook descriptions such as Virchow's node (prominent left supraclavicular node) and Sister Mary Joseph's nodule (periumbilical nodule) are rarely seen in primary care.

A meta-analysis of 15 studies with 57 363 patients found that "alarm" features (box 1) had a pooled sensitivity of 67% (54% to 83%), pooled specificity of 66% (55% to 79%),

Common conditions that can mimic the symptoms of gastric cancer

Differential diagnosis	Features suggestive of cancer	Differentiating investigations
Benign oesophageal stricture	No history of gastro-oesophageal reflux disease	Endoscopy and biopsy
Peptic ulcer disease	Overt gastrointestinal bleeding, weight loss, early satiety, palpable masses or lymphadenopathy, jaundice, progressive dysphagia, recurrent vomiting	Endoscopy and biopsy; patients with peptic ulcers should undergo repeat endoscopy after treatment to assess healing
	Family history of cancer	
	Age of symptom onset >55 years	
Achalasia*	Duration of symptoms <6 months	Oesophageal manometry, endoscopy, and biopsy*
	Age at presentation >60 years	
	Substantial weight loss relative to symptom duration	

*Gastro-oesophageal cancer that initially presents with the clinical and investigative findings of achalasia is known as pseudoachalasia.

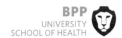

BOX 1 ALARM FEATURES SUGGESTIVE OF GASTRIC CANCER[26]

- New onset dyspepsia (in patients aged >55 years)
- Family history of upper gastrointestinal cancer
- Unintended weight loss
- Upper or lower gastrointestinal bleeding
- Progressive dysphagia
- Odynophagia
- Unexplained iron deficiency anaemia
- Persistent vomiting
- Palpable mass or lymphadenopathy
- Jaundice

BOX 2 AMERICAN JOINT COMMITTEE ON CANCER (AJCC) CANCER STAGING, 2010

Primary tumour (T)

- TX: primary tumour cannot be assessed
- T0: no evidence of primary tumour
- Tis: carcinoma in situ, intra-epithelial tumour
- T1: tumour invades lamina propria, muscularis mucosae, or submucosa
- T2: tumour invades muscularis propria
- T3: tumour penetrates subserosal connective tissue
- T4: tumour invades serosa (visceral peritoneum) or adjacent structures

Regional lymph nodes (N)

- NX: regional lymph node(s) cannot be assessed
- N0: no regional lymph node metastases
- N1: metastasis in 1-2 regional lymph nodes
- N2 = metastasis in 3-6 regional lymph nodes
- N3: metastasis in ≥7 regional lymph nodes

Distant metastasis (M)

- M0: no distant metastasis
- M1: distant metastasis

Stage grouping

- Stage 0: Tis N0 M0
- Stage IA: T1 N0 M0
- Stage IB: T2 N0 M0; T1 N1 M0
- Stage IIA: T3 N0 M0; T2 N1 M0; T1 N2 M0
- Stage IIB: T4a N0 M0; T3 N1 M0; T2 N2 M0; T1 N3 M0
- Stage IIIA: T4a N1 M0; T3 N2 M0; T2 N3 M0
- Stage IIIB: T4b N0 M0; T4b N1 M0; T4a N2 M0; T3 N3 M0
- Stage IIIC: T4b N2 M0; T4b N3 M0; T4a N3 M0
- Stage IV: any T any N M1

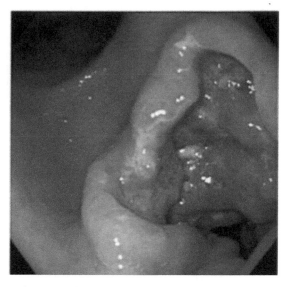

Fig 2 Endoscopic image of an advanced ulcerated gastric tumour

referral to a specialist upper gastrointestinal surgery unit is warranted.

How is gastric cancer diagnosed?

Endoscopy and biopsy of primary tumour

British consensus guidelines recommend that the diagnosis is made by visualising a mass on endoscopy and by histological confirmation using at least six biopsy samples from the mass and adjacent tissue (fig 2).[28] If the biopsy result of a suspicious lesion is negative, a repeat biopsy is needed. Pathological examination may include immunohistochemistry for HER2/neu, which is overexpressed in a subset of gastric cancers,[29] because targeted treatment may be an option for these tumours.[30]

Staging of confirmed gastric cancer

Recent advances in imaging have enabled more accurate staging, and fewer patients with advanced or incurable disease are now referred for aggressive treatment. A meta-analysis of 54 studies of 5601 patients suggested that endoscopic ultrasonography had a sensitivity and specificity of 86% and 91% for T stage tumours and 69% and 84% for N stage tumours, respectively (box 2).[31] However, owing to the limited capacity of this technique for staging mucosal disease, current UK guidelines advocate its use only for gastro-oesophageal junction tumours and selected gastric cancers.[28]

A meta-analysis of 33 patients showed that computed tomography of the abdomen detected liver metastases with a sensitivity of 74% (59% to 85%) and specificity of 99% (97% to 100%) and peritoneal metastases with a sensitivity of 33% (16% to 56%) and specificity of 99% (98% to 100%). Computed tomography of the chest is indicated only in patients with proximal or gastro-oesophageal junction tumours. Positron emission tomography combined with computed tomography has become increasingly available in tertiary centres. A recent prospective cohort study of 113 patients found that this technique detected metastatic disease with a sensitivity of 35% (19% to 55%) and specificity of 99% (93% to 100%).[32]

When imaging investigations are negative, staging laparoscopy should be used to detect peritoneal and metastatic disease under 5 mm in diameter, which may be missed even with high quality radiological imaging.

and a pooled positive likelihood ratio of 2.74 (1.47 to 5.24).[27] The National Cancer Institute study suggested that although these symptoms have limited predictive value, their identification will probably remain part of dyspepsia management strategies in the United Kingdom[28] and US[26] until better approaches emerge.

The table lists the common differential diagnoses of gastric cancer.

Who should be referred for further investigations?

UK consensus guidelines in 2011 recommended that patients aged 55 years or more with new onset dyspepsia and all those with alarm symptoms should undergo urgent (within two weeks) upper gastrointestinal endoscopy.[28] If macroscopic signs of tumour (ulceration, masses, or mucosal changes) are found on endoscopy, immediate

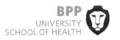

Laparoscopy also enables peritoneal cytology and biopsies to be obtained from suspicious lesions and should be considered before definitive treatment. A retrospective review of 511 patients found that staging laparoscopy effectively changed treatment decisions in 28.0% of patients with gastric cancer after computed tomography and endoscopic ultrasonography.[33]

What is the approach to making a decision about treatment?

Thorough oncological staging and preoperative evaluation of fitness are vital for patients with invasive gastric cancer. Tumours that show local invasion (T4) or distant metastases (M1) are typically not amenable to curative treatment. The patient's fitness is determined by physical activity status, biological age, and comorbidities. It can be measured objectively by lung function and cardiopulmonary exercise testing. Final treatment recommendations are made at a multidisciplinary team meeting involving experienced surgeons, radiologists, pathologists, and oncologists. The final decision should be made together with the patient after the clinician carefully explains the recommended treatment.

Treatment with intent to cure—what are the options?

Surgical resection

Current UK and US guidelines recommend that all medically fit patients with regionally confined disease undergo primary surgical resection for up to stage IA tumours and surgery after neoadjuvant therapy for stage II-III tumours.[28] [34] The extent of surgical resection usually depends on tumour location. Although total gastrectomy is routinely performed for proximal tumours, multicentre randomised controlled trials have shown similar survival rates after subtotal gastrectomy for distal tumours.[35 36]

The extent of lymph node dissection is a key consideration during surgery. Recent randomised controlled trials have advocated D2 lymph node dissection (perigastric nodes and nodes along the coeliac trunk) over D1 dissection (perigastric nodes only) because D2 dissection results in lower rates of locoregional recurrence and cancer related death, despite increased rates of early morbidity and mortality.[37 38] Most high volume centres currently perform modified (spleen preserving) D2 dissections.

Randomised trials of minimally invasive gastrectomy versus open surgery suggest that long term outcomes are similar, although laparoscopic procedures offer better pain control and are associated with reduced blood loss and postoperative complication rates.[39 40]

A prospective study of 827 patients found that robotic gastrectomy produced better short term and comparable oncological outcomes compared with laparoscopic gastrectomy.[41]

Early gastric cancer (T1a) can be treated with endoscopic mucosal resection if it is confined to the mucosa, less than 2 cm in diameter, of low or moderate differentiation, and exhibits no ulceration or lymphovascular involvement.[28 42]

Neoadjuvant and adjuvant treatment

Systemic treatment is given before definitive surgery (neoadjuvant) or after resection (adjuvant) to treat micrometastases and improve outcome. The pivotal Medical Research Council Adjuvant Gastric Infusional Chemotherapy (MAGIC) trial randomised 503 patients with cancer of the gastro-oesophageal junction or gastric body to surgery alone or three preoperative cycles of chemotherapy (epirubicin, cisplatin, 5-fluorouracil), followed when possible by three cycles after surgery.[43] Chemotherapy resulted in a significantly greater five year survival than surgery alone (36% v 23%; P=0.009), indicating significant benefit for patients with stage 2 disease or higher, although the necessity for six cycles was unresolved. This has become the standard of care for resectable gastric cancer in the UK. A later multi-centre randomised trial in patients with advanced disease, which found that oxaliplatin can replace cisplatin and that oral fluoropyrimidine capecitabine can replace the inconvenient 5-fluorouracil infusion, has resulted in wider neoadjuvant use of these agents.[44]

Adjuvant chemoradiation also showed benefit in a randomised trial of 556 patients with resected adenocarcinoma of the stomach or gastro-oesophageal junction, who were randomly assigned to surgery plus postoperative chemoradiation (fluorouracil/calcium folinate for five days then 4500 cGy radiation at 180 cGy/day, five days a week for five weeks) or surgery alone.[45] One month after completing radiotherapy, two five day cycles of fluorouracil plus calcium folinate were given. The median survival of the adjuvant chemoradiation group was 36 months compared with 27 months in the surgery alone group (P=0.005). The trial was criticised for poor survival in the surgery alone arm, with only 10% of patients in the surgery arm receiving a D2 resection and D0 resection in more than 50% of patients. In addition, toxicity was high, and this regimen—although used in the US—has not been widely adopted in the UK.

A meta-analysis of adjuvant chemotherapy trials suggests that such treatment is beneficial, although the size of the effect is small and the optimal agents are unclear. Adjuvant chemotherapy was associated with a significant benefit on overall survival (hazard ratio 0.82, 0.76 to 0.90; P <0.001) and disease-free survival (0.82, 0.75 to 0.90; P<0.001), with five year overall survival increasing from 49.6% to 55.3% with chemotherapy.[46]

Patients who undergo chemotherapy for gastric cancer may develop fatigue, nausea, vomiting, alopecia, neuropathy, and other side effects specific to the agents used.[43 44] Neutropenic sepsis is potentially life threatening and may present with fever alone. Its recognition and management are crucial in the primary care setting.[47]

Where to have surgery for gastric cancer?

In recent years, cancer services have become centralised to high volume units, and studies have shown improved in-hospital outcomes when centres and surgeons are experienced at major cancer surgery.[48] Prospective nationwide data from the American College of Surgeons' national surgical quality improvement programme attributed the lower mortality rates at high volume centres to better management of postoperative complications.[49] Large prospective studies suggest that, although postoperative mortality and mid-term survival are better in high volume centres,[50] long term survival and recurrence may be independent of hospital volume.[51]

What does palliative care involve and what are the considerations?

Up to half of all patients with gastric cancer present with incurable disease and require palliative treatment.[28] Best supportive care aims to prevent or alleviate symptoms such as bleeding, obstruction, pain, nausea, and vomiting and

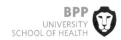

to improve quality of life for patients and caregivers. This should be a key focus of the multidisciplinary team, taking into account performance status and patient preference, with early direct involvement of the palliative care team and clinical nurse specialists.

Treatment of advanced disease

Chemotherapy and chemoradiotherapy
Randomised trials have shown that chemotherapy improves quality of life over best supportive care alone in patients with metastatic gastric cancer.[52] [53] In the UK, the epirubicin, cisplatin, and 5-fluorouracil regimen or variants including oxaliplatin and capecitabine are most widely used. In the REAL-2 study, which compared similar regimens, median survival was 9.3-11.2 months.[44]

A randomised Korean trial of patients after initial chemotherapy showed a small survival benefit from second line treatment with taxane or irinotecan based chemotherapy—5.3 months for 33 patients in the chemotherapy arm and 3.8 months in 69 patients in the best supportive care arm (hazard ratio 0.657, 0.485 to 0.891; one sided P=0.007).[52] Patient preference, performance status, and potential side effects must be factored into decisions to administer such treatment.

A fifth of patients with gastric cancer have tumours with amplification of HER2 (erbB2).[54] The randomised ToGA (Trastuzumab with Chemotherapy in HER2-Positive Advanced Gastric Cancer) study of 594 patients showed that targeted treatment with herceptin (trastuzumab) plus chemotherapy (cisplatin with capecitabine or 5-fluorouracil) was superior to chemotherapy alone, with a median survival of 13.8 versus 11.1 months, respectively (P=0.0048).[54] For patients whose tumours showed high HER2 expression, median overall survival was 16.0 months (15 to 19) in those assigned to trastuzumab plus chemotherapy versus 11.8 months (10 to 13) in those assigned to chemotherapy alone. The ToGA trial established this treatment as standard for HER2 positive patients with advanced cancer.

Palliative surgery
Palliative gastrectomy may benefit patients with obstruction of the gastric outlet secondary to antral tumours, or for incomplete dysphagia caused by tumours of the cardia. The decision to manage patients palliatively should not limit the extent of surgery; a large retrospective study has shown that more radical procedures may improve survival and quality of life in eligible patients.[55] A gastrojejunostomy, which can often be performed laparoscopically, and endoscopic stenting can be performed in those who are not eligible for first line surgical procedures.

How should patients be followed up after treatment?
Routine blood tests are needed to monitor bone marrow function during chemotherapy, and nutritional monitoring is recommended after surgery (for example, vitamin B12 monitoring after proximal or total gastrectomy). Despite the lack of randomised evidence evaluating follow-up strategies,[28] most UK based tertiary centres review patients every four months for three years, and annually thereafter; with radiographic imaging and endoscopy performed as clinically indicated. Patients with recurrent disease may benefit from surgery if complete resection is possible, although most patients undergo salvage chemotherapy, provided they have adequate performance status.[56]

Can gastric cancer be prevented?
Primary prevention
A meta-analysis of seven randomised trials conducted in high risk regions for gastric cancer (six in Asia) showed that eradication of H pylori reduced the risk of gastric cancer from 1.7% to 1.1% (relative risk 0.65, 0.43 to 0.98).[57] An intention to treat analysis of a recent Chinese randomised trial of 3365 participants found that a two week course of omeprazole and amoxicillin reduced the incidence of gastric cancer by 39% within 15 years of randomisation, with similar but not significant reductions in mortality from gastric cancer.[58] The cost effectiveness of H pylori vaccination as long term prophylaxis against gastric cancer in the US has been extrapolated by simulation studies,[59] but evidence for the benefit of H pylori eradication in low risk regions is lacking.

A meta-analysis of case-control studies (14 442 cases and 73 918 controls) found that people who had ever smoked had a 43% greater risk of developing gastric cancer (odds ratio 1.43, 1.24 to 1.66) than never smokers, whereas current smokers had a 57% greater risk (1.57, 1.24 to 2.01).[60] This suggests that efforts to prevent cigarette smoking, and help people quit, would reduce the incidence of gastric cancer.

Secondary prevention
A multi-centre open label randomised controlled trial of 544 patients found that eradication of H pylori (with lansoprazole, amoxicillin, and clarithromycin) after endoscopic resection for early gastric cancer decreased the risk of developing metachronous gastric carcinoma (hazard ratio 0.339, 0.157 to 0.729; P=0.003) at three years' follow-up.[61] It recommended prophylactic eradication of H pylori after endoscopic resection of early gastric cancer to prevent the development of metachronous gastric carcinoma.

Is there a role for screening?
Screening for early gastric cancer requires the presence of an easily identifiable group with a high absolute risk. One such group might be middle aged male smokers with a history of Helicobacter pylori infection or other pre-malignancy, such as Barrett's oesophagus. However, absolute risk also takes into account the incidence of cancer. The large numbers of potentially high risk people and the low incidence of gastric cancer make screening programmes unfeasible in all regions but those with a high incidence of gastric cancer (such as Japan and Chile).[62] In such regions, serological screening techniques involving pepsinogens, gastrin-17 and anti-H pylori (or anti-Cag-A, or both) antibodies are being evaluated, in addition to photofluorography and endoscopy.[63] [64] Nanomaterial based breath testing has also recently been evaluated as a screening tool—a pilot study to a large multicentre trial found that this test has a sensitivity of 89% and specificity of 90% in distinguishing gastric cancer from benign gastric disease.[65]

Is the prognosis for patients with gastric cancer improving?
A single centre Korean study of 12 026 patients with gastric cancer found that the five year overall survival rate increased from 64.0% to 73.2% (P<0.001) from 1986 to 2006.[66] A large European study of 10 cancer registries across seven countries showed similar improvements but also detected marked variation in survival rates (28.0-44.3%) between certain countries, which could not be explained by operative mortality alone.[67]

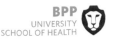

Greater access to care; better diagnostic techniques for early detection; more rational surgical strategies; lower complication rates; advances in anaesthesia, perioperative care, and nutritional care; and wider use of systemic chemotherapy have been deemed responsible for such improvements in prognosis. These factors may also partly explain the discrepancies in postoperative survival rates across the world, although quantitative data are lacking for this.[66] [67]

What treatment strategies lie on the horizon?

Novel targeted biological agents are being investigated in the treatment of gastric cancer. The role of anti-angiogenic agents such as bevacizumab (a monoclonal antibody targeting vascular endothelial growth factor) combined with chemotherapy is the subject of a randomised trial.[68] No targeted small molecules or antibodies have yet shown benefit in the management of gastric cancer, but greater understanding of the underlying molecular basis of the disease will undoubtedly suggest strategies for treatment in the future.

Contributors: SGT conceived the review, extracted evidence, and drafted the manuscript. MAC, DH, and MM coauthored the article (including article direction, interpreting the literature, and editing the manuscript). MM is guarantor.

Funding: Supported by the National Institute for Health Research University College London Hospitals Biomedical Research Centre. DH was supported by CRUK grant C2259/A16569.

Competing interests: We have read and understood the BMJ Group policy on declaration of interests and declare the following interests: None.

Provenance and peer review: Not commissioned; externally peer reviewed.

1 Ferlay J, Shin HR, Bray F, Forman D, Mathers C, Parkin DM. Estimates of worldwide burden of cancer in 2008: GLOBOCAN 2008. *Int J Cancer*2010;127:2893-917.

2 Coupland VH, Allum W, Blazeby JM, Mendall MA, Hardwick RH, Linklater KM, et al. Incidence and survival of oesophageal and gastric cancer in England between 1998 and 2007, a population-based study. *BMC Cancer*2012;12:11.

3 Jemal A, Bray F, Center MM, Ferlay J, Ward E, Forman D. Global cancer statistics. *CA Cancer J Clin*2011;61:69-90.

4 Guggenheim DE, Shah MA. Gastric cancer epidemiology and risk factors. *J Surg Oncol*2013;107:230-6.

5 Anderson WF, Camargo MC, Fraumeni JF Jr, Correa P, Rosenberg PS, Rabkin CS. Age-specific trends in incidence of noncardia gastric cancer in US adults. *JAMA*2010;303:1723-8.

6 Crew KD, Neugut AI. Epidemiology of gastric cancer. *World J Gastroenterol*2006;12:354-62.

7 Office for National Statistics. Cancer statistics registrations: registrations of cancer diagnosed in 2008, England. Series MB1 no 39. 2010. www.ons.gov.uk/ons/rel/vsob1/cancer-statistics-registrations--england--series-mb1-/no--39--2008/index.html .

8 Bertuccio P, Chatenoud L, Levi F, Praud D, Ferlay J, Negri E, et al. Recent patterns in gastric cancer: a global overview. *Int J Cancer*2009;125:666-73.

9 International Agency for Research on Cancer. Pathology and genetics of tumours of the digestive system. 2000. www.iarc.fr/en/publications/pdfs-online/pat-gen/bb2/bb2-cover.pdf

10 Cavaleiro-Pinto M, Peleteiro B, Lunet N, Barros H. Helicobacter pylori infection and gastric cardia cancer: systematic review and meta-analysis. *Cancer Causes Control*2011;22:375-87.

11 Ladeiras-Lopes R, Pereira AK, Nogueira A, Pinheiro-Torres T, Pinto I, Santos-Pereira R, et al. Smoking and gastric cancer: systematic review and meta-analysis of cohort studies. *Cancer Causes Control*2008;19:689-701.

12 Smyth EC, Capanu M, Janjigian YY, Kelsen DK, Coit D, Strong VE, et al. Tobacco use is associated with increased recurrence and death from gastric cancer. *Ann Surg Oncol*2012;19:2088-94.

13 Sjodahl K, Lu Y, Nilsen TI, Ye W, Hveem K, Vatten L, et al. Smoking and alcohol drinking in relation to risk of gastric cancer: a population-based, prospective cohort study. *Int J Cancer*2007;120:128-32.

14 Tramacere I, Negri E, Pelucchi C, Bagnardi V, Rota M, Scotti L, et al. A meta-analysis on alcohol drinking and gastric cancer risk. *Ann Oncol*2012;23:28-36.

15 Duell EJ, Travier N, Lujan-Barroso L, Clavel-Chapelon F, Boutron-Ruault MC, Morois S, et al. Alcohol consumption and gastric cancer risk in the European Prospective Investigation into Cancer and Nutrition (EPIC) cohort. *Am J Clin Nutr*2011;94:1266-75.

16 World Cancer Research Fund. Food, nutrition, physical activity, and the prevention of cancer: a global perspective. 2007. www.dietandcancerreport.org/cancer_resource_center/downloads/Second_Expert_Report_full.pdf

17 Shikata K, Kiyohara Y, Kubo M, Yonemoto K, Ninomiya T, Shirota T, et al. A prospective study of dietary salt intake and gastric cancer incidence in a defined Japanese population: the Hisayama study. *Int J Cancer*2006;119:196-201.

18 Kim J, Park S, Nam BH. Gastric cancer and salt preference: a population-based cohort study in Korea. *Am J Clin Nutr*2010;91:1289-93.

19 Park B, Shin A, Park SK, Ko KP, Ma SH, Lee EH, et al. Ecological study for refrigerator use, salt, vegetable, and fruit intakes, and gastric cancer. *Cancer Causes Control*2011;22:1497-502.

20 Larsson SC, Bergkvist L, Wolk A. Fruit and vegetable consumption and incidence of gastric cancer: a prospective study. *Cancer Epidemiol Biomarkers Prev*2006;15:1998-2001.

21 Vannella L, Lahner E, Osborn J, Annibale B. Systematic review: gastric cancer incidence in pernicious anaemia. *Aliment Pharmacol Ther*2013;37:375-82.

22 Fitzgerald RC, Hardwick R, Huntsman D, Carneiro F, Guilford P, Blair V, et al. Hereditary diffuse gastric cancer: updated consensus guidelines for clinical management and directions for future research. *J Med Genet*2010;47:436-44.

23 Pharoah PD, Guilford P, Caldas C. Incidence of gastric cancer and breast cancer in CDH1 (E-cadherin) mutation carriers from hereditary diffuse gastric cancer families. *Gastroenterology*2001;121:1348-53.

24 Lynch HT, Grady W, Suriano G, Huntsman D. Gastric cancer: new genetic developments. *J Surg Oncol*2005;90:114-33; discussion 33.

25 Capelle LG, Van Grieken NC, Lingsma HF, Steyerberg EW, Klokman WJ, Bruno MJ, et al. Risk and epidemiological time trends of gastric cancer in Lynch syndrome carriers in the Netherlands. *Gastroenterology*2010;138:487-92.

26 Talley NJ, Vakil NB, Moayyedi P. American gastroenterological association technical review on the evaluation of dyspepsia. *Gastroenterology*2005;129:1756-80.

27 Vakil N, Moayyedi P, Fennerty MB, Talley NJ. Limited value of alarm features in the diagnosis of upper gastrointestinal malignancy: systematic review and meta-analysis. *Gastroenterology*2006;131:390-401; quiz 659-60.

28 Allum WH, Blazeby JM, Griffin SM, Cunningham D, Jankowski JA, Wong R. Guidelines for the management of oesophageal and gastric cancer. *Gut*2011;60:1449-72.

29 Gravalos C, Jimeno A. HER2 in gastric cancer: a new prognostic factor and a novel therapeutic target. *Ann Oncol*2008;19:1523-9.

30 National Institute for Health and Care Excellence. Trastuzumab for the treatment of HER2-positive metastatic gastric cancer. TA208. 2010. http://guidance.nice.org.uk/TA208.

31 Mocellin S, Marchet A, Nitti D. EUS for the staging of gastric cancer: a meta-analysis. *Gastrointest Endosc*2011;73:1122-34.

32 Smyth E, Schoder H, Strong VE, Capanu M, Kelsen DP, Coit DG, et al. A prospective evaluation of the utility of 2-deoxy-2-[(18) F]fluoro-D-glucose positron emission tomography and computed tomography in staging locally advanced gastric cancer. *Cancer*2012;118:5481-8.

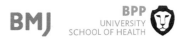

33 de Graaf GW, Ayantunde AA, Parsons SL, Duffy JP, Welch NT. The role of staging laparoscopy in oesophagogastric cancers. *Eur J Surg Oncol*2007;33:988-92.

34 National Comprehensive Cancer Network. Gastric cancer. Version 2. 2013. www.nccn.org/professionals/physician_gls/pdf/gastric.pdf.

35 Bozzetti F, Marubini E, Bonfanti G, Miceli R, Piano C, Gennari L. Subtotal versus total gastrectomy for gastric cancer: five-year survival rates in a multicenter randomized Italian trial. Italian Gastrointestinal Tumor Study Group. *Ann Surg*1999;230:170-8.

36 Gouzi JL, Huguier M, Fagniez PL, Launois B, Flamant Y, Lacaine F, et al. Total versus subtotal gastrectomy for adenocarcinoma of the gastric antrum. A French prospective controlled study. *Ann Surg*1989;209:162-6.

37 Songun I, Putter H, Kranenbarg EM, Sasako M, van de Velde CJ. Surgical treatment of gastric cancer: 15-year follow-up results of the randomised nationwide Dutch D1D2 trial. *Lancet Oncol*2010;11:439-49.

38 Sasako M, Sano T, Yamamoto S, Kurokawa Y, Nashimoto A, Kurita A, et al. D2 lymphadenectomy alone or with para-aortic nodal dissection for gastric cancer. *N Engl J Med*2008;359:453-62.

39 Kim HH, Hyung WJ, Cho GS, Kim MC, Han SU, Kim W, et al. Morbidity and mortality of laparoscopic gastrectomy versus open gastrectomy for gastric cancer: an interim report—a phase III multicenter, prospective, randomized Trial (KLASS Trial). *Ann Surg*2010;251:417-20.

40 Ohtani H, Tamamori Y, Noguchi K, Azuma T, Fujimoto S, Oba H, et al. A meta-analysis of randomized controlled trials that compared laparoscopy-assisted and open distal gastrectomy for early gastric cancer. *J Gastrointest Surg*2010;14:958-64.

41 Woo Y, Hyung WJ, Pak KH, Inaba K, Obama K, Choi SH, et al. Robotic gastrectomy as an oncologically sound alternative to laparoscopic resections for the treatment of early-stage gastric cancers. *Arch Surg*2011;146:1086-92.

42 Bennett C, Wang Y, Pan T. Endoscopic mucosal resection for early gastric cancer. *Cochrane Database Syst Rev*2009;4:CD004276.

43 Cunningham D, Allum WH, Stenning SP, Thompson JN, Van de Velde CJ, Nicolson M, et al. Perioperative chemotherapy versus surgery alone for resectable gastroesophageal cancer. *N Engl J Med*2006;355:11-20.

44 Cunningham D, Starling N, Rao S, Iveson T, Nicolson M, Coxon F, et al. Capecitabine and oxaliplatin for advanced esophagogastric cancer. *N Engl J Med*2008;358:36-46.

45 Macdonald JS, Smalley SR, Benedetti J, Hundahl SA, Estes NC, Stemmermann GN, et al. Chemoradiotherapy after surgery compared with surgery alone for adenocarcinoma of the stomach or gastroesophageal junction. *N Engl J Med*2001;345:725-30.

46 Paoletti X, Oba K, Burzykowski T, Michiels S, Ohashi Y, Pignon JP, et al. Benefit of adjuvant chemotherapy for resectable gastric cancer: a meta-analysis. *JAMA*2010;303:1729-37.

47 National Institute for Health and Care Excellence. Neutropenic sepsis: prevention and management of neutropenic sepsis in cancer patients. CG151. 2012. http://publications.nice.org.uk/neutropenic-sepsis-prevention-and-management-of-neutropenic-sepsis-in-cancer-patients-cg151.

48 Coupland VH, Lagergren J, Luchtenborg M, Jack RH, Allum W, Holmberg L, et al. Hospital volume, proportion resected and mortality from oesophageal and gastric cancer: a population-based study in England, 2004-2008. *Gut*2013;62:961-6.

49 Ghaferi AA, Birkmeyer JD, Dimick JB. Variation in hospital mortality associated with inpatient surgery. *N Engl J Med*2009;361:1368-75.

50 Dikken JL, Dassen AE, Lemmens VE, Putter H, Krijnen P, van der Geest L, et al. Effect of hospital volume on postoperative mortality and survival after oesophageal and gastric cancer surgery in the Netherlands between 1989 and 2009. *Eur J Cancer*2012;48:1004-13.

51 Enzinger PC, Benedetti JK, Meyerhardt JA, McCoy S, Hundahl SA, Macdonald JS, et al. Impact of hospital volume on recurrence and survival after surgery for gastric cancer. *Ann Surg*2007;245:426-34.

52 Wagner AD, Unverzagt S, Grothe W, Kleber G, Grothey A, Haerting J, et al. Chemotherapy for advanced gastric cancer. *Cochrane Database Syst Rev*2010;3:CD004064.

53 Kang JH, Lee SI, Lim do H, Park KW, Oh SY, Kwon HC, et al. Salvage chemotherapy for pretreated gastric cancer: a randomized phase III trial comparing chemotherapy plus best supportive care with best supportive care alone. *J Clin Oncol*2012;30:1513-8.

54 Bang YJ, Van Cutsem E, Feyereislova A, Chung HC, Shen L, Sawaki A, et al. Trastuzumab in combination with chemotherapy versus chemotherapy alone for treatment of HER2-positive advanced gastric or gastro-oesophageal junction cancer (ToGA): a phase 3, open-label, randomised controlled trial. *Lancet*2010;376:687-97.

55 Zhang JZ, Lu HS, Huang CM, Wu XY, Wang C, Guan GX, et al. Outcome of palliative total gastrectomy for stage IV proximal gastric cancer. *Am J Surg*2011;202:91-6.

56 Song KY, Park SM, Kim SN, Park CH. The role of surgery in the treatment of recurrent gastric cancer. *Am J Surg*2008;196:19-22.

57 Fuccio L, Zagari RM, Eusebi LH, Laterza L, Cennamo V, Ceroni L, et al. Meta-analysis: can Helicobacter pylori eradication treatment reduce the risk for gastric cancer? *Ann Intern Med*2009;151:121-8.

58 Ma JL, Zhang L, Brown LM, Li JY, Shen L, Pan KF, et al. Fifteen-year effects of Helicobacter pylori, garlic, and vitamin treatments on gastric cancer incidence and mortality. *J Natl Cancer Inst*2012;104:488-92.

59 Rupnow MF, Chang AH, Shachter RD, Owens DK, Parsonnet J. Cost-effectiveness of a potential prophylactic Helicobacter pylori vaccine in the United States. *J Infect Dis*2009;200:1311-7.

60 La Torre G, Chiaradia G, Gianfagna F, De Lauretis A, Boccia S, Mannocci A, et al. Smoking status and gastric cancer risk: an updated meta-

analysis of case-control studies published in the past ten years. *Tumori*2009;95:13-22.

61 Fukase K, Kato M, Kikuchi S, Inoue K, Uemura N, Okamoto S, et al. Effect of eradication of Helicobacter pylori on incidence of metachronous gastric carcinoma after endoscopic resection of early gastric cancer: an open-label, randomised controlled trial. *Lancet*2008;372:392-7.

62 Lagergren J, Ye W, Bergstrom R, Nyren O. Utility of endoscopic screening for upper gastrointestinal adenocarcinoma. *JAMA*2000;284:961-2.

63 Rugge M. Secondary prevention of gastric cancer. *Gut*2007;56:1646-7.

64 Kato M, Asaka M. Recent development of gastric cancer prevention. *Jpn J Clin Oncol*2012;42:987-94.

65 Xu ZQ, Broza YY, Ionsecu R, Tisch U, Ding L, Liu H, et al. A nanomaterial-based breath test for distinguishing gastric cancer from benign gastric conditions. *Br J Cancer*2013;108:941-50.

66 Ahn HS, Lee HJ, Yoo MW, Jeong SH, Park DJ, Kim HH, et al. Changes in clinicopathological features and survival after gastrectomy for gastric cancer over a 20-year period. *Br J Surg*2011;98:255-60.

67 Lepage C, Sant M, Verdecchia A, Forman D, Esteve J, Faivre J. Operative mortality after gastric cancer resection and long-term survival differences across Europe. *Br J Surg*2010;97:235-9.

68 Van Cutsem E, de Haas S, Kang YK, Ohtsu A, Tebbutt NC, Ming Xu J, et al. Bevacizumab in combination with chemotherapy as first-line therapy in advanced gastric cancer: a biomarker evaluation from the AVAGAST randomized phase III trial. *J Clin Oncol*2012;30:2119-27.

Related links

bmj.com
- Get Cleveland Clinic CME credits for this article

bmj.com/archive
Previous articles in this series
- The diagnosis and management of gastric cancer (BMJ 2013;347:f6367)
- An introduction to advance care planning in practice (BMJ 2013;347:f6064)
- Post-mastectomy breast reconstruction (BMJ 2013;347:f5903)
- Identifying brain tumours in children •and young adults (BMJ 2013;347:f5844)
- Gout (BMJ 2013;347:f5648)

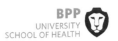

Ductal carcinoma in situ of the breast

Nicola L P Barnes specialist registrar breast surgery[1], Jane L Ooi consultant breast and oncoplastic surgeon[1], John R Yarnold professor of clinical oncology[2], Nigel J Bundred professor of surgical oncology[3]

[1]Breast Unit, Royal Bolton Hospital, Bolton BL4 0JR, UK

[2]Radiotherapy Unit, Institute of Cancer Research and Royal Marsden Hospital, London, UK

[3]Department of Surgical Oncology, South Manchester University Hospital, Manchester, UK

Correspondence to: N L P Barnes nicolabarnes@doctors.org.uk

Cite this as: BMJ 2012;344:e797

‹DOI› 10.1136/bmj.e797
http://www.bmj.com/content/344/bmj.e797

Ductal carcinoma in situ (DCIS) is a preinvasive (also termed non-invasive) breast cancer, where proliferations of malignant ductal epithelial cells remain confined within intact breast ducts (fig 1). DCIS is a precursor lesion that has the potential to transform into an invasive cancer over a timescale that may be a few years or decades long. The development of its ability to invade and metastasise is as yet unquantifiable and is attributed to the accumulation of somatic mutations in premalignant cells. Treatment aims to prevent DCIS from progressing to invasive breast cancer.

DCIS was rarely diagnosed before the introduction of national screening programmes but is now common, accounting for 20% of screen detected cancers in the United Kingdom.[1] Treatment usually comprises surgery (mastectomy or wide local excision), with or without adjuvant radiotherapy. However, it is possible that a subset of these lesions would never progress to invasive breast cancer over the lifetime of the patient if left untreated, and in this (as yet undefined) population traditional management may represent overtreatment. Deciding on appropriate personalised treatment for individual patients diagnosed with DCIS is an ongoing challenge, because the optimum management remains controversial. We review relevant randomised controlled trials, meta-analyses, preclinical, and clinical studies to provide the reader with an overview of the evidence base underpinning current management of patients with DCIS and to highlight controversies and unanswered research questions.

How does DCIS develop?

The natural course of DCIS is poorly understood. It is categorised into low grade, intermediate grade, and high grade disease according to combinations of cell morphology, architecture, and the presence of necrosis. High grade DCIS has pleomorphic, irregularly spaced, large nuclei that vary in size and have irregular nuclear contours, coarse chromatin, prominent nucleoli, and frequent mitoses. Low grade DCIS has monomorphic, evenly spaced cells with rounded centrally placed nuclei, inconspicuous nucleoli, infrequent mitoses, and rarely necrosis of individual cells. Intermediate grade DCIS lies within these extremes—the nuclei are typically larger than in low grade DCIS and show moderate pleomorphism.[2] The developmental pathway of low grade and intermediate grade DCIS is thought to differ from that of high grade disease. Low grade tumours show a loss in the 16q chromosome, whereas high grade disease more often shows 17q gain.[3] Atypical ductal hyperplasia is thought to be a precursor lesion of low grade DCIS and has a similar fivefold increased risk of subsequent invasive cancer. High grade DCIS has no obvious precursor lesion. Low grade DCIS, if it progresses, tends to develop into low grade invasive cancer, whereas high grade DCIS progresses to high grade invasive disease.

Risk factors for developing DCIS include a family history of breast cancer, nulliparity, older age at birth of first child, and positivity for BRCA1 and BRCA2.[4][5] Since the publication of the Women's Health Initiative and the Million Women Study,[6][7] the association between invasive breast cancer and combined oestrogen and progesterone hormone replacement therapy has been well documented. However, hormone replacement therapy did not significantly increase the risk of developing DCIS in these two studies. In the Women's Health Initiative study there were 47 cases of DCIS in the hormone replacement therapy group versus 37 cases in the control group (hazard ratio 1.18; weighted P=0.09).[6] The Million Women study did not report an association with DCIS. A large surveillance study published in 2009 found that atypical ductal hyperplasia (and by implication, low grade DCIS) has become less common since women stopped using hormone replacement therapy.[8] This suggests that, although hormone replacement therapy may not increase the risk of developing DCIS, it may promote the growth of pre-existing populations of oestrogen receptor positive DCIS progenitor cells.

When considering referral to a family history clinic, a case of DCIS in the family should count towards the indicators for genetic testing in the same way that an invasive cancer does. Non-screen detected DCIS is rare in the UK, and a diagnosis of DCIS in a first degree relative under screening age may also warrant consideration of family history risk assessment.

How might DCIS present?

More than 90% of cases of DCIS are detected at screening while asymptomatic. About 6% of all symptomatic breast cancers are preinvasive.[1] Some patients present with Paget's disease of the nipple (an eczematous-type nipple lesion that does not resolve with topical steroid treatment), nipple discharge (which is usually from a single duct and either blood stained or clear), or a palpable mass. DCIS that

---

SOURCES AND SELECTION CRITERIA

We searched Medline and PubMed for meta-analyses, randomised controlled trials, and original peer reviewed articles, using ductal carcinoma in situ, DCIS, preinvasive, non-invasive, treatment, radiotherapy, endocrine therapy, and psychosocial as main search terms. Only papers written in English were selected and we obtained the full text for each. We searched the Cochrane database for relevant reviews and www.Clinicaltrials.gov for current research.

SUMMARY POINTS

- Ductal carcinoma in situ (DCIS) is a preinvasive breast cancer—malignant cells are confined within an intact ductal basement membrane
- Most cases (90%) are asymptomatic and detected at screening, but it can present as Paget's disease of the nipple, nipple discharge, or a lump
- Treatment aims to prevent invasive disease
- Oestrogen receptor status tends to be preserved in recurrences or disease progression; this has implications for adjuvant treatment and reducing risk of recurrence
- The optimum treatment is unclear, and urgent clarification is needed
- Women with DCIS should have the option of entering high quality randomised controlled trials

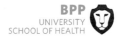
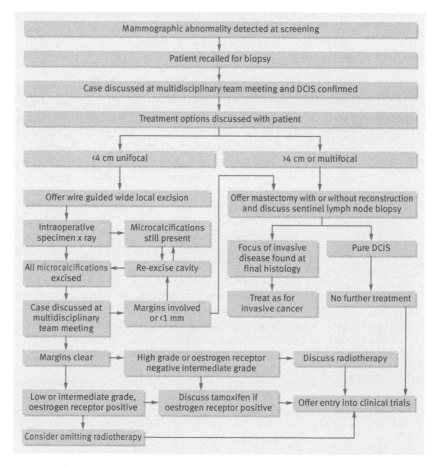

| Normal duct | DCIS | Invasive cancer |

Fig 1 Difference between normal, ductal carcinoma in situ (DCIS), and invasive disease

presents with clinical signs is more likely to be extensive or to have an invasive component.

Men can also develop DCIS and tend to present with symptoms of blood stained nipple discharge or a retroareolar mass. The standard treatment for men is mastectomy with excision of the nipple-areola complex. DCIS accounts for about 5% of breast cancers in men,[9] but the proportion of men who would progress to invasive cancer if DCIS was not treated is unknown.

How is DCIS diagnosed and treated?

At screening mammography, malignant looking microcalcifications are the most common abnormality. Architectural distortion, ill defined masses, nodules, or ductal asymmetry can also indicate underlying DCIS. Figure 2 shows a flow chart of a typical screen detected treatment pathway. Women with an abnormal mammogram will be recalled for an image guided biopsy, under local anaesthetic, with either a 14 gauge core biopsy gun or vacuum assisted biopsy device. If the area of abnormality is extensive, multiple cores of different areas can be taken,

to try to increase the chance of detecting a coexistent invasive tumour. Core biopsy and vacuum assisted biopsy are preferable to fine needle aspiration, which cannot discriminate between in situ and invasive cancer because it provides no information on the basement membrane. A recent meta-analysis showed that, compared with 14 gauge core biopsy, use of an 11 gauge vacuum assisted biopsy device halves the risk of missing a coexisting invasive cancer (P=0.006).[10] Other factors associated with missing associated invasive disease include having a high grade lesion (P<0.001), an imaging size greater than 20 mm (P,0.001), a breast imaging reporting and data system (BI-RADS) score of 4 or 5 (P for trend=0.005), a mass visible at mammography (v calcification only, P<0.001), and a palpable abnormality (P<0.001).[10]

For symptomatic cases the diagnostic pathway will depend on presentation—core biopsy for a palpable lump, punch biopsy for Paget's disease of the nipple, and smear cytology to look for malignant cells for nipple discharge. Microdochectomy (removal of just the symptomatic breast duct(s)) or total duct excision will need to be performed if

Fig 2 Typical screen detected treatment pathway for ductal carcinoma in situ (DCIS)

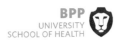

the only symptom is persistent clear or bloody discharge to exclude underlying DCIS (or invasive disease).

The breast surgeon and breast care nurse will then counsel the patient on the surgical options. One option is breast conserving surgery by means of wide local excision, usually using wire localisation (a wire inserted stereotactically, under mammographic guidance; more than one wire may be needed to bracket large areas). This allows the surgeon to excise the lesion accurately. The patient will be offered mastectomy if the area of DCIS is extensive or breast size in relation to lesion size does not allow for cosmetically or surgically acceptable wide local excision, and occasionally because of patient preference. National Institute for Health and Clinical Excellence (NICE) guidance suggests that sentinel lymph node biopsy (to stage the axilla) should be performed at the time of mastectomy for lesions greater than 4 cm because of the small incidence of occult invasive disease in extensive DCIS.[11] Axillary surgery is not indicated alongside wide local excision.

Women with extensive DCIS, if medically fit, are excellent candidates for immediate breast reconstruction. In the UK, about 35% of women with DCIS have a mastectomy and 72% have wide local excision.[1]

After wide local excision, the specimen is x rayed to ensure that all suspicious microcalcifications have been removed. After mastectomy, the histopathologist may request imaging of specimen slices to aid detection of the disease and its extent.

After surgery, the case will be discussed at a multidisciplinary team meeting (comprising radiologists, pathologists, oncologists and surgeons) to ensure that margins are clear histologically and radiologically. The optimum margin width is controversial, but a circumferential margin of at least 1 mm is generally accepted. If margins are close (<1 mm) or involved after wide local excision, cavity re-excision or mastectomy should be offered to achieve clear margins.

What other investigative tools are useful in diagnosis and treatment?

Ductoscopy is not used routinely in the management of DCIS and is currently mainly a research tool. However, direct visualisation of the ductal system is an appealing option for a disease that is located purely within the ducts and may be especially useful for cases of nipple discharge. Instillation of chemotherapy agents directly into the ducts is also a theoretical possibility,[12] and this feature may be exploited in the future.

There is increasing evidence that magnetic resonance imaging may have an important role in the clinical assessment of the extent of DCIS.[13] Several ongoing trials are looking at the use of magnetic resonance imaging in the diagnosis and treatment planning of DCIS. This technique may be able identify occult multifocal or contralateral disease in patients with DCIS, but there is still some concern that overestimation of the extent of disease may lead to wider than necessary margins or unnecessary mastectomy, in addition to identifying high numbers of contralateral lesions that turn out to be benign.

What adjuvant treatments can be used in DCIS?

No further treatment is needed after mastectomy for pure DCIS. However, after breast conserving surgery the optimum adjuvant treatment is uncertain. Large randomised controlled trials (RCTs) have looked at the use of radiotherapy and tamoxifen as adjuvant treatments for DCIS.

Radiotherapy

Four RCTs have looked at using adjuvant radiotherapy after breast conserving surgery for DCIS—EORTC 10853,[14] NSABP B-17,[15] UK/ANZ DCIS,[16] and SweDCIS,[17] with a subsequent Cochrane review.[18] All of the trials showed a significant reduction in DCIS and invasive recurrence after radiotherapy (all used 50 Gy, standard fractionation, and no tumour bed boost dose), and all have long term follow-up (8-10 years). Radiotherapy also significantly reduced ipsilateral recurrence from 15-20% to 5-9% at five years and from 24% to 12% at 10 years of follow-up.[14 15 16 17] On pooling the trial results in the Cochrane review, ipsilateral invasive recurrence was halved at 10 years across the trials (hazard ratio 0.50, 95% confidence interval 0.32 to 0.76; P=0.0001).[18] About 50% of the recurrences over all the trials were invasive cancer, and 50% further DCIS.

The Cochrane review looked at the subgroups of age above or below 50 years, presence or absence of comedo necrosis (areas of necrotic debris within the DCIS), and size greater than or less than 10 mm; all subgroups benefited from the addition of radiotherapy, with recurrence rates approximately halving. Older (>50 years) patients had greater benefit from radiotherapy than younger ones (0.35 (>50) v 0.67 (<50)).[18] None of these trials was prospectively designed for these subgroup analyses, so the results should be interpreted with caution. The NSABP B-17 trial recently published long term (>10 year follow-up) results, which showed that recurrence of an invasive tumour in the ipsilateral breast was associated with a slightly increased risk of death (1.75, 1.45 to 2.96; P<0.001), whereas recurrence of DCIS was not.[19] Twenty two of the 39 deaths were attributed to breast cancer.[19] Such an effect was not seen in the 10 year follow-up of the UK/ANZ DCIS trial, which showed no increased risk of death after wide local excision alone.[16]

In practice, the trial results show that nine women require treatment with radiotherapy to prevent one ipsilateral recurrence (50% of recurrences are further DCIS).[18] Clinicians can therefore advise patients that for every 100 women who opt for radiotherapy, five to 10 fewer invasive breast cancers develop. Most of the invasive cancers that do occur are detected at surveillance mammography and will probably be small, subclinical, of early stage, and cured by further treatment (mastectomy, endocrine therapy, or chemotherapy, or a combination thereof). Having a recurrence of any type will not strike most women as a trivial risk, but they will need to be carefully counselled about their risk-benefit profile, especially because patients randomised to radiotherapy in the UZ/ANZ DCIS trial had an increase in death from cardiovascular disease (P=0.008), although numbers were small.[16]

Tamoxifen

Two large RCTs have looked at using tamoxifen in addition to radiotherapy after breast conserving surgery. Neither trial tested oestrogen receptor (ER) status at the time of diagnosis, so trial entrants were both ER positive and negative. The NSABP B-24 trial found that the addition of tamoxifen to radiotherapy decreased subsequent invasive cancer from 7% to 4% at five years.[20] This effect was maximal in younger women (<50) and at retrospective review was shown to be of benefit only in ER positive cases.[21] At long

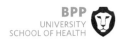

RISK FACTORS FOR RECURRENCE OF DUCTAL CARCINOMA IN SITU

- Involved or close (<1 mm) excision margins after breast conserving surgery
- High grade or poorly differentiated disease
- Comedo necrosis
- Younger age at diagnosis (<40 years)
- Oestrogen receptor negative disease
- Symptomatic presentation

---

term review, the addition of tamoxifen to radiotherapy reduced recurrence of an invasive tumour in the ipsilateral breast (at median follow-up of 163 months) by 32% (0.68, 0.49 to 0.95; P=0.025).[19] The UK/ANZ DCIS trial showed that tamoxifen reduced recurrent ipsilateral DCIS (0.70, 0.51 to 0.86; P=0.003) and contralateral tumours (0.44, 0.25 to 0.77; P=0.005), but it did not show a significant effect on ipsilateral invasive disease (0.95, 0.66 to 1.38; P=0.8), at a median follow-up of 12.7 years.[16] However, the ER status of these patients was unknown. In this trial tamoxifen was more effective in low grade and intermediate grade tumours than in high grade ones; this is probably because low grade DCIS tends to be nearly 100% ER positive, with only 60% of high grade cases expressing ER.[22] The UK/ANZ DCIS trial authors suggested that the variation in findings between the two trials may have resulted from around 34% of women in the NSABP B-24 trial being under 50 years,[20] whereas more than 90% of women in the UK trial were over 50.[16] Tamoxifen had no significant effects on mortality in either trial.

The IBIS-II study and the NSABP B-35 trial are investigating the use of aromatase inhibitors as adjuvant treatment in DCIS. The MAP.3 trial, which looked at the aromatase inhibitor exemestane as preventive treatment in postmenopausal women, showed that exemestane reduced the number of further breast events in women who had undergone mastectomy for DCIS, although the numbers of events were small.[23]

What is the potential of DCIS to become invasive, and could we be overtreating it?

Pure DCIS poses no threat to life. The goal of treating DCIS is to prevent invasive cancer. The introduction of national breast screening programmes was partly based on the premise that the detection and treatment of DCIS would, after a lag phase, result in a decrease in the incidence of invasive breast cancer. However, such a decrease has not occurred,[24] and this has led to speculation that we may be overtreating women with low risk DCIS that may never progress to invasive disease or pose a threat to life. It has been suggested that DCIS should be reclassified as a "ductal intraepithelial neoplasia,"[25] to distance it from invasive disease. This has not been generally adopted. An investigator initiated clinical trial studying the effect of preoperative endocrine treatment in DCIS found marked morphological changes, decreased proliferation, and changes in protein expression in DCIS after neoadjuvant endocrine treatment. The authors suggested that selected cases of DCIS could be treated by endocrine therapy alone (if ER positive)[26] or even "watchful waiting" with no intervention at all.[24]

This hypothesis is backed up by the previously discussed study on atypical ductal hyperplasia, which showed that this disease (and by implication, low grade DCIS) has become less common since women stopped using hormone replacement therapy.[8] Low grade DCIS is highly oestrogen dependent and unlikely to progress to invasive disease once the oestrogenic drive is removed, either postmenopausally or by the use of aromatase inhibitors. Postmenopausal women comprise the bulk of the screening population, and the recent MAP.3 trial suggests that exemestane reduces the development of DCIS in a prevention setting.[23] It is ER positive cases of low risk DCIS that, in theory, may not need surgical treatment. However, accurate and confident definition of these "low risk" groups, if they exist, is still elusive and the existing evidence shows that overall invasive recurrence rates are as high as 10-20% after surgery alone at 15 years.[16] [19]

ER negative DCIS has a higher recurrence rate and is not affected by endocrine treatment, so effective local control is essential. There tends to be receptor preservation between DCIS and its subsequent recurrence. ER negative DCIS tends to recur as ER negative DCIS or ER negative invasive disease. This has implications when considering adjuvant treatment and reducing the risk of recurrence. If ER negative DCIS recurs as invasive cancer it invariably needs chemotherapy.

Genotyping might help identify high risk and low risk patients, as it does for invasive disease. Genomic Health has recently released the Oncotype DX Breast Cancer Assay for DCIS—an assay of 21 cancer related genes—which they state can estimate the likelihood of local recurrence (DCIS or invasive carcinoma) at 10 years (www.oncotypedx.com/en-US/Breast/HealthcareProfessional/DCIS.aspx). Its clinical applicability will become apparent only with time.

Which women are at risk of recurrence after treatment for DCIS?

After a diagnosis of DCIS, NICE guidance suggests that patients should be offered annual mammography for five years (or until they reach screening age) and then return to the national screening programme.[11]

After mastectomy the risk of recurrence is low, at about 1%, although ipsilateral recurrences are mostly invasive disease. This is probably because follow-up imaging is not routinely performed on the ipsilateral side after mastectomy, so any skin flap or chest wall disease is seen only when it becomes palpable, at which point it is likely to be invasive.

The overall risk after wide local excision alone with no attention to margin status is higher, at about 25%.[15] [27]

Score	1	2	3
Size (mm)	≤15	16-40	>40
Margin (mm)	≥10	1-9	<1
Class	Grade 1/2 no necrosis	Grade 1/2 no necrosis	Grade 3
Age (years)	>60	40-60	<40

Scores for each category are added up to give an overall score from 3 to 12, which is then referenced to a recurrence prediction and management suggestion table

Score	Treatment
4-6	Wide local excision
7: margins ≥3 mm	Wide local excision
7: margins <3 mm	Wide local excision and radiotherapy
8: margins ≥3 mm	Wide local excision and radiotherapy
8: margins <3 mm	Mastectomy
9: margins ≥5 mm	Wide local excision and radiotherapy
9: margins <5 mm	Mastectomy
10-12	Mastectomy

Fig 3 Van Nuys prognostic index

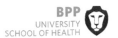

Recurrences are split equally between further DCIS and invasive disease. The woman's individual risk of recurrence—most importantly invasive recurrence and subsequent risk of death—should guide any offers of adjuvant treatments after breast conserving surgery.

Key risk factors for recurrence have been identified in the main RCTs in DCIS. The most important and modifiable risk factor is involved margins at breast conserving surgery and failure to remove all suspicious microcalcifications. Younger age at diagnosis (<40 years), high grade disease, and the presence of comedo necrosis are also important[15] [20] [27] [28] [29] (box). The University of Southern California/Van Nuys prognostic index is an American scoring system that brings together some of these risk factors. It was designed to achieve a less than 20% recurrence rate at 12 years (fig 3).[30] It has not yet been independently validated, however, and its effect on a UK screening population, where most tumours are small (<2 cm), is limited. It has not been shown to be prognostic for this screen detected population,[31] so its use is not encouraged in these patients.[31]

Breast cancer stem cells could contribute to recurrence of DCIS. These cells can self renew, proliferate, and avoid apoptosis. Aberrant activation of cell signalling pathways involved in stem cell self renewal (such as the Notch protein) might contribute to the recurrence of DCIS by allowing the cells to survive and proliferate.[32] These pathways are also under investigation as potential therapeutic targets.

What is the psychosocial impact of a diagnosis of DCIS?

The perceived risk of recurrence after treatment for DCIS is often higher than the actual risk. A study of 487 women with DCIS, treated with both mastectomy and breast conserving surgery, showed that 39% of women thought they had at least a moderate (25-30%) likelihood of developing invasive cancer in the next five years and 28% thought there was a moderate likelihood of DCIS spreading to other parts of their body.[33] A recent descriptive qualitative study highlighted that women can find it especially difficult to accept the perceived paradox between having a "precancerous" condition and the extensive surgery that is sometimes needed. Women more easily accepted the need for wide local excision than for mastectomy.[34] In the same study, some of the women did not like the term "precancerous"—they found it unhelpful and thought that it lessened the importance of the diagnosis. Women also found the need to continually justify having their treatment to themselves and others and found it difficult to explain their diagnosis.[34] This is an area where the support, counselling, and information provided by breast care nurses is invaluable.

The potential of audit data to inform future practice

The Sloane project is a prospective UK based audit on screen detected DCIS, lobular carcinoma in situ, atypical ductal hyperplasia, and atypical lobular hyperplasia. The main aim of the project is to record the current management of non-invasive breast disease and atypical hyperplasia in the UK by collecting information on the radiological and pathological features of cases, surgical and adjuvant treatment, and recurrences. It will hopefully help to answer questions about the diagnosis, treatment, and clinical outcomes of these diseases. It is the largest audit of its kind, and currently 10 732 cases have been submitted by participating UK breast screening units. Although the addition of new cases is anticipated to end in April 2012, the collection of data on future events for cases already in the audit will hopefully continue into the foreseeable future.

What does the future hold?

There is no agreed practice in the UK or elsewhere for the use of radiotherapy or tamoxifen after breast conserving surgery for DCIS, so there is no clear standard of care. Two very different approaches could potentially be considered—evidence suggests that all women benefit from radiotherapy after breast conserving surgery, yet some experts suggest that we should be considering (at the most extreme) "watchful waiting." Current practice seems to be somewhere in the middle, with patients being offered surgery, and to a variable and unstandardised extent, radiotherapy and tamoxifen. We urgently need to be able to distinguish between "low risk" women who could be safely treated with surgical excision alone, hormonal therapy alone, or possibly "watchful waiting" and "high risk" patients who need all available adjuvant treatment. This can be achieved only with a randomised controlled trial of active treatment versus active monitoring, stratified according to DCIS grade. Women with DCIS should therefore have the option of entering into high quality randomised controlled trials that will help to determine optimum treatment.

We thank the Sloane Project management team for up to date information on the Sloane Project numbers. JRY acknowledges NHS funding to the NIHR Biomedical Research Centre. NJB acknowledges funding from the NIHR Programme and Cancer Research UK.

Contributors: NLPB planned and drafted the article, JLO and JRY revised the article, and NJB planned and revised the article. NLPB is guarantor.

Funding: None received.

Competing interests: All authors have completed the ICMJE uniform disclosure form at www.icmje.org/coi_disclosure.pdf (available on request from the corresponding author) and declare: no support from any organisation for the submitted work; no financial relationships with any organisations that might have an interest in the submitted work in the previous three years; no other relationships or activities that could appear to have influenced the submitted work.

Provenance and peer review: Not commissioned; externally peer reviewed.

1 NHS cancer screening programmes. All breast cancer report. An analysis of all symptomatic and screen detected breast cancers diagnosed in 2006. NHS breast screening programme Oct 2009.
2 NHS Breast Screening Programme. Pathology reporting of breast disease. National Pathology Co-ordinating Group. Publication no 58, 2005.
3 Hwang ES, DeVries S, Chew KL, Moore DH 2nd, Kerlikowske K, Thor A, et al. Patterns of chromosomal alterations in breast ductal carcinoma in situ. Clin Cancer Res2004;10:5160-7.
4 Claus EB, Stowe M, Carter D. Breast carcinoma in situ: risk factors and screening patterns. J Natl Cancer Inst 2001;93:1811-7.
5 Claus EB, Petruzella S, Matloff E, Carter D. Prevalence of BRCA1 and BRCA2 mutations in women diagnosed with ductal carcinoma in situ. JAMA2005;293:964-9.
6 Chlebowski RT, Hendrix SL, Langer RD, Stefanick ML, Gass M, Lane D, et al; WHI Investigators. Influence of estrogen plus progestin on breast cancer and mammography in healthy postmenopausal women: the Women's Health Initiative Randomized Trial. JAMA2003;289:3243-53.
7 Beral V; Million Women Study Collaborators. Breast cancer and hormone-replacement therapy in the Million Women Study. Lancet2003;362:419-27.
8 Menes TS, Kerlikowske K, Jaffer S, Seger D, Miglioretti DL. Rates of atypical ductal hyperplasia have declined with less use of postmenopausal hormone treatment: findings from the Breast Cancer Surveillance Consortium. Cancer Epidemiol Biomarkers Prev2009;18:2822-8.
9 Pappo I, Wasserman I, Halevy A. Ductal carcinoma in situ of the breast in men: a review. Clin Breast Cancer2005;6:310-4.
10 Brennan ME, Turner RM, Ciatto S, Marinovich ML, French JR, Macaskill P, et al. Ductal carcinoma in situ at core-needle biopsy: meta-analysis of underestimation and predictors of invasive breast cancer. Radiology2011;260:119-28.
11 National Institute for Health and Clinical Excellence. Early and locally advanced breast cancer diagnosis and treatment. CG80. 2009. www.nice.org.uk/CG80.

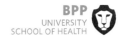

TIPS FOR NON-SPECIALISTS

- Refer patients with persistent eczematous changes of the nipple to a breast clinic for exclusion of Paget's disease of the nipple
- Stress to the patient that a diagnosis of pure ductal carcinoma in situ (DCIS) has no direct impact on mortality
- Medically fit women who need a mastectomy for DCIS are often excellent candidates for immediate reconstruction, which should be offered to all appropriate patients
- Women may be confused about their optimum treatment. Explain treatment options and up to date research findings carefully, taking time to ensure that the patient understands
- Inclusion in ongoing clinical trials should be offered to all suitable patients

QUESTIONS FOR FUTURE RESEARCH

- How can we identify women with "low risk" disease who do not need treatment and those at "high risk" who need maximal treatment?
- Can genotyping of ductal carcinoma in situ (DCIS) help predict risk of progression to invasive disease or recurrence after initial treatment?
- Will magnetic resonance imaging aid diagnosis and follow-up of patients with DCIS?
- Can ductoscopy be used in the diagnosis and treatment of DCIS?

ONGOING RESEARCH

- IBIS-II trial: Investigating the benefit of tamoxifen versus the aromatase inhibitor anastrozole (or placebo) in postmenopausal women after breast conserving surgery for ductal carcinoma in situ (DCIS) (in active follow-up)
- ICICLE trial: Trying to identify genes that increase the risk of developing DCIS in addition to which women with DCIS are at risk of developing invasive disease if left untreated
- NSABP B-35 trial: Comparing anastrozole with tamoxifen for postmenopausal women with DCIS after lumpectomy and radiotherapy (in active follow-up)
- NSABP B-43 trial: Comparing trastuzumab (Herceptin) with radiotherapy or radiotherapy alone for women with HER2 positive DCIS treated by lumpectomy (still recruiting)
- The Memorial Sloan-Kettering Cancer Centre (USA) is conducting a trial of breast magnetic resonance imaging as a preoperative tool for DCIS
- The National Cancer Institute in France is evaluating the diagnostic performance of magnetic resonance imaging with or without biopsy to optimise the resection of DCIS
- The Mayo Clinic (USA) is looking at molecular breast imaging in patients with suspected DCIS
- The National Cancer Institute/University of Pennsylvania is undertaking a phase I/II study of vaccines made from the patient's white blood cells mixed with peptides (which may help the body mount an effective immune response against tumour cells) in patients with DCIS

ADDITIONAL EDUCATIONAL RESOURCES

Resources for healthcare professionals

- The Sloane Project (www.sloaneproject.co.uk)—UK wide prospective audit of screen detected non-invasive and atypical hyperplasia of the breast
- National Institute for Health State of the Science Conference on Diagnosis and Management of DCIS report 2009 (www.consensus.nih.gov)—Summary statement from the meeting
- 2009 National Institutes for Health state-of-the-science meeting on ductal carcinoma in situ: management and diagnosis. *J Natl Cancer Inst Monogr* 2010;41:111-222
- Goodwin A, Parker S, Ghersi D, Wilcken N. Post-operative radiotherapy for ductal carcinoma in situ of the breast. *Cochrane Database Syst Rev* 2009;21:CD000563

Resources for patients

- National Breast and Ovarian Cancer Centre. Understanding ductal carcinoma in situ (DCIS) and deciding about treatment (www.psych.usyd.edu.au/cemped/docs/dcisgw.pdf)—A communication aid booklet for women with DCIS
- Health Talk On Line (www.healthtalkonline.org)—Large database of patient interviews, where real patients talk about their experiences in dealing with a wide range of health topics including DCIS
- MacMillan Cancer Support (www.macmillan.org.uk)—Comprehensive website of cancer information and support
- Cancer Prevention Institute of California (www.dcis.info)—Information on DCIS

12 Tang S, Twelves D, Isacke C, Gui G. Mammary ductoscopy in the current management of breast disease. *Surg Endosc* 2010;25:1712-22.
13 Lehman CD. Magnetic resonance imaging in the evaluation of ductal carcinoma in situ. *J Natl Cancer Monogr* 2010;2010:150-1.
14 Bijker N, Meijnen P, Peterse JL, Bogaerts J, Van Hoorebeeck I, Julien JP, et al. Breast-conserving treatment with or without radiotherapy in ductal carcinoma in situ: ten-year results of EORTC randomized phase III trial 10853. *J Clin Oncol* 2006;243:381-7.
15 Fisher ER, Dignam J, Tan-Chiu E, Costantino J, Fisher B, Paik S, et al. Pathologic findings from the National Surgical Adjuvant Breast Project (NSABP) eight year update of protocol B17: intraductal carcinoma. *Cancer* 1999;86:429-38.
16 Cuzick J, Sestaka I, Pinder SE, Ellis IO, Forsyth S, Bundred NJ, et al. Effect of tamoxifen and radiotherapy in women with locally excised ductal carcinoma in situ: long-term results from the UK/ANZ DCIS trial. *Lancet Oncol* 2010;12:21-9.
17 Emdin SO, Granstrand B, Ringberg A, Sandelin K, Arnesson LG, Nordgren H, et al. SweDCIS: radiotherapy after sector resection for ductal carcinoma in situ of the breast. Results of a randomised trial in a population offered mammography screening. *Acta Oncol* 2006;45:536-43.
18 Goodwin A, Parker S, Ghersi D, Wilcken N. Post-operative radiotherapy for ductal carcinoma in situ of the breast. *Cochrane Database Syst Rev* 2009;21:CD000563.
19 Wapnir IL, Dignam JJ, Fisher B, Mamounas EP, Anderson JJ, Julien TB, et al. Long-term outcomes of invasive ipsilateral breast tumor recurrences after lumpectomy in NSABP B-17 and B-24 randomized clinical trials for DCIS. *J Natl Cancer Inst* 2011;103:478-88.
20 Fisher B, Dignam J, Wolmark N, Wickerman DC, Fisher ER, Mamounas EP, et al. Tamoxifen in the treatment of intraductal breast cancer: national surgical adjuvant breast and bowel project B-24 randomised controlled trial. *Lancet* 1999;353:1993-2000.
21 Allred DC, Bryant J, Land S, Paik S, Fisher E, Julien T, et al. Estrogen receptor expression as a predictive marker of the effectiveness of tamoxifen in the treatment of intraductal breast cancer: findings of the NSABP protocol B-24 [abstract]. *Breast Cancer Res Treat* 2002;76(suppl 1):S36.
22 Barnes NL, Boland GP, Davenport A, Knox WF, Bundred NJ. Relationship between hormone receptor status and tumour size, grade and comedo necrosis in ductal carcinoma in situ. *Br J Surg* 2005;92:429-34.
23 Goss PE, Ingle JN, Alés-Martínez JE, Cheung AM, Chlebowski RT, Wactanski-Wende J, et al; NCIC CTG MAP.3 Study Investigators. Exemestane for breast-cancer prevention in postmenopausal women. *N Engl J Med* 2011;364:2381-91.
24 Ozanne EM, Shieh Y, Barnes J, Bouzan C, Hwang ES, Esserman LJ. Characterizing the impact of 25 years of DCIS treatment. *Breast Cancer Res Treat* 2011;129:165-73.
25 Graff S. Ductal carcinoma in situ: should the name be changed? *J Natl Cancer Inst* 2010;102:6-8.
26 Chen YY, DeVries S, Anderson J, Lessing J, Swain R, Cin K, et al. Pathologic and biologic response to preoperative endocrine therapy in patients with ER-positive ductal carcinoma in situ. *BMC Cancer* 2009;9:285.
27 Julien J, Bijker N, Fentiman I, Peterse JL, Delledonne V, Rouanet P, et al. Radiotherapy in breast-conserving treatment for ductal carcinoma in situ: first results of the EORTC randomized phase III trial 10853. *Lancet* 2000;355:528-33.
28 Bijker N, Peterse JL, Duchateau L, Julien JP, Fentiman IS, Duval C, et al. Risk factors for recurrence and metastasis after breast conserving therapy for ductal carcinoma in situ: analysis of EORTC trial. *J Clin Oncol* 2001;19:2263-71.
29 Houghton J, George WD, Cuzick J, Duggan C, Fentiman IS, Spittle M. Radiotherapy and tamoxifen in women with completely excised ductal carcinoma in situ of the breast in the UK, Australia, and New Zealand: randomised controlled trial. *Lancet* 2003;362:95-102.
30 Silverstein MJ, Lagios MD. Choosing treatment for patients with DCIS: fine tuning the University of Southern California/Van-Nuys prognostic index. *J Natl Cancer Inst Monogr* 2010;41:193-6.
31 Boland GP, Chan KC, Knox WF, Roberts SA, Bundred NJ. Value of the Van Nuys prognostic index in prediction of recurrence o ductal carcinoma in situ after breast-conserving surgery. *Br J Surg* 2003;90:426-32.
32 Harrison H, Farnie G, Howell SJ, Rock RE, Stylianou S, Brennan KR, et al. Regulation of breast cancer stem cell activity by signaling through the Notch4 receptor. *Cancer Res* 2010;70:709-18.
33 Partridge A, Adloff K, Blood E, Dees EC, Kaelin C, Golshan M, et al. Risk perceptions and psychosocial outcomes of women with ductal carcinoma in situ: longitudinal results from a cohort study. *J Natl Cancer Inst* 2008;100:243-51.
34 Kennedy F, Harcourt D, Rumsey N. The shifting nature of women's experiences and perceptions of ductal carcinoma in situ. *Journal of Advanced Nursing* 2012;68:856-67.

Related links

bmj.com
- Managing retinal vein occlusion (2012;344:e499)
- New recreational drugs and the primary care approach to patients who use them (2012;344:e288)
- Diagnosis and management of Raynaud's phenomenon (2012;344:e289)
- Improving healthcare access for people with visual impairment and blindness (2012;344:e542)

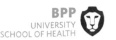

Management of breast cancer—Part I

Nicholas C Turner oncologist [1,2], Alison L Jones oncologist[1,3]

[3]University College London Hospitals NHS Foundation Trust, London

[1]Department of Medical Oncology, Royal Free Hospital NHS Foundation Trust, London NW3 2QG

[2]Breakthrough Breast Cancer Research Centre, Institute of Cancer Research, London

Correspondence to: A L Jones alison.jones@royalfree.nhs.uk

Cite this as: BMJ 2008;337:a421

<DOI> 10.1136/bmj.a421
http://www.bmj.com/content/337/bmj.a421

Breast cancer remains the second most common cause of cancer related death in women in the United Kingdom, with over 12000 deaths a year. However, substantial progress is being made: deaths from breast cancer in the Western world have fallen by over 25% in the past two decades,[1] reflecting substantial improvements in management (fig 1). Incidence in Great Britain has risen by 50% over the past three decades, reflecting not only changes in population demographics and environmental factors but also an increase in diagnosis as a result of screening. Over a similar time period mortality has fallen.

We review here the recent advances in the prevention, screening, and treatment of breast cancer and the recent efforts to individualise treatment. The review is published in two parts; in the second part we will review advances in the systemic treatment of breast cancer and how an increasing understanding of the biology of breast cancer is beginning to change the way we treat the disease.

Primary prevention

What risk factors may be avoidable?

Progress in primary prevention has come from improved understanding of the causes of breast cancer; identification of modifiable risk factors such as avoidance of post-menopausal obesity, increased exercise, reducing alcohol intake; and encouragement to breast feed (see www.breakthrough.org.uk and www.cancer.gov, which review these issues comprehensively). No conclusive evidence exists of risk from specific dietary components,[2] such as dairy products and fat, other than that mediated through the link with obesity. Similarly, randomised studies examining reduced dietary fat in secondary prevention, after treatment for early breast cancer, have found no consistent effect on recurrence of breast cancer.[3] [4]

SOURCES AND SELECTION CRITERIA

We obtained references from PubMed after searching with the term "breast cancer" and limiting our search to clinical trials. All reductions in risk are quoted as relative risk reductions unless otherwise stated.

SUMMARY POINTS

- Breast cancer mortality is falling in the Western world as a result of advances in treatment, but it remains a leading cause of death owing to the high and increasing incidence

- Several risk factors may present opportunities to lower risk, such as prolonged use of combined hormone replacement therapy and lifestyle factors

- Tamoxifen or raloxifene taken for five years prevents a third of breast cancers, but with no evidence of a reduction in deaths from breast cancer

- For women at high risk of breast cancer, screening with magnetic resonance imaging is significantly more sensitive than mammography

- Advances in surgery continue to decrease morbidity through use of sentinel lymph node biopsy and oncoplastic surgery

- Adjuvant radiotherapy for many women can now be given over shorter periods, with similar efficacy and side effects

---

Prolonged exposure to exogenous oestrogen has now been confirmed as a risk factor for post-menopausal women. The women's health initiative, followed by the million women study, confirmed that hormone replacement therapy with combined oestrogen and progestogen doubled the risk of breast cancer,[5] whereas oestrogen-only therapy increased the risk by 30%.[5] The use of combined therapy represents a potentially key modifiable factor, and in the United States the incidence of breast cancer fell significantly after many women stopped taking long term hormone replacement therapy.[6]

Interest has been expressed in the interaction between environmental risk factors and genetic predisposition.[7] Some risk factors probably have a higher impact in some genetic backgrounds than in others. Large cohort studies are under way that will help identify these interactions, including the UK breakthrough generations study (www.breakthroughgenerations.org.uk).

Can drugs be used to prevent breast cancer?

On the basis of the evidence linking cumulative oestrogen exposure to breast cancer, randomised studies of chemoprevention were started over 20 years ago, initially with tamoxifen, a selective oestrogen receptor modulator. These studies recruited women considered to be at higher risk of developing breast cancer because of their family history or their Gail risk score (a score of risk of breast cancer). They found that tamoxifen taken for five to eight years reduced the risk of developing invasive breast cancer by 38%.[8] Whether this would also apply to women without risk factors is less clear. Another selective oestrogen receptor modulator, raloxifene, was noted to reduce the risk of breast cancer in women not selected for breast cancer risk, in a study of osteoporosis treatment.[9] A subsequent randomised trial of nearly 20000 post-menopausal women at risk of breast cancer found that the preventive effect of raloxifene was similar to that of tamoxifen.[10]

Despite the reduction in breast cancer incidence with tamoxifen and raloxifene, there has been no improvement in breast cancer specific mortality or in overall survival,[8] [10] although these studies were not powered to detect a small effect on mortality.[8] Tamoxifen was associated with side effects with a small increase in the incidence of endometrial cancer, venous thromboembolism, stroke, and cataracts; however, these were less frequent with raloxifene[10] and are uncommon in younger women. The failure to improve survival may reflect the types of cancer prevented by selective oestrogen receptor modulators (only the less aggressive oestrogen receptor positive breast cancers,[8] many of which would have been cured on presentation). These limited benefits with selective oestrogen receptor modulators have led to their approval for breast cancer prevention in the United States but not in Europe. The preventive effects of aromatase inhibitors are currently being examined in the second international breast cancer intervention study (IBIS II).

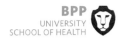
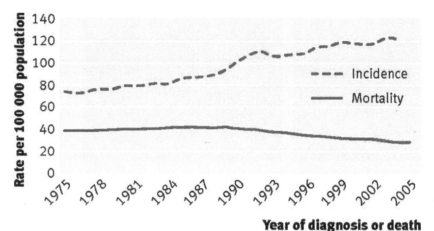

Fig 1 Age standardised (European) incidence and mortality rates of breast cancer in women in Great Britain, 1975-2005. Adapted from Cancer Research UK (http://info.cancerresearchuk.org/cancerstats/types/breast/)

What evidence exists for prevention in high risk groups?

Women with germline mutations in the genes BRCA1 and BRCA2 have a lifetime risk of developing breast cancer of up to 80%, and advances in breast cancer genetics have led to the recent identification of several new predisposition genes.[11] In addition, women who received thoracic irradiation for Hodgkin's disease after menarche and before age 30 have a substantial increased risk of breast cancer.[12] Whether the preventive strategies discussed above reduce risk for high risk groups (especially those with different genetic backgrounds) is uncertain.

Preventive strategies that have been investigated specifically in women with mutations of the genes BRCA1 and BRCA2 include:

- Tamoxifen: insufficient women with BRCA1 and BRCA2 mutations were included in the tamoxifen studies for meaningful conclusions to be drawn.[13] No data have been reported with raloxifene
- Bilateral oophorectomy, as well as reducing risk of ovarian cancer by up to 85% reduces the risk of breast cancer by 50%.[14]
- Bilateral risk reducing mastectomy cuts the risk of breast cancer by 90%[15] (some breast tissue is left behind after mastectomy).

Recently the uptake of these strategies has been reported in a study of over 2600 women with BRCA1 and BRCA2 mutations from nine different countries at a median of 3.9 years after genetic testing: 57% of women had a prophylactic oophorectomy, 18% had a risk reducing mastectomy, and 9% (who had not had a risk reducing mastectomy) had hormonal chemoprevention.[16] Just under half of women with known BRCA1 and BRCA2 mutations had not taken up a preventive strategy and relied on radiological screening alone.

Screening

How beneficial is mammography?

A Cochrane review concluded that mammographic screening reduces the risk of dying of breast cancer by about 15%,[17] at the expense of a 30% increase in diagnosis. About 2000 women need to be screened for 10 years to prevent a single death from breast cancer.[17] Over the same period 10 women will be diagnosed with breast cancer that would otherwise have remained clinically occult, never to be diagnosed. However, no consensus exists over the benefit of mammographic screening, and other analyses have

concluded that mammography is more effective than the Cochrane review suggested, and these quote reductions in mortality of up to 35%.[18] Across Europe and the United States no consensus exists on the age for starting screening or on frequency.

Is magnetic resonance imaging an advance on mammography?

Contrast enhanced magnetic resonance imaging has been shown to be more sensitive than mammography in detecting invasive breast cancers in high risk populations.[14] In the UK MARIBS study of women with a strong family history of breast cancer, the sensitivity of annual mammography was estimated at 40%, compared with 77% for magnetic resonance imaging and 94% for combined magnetic resonance imaging and mammography.[19] Concerns have been expressed about the specificity of magnetic resonance imaging (83% alone and 77% for combined, compared with 93% for mammography).[19] Magnetic resonance imaging is also more sensitive at identifying the non-invasive early stages of breast cancer (ductal carcinoma in situ); in one study it detected 92% of cases before surgery whereas mammography detected 56%.[20]

In the UK, the National Institute for Health and Clinical Excellence (NICE) has advised annual screening with magnetic resonance imaging for high risk women from age 30 (or age 20 with germline P53 mutations).[14] Magnetic resonance imaging for breast screening, however, presents substantial financial and resource concerns, which have yet to be fully resolved in the UK. Moreover, the impact on breast cancer mortality of screening with magnetic resonance imaging is unknown.

Local treatment of early stage disease

The diagnosis of breast cancer by triple assessment (clinical, radiological, and pathological, increasingly with core biopsy) is established in the context of multidisciplinary management. Magnetic resonance imaging is useful in selected cases to define tumour extent, especially in invasive lobular breast cancer, and to detect multifocal disease before surgery and assess the contralateral breast (fig 2). Functional imaging with positron emission tomography using fluorodeoxyglucose (FDG-PET) is accepted in the staging of many cancers but is not routinely used in breast cancer at diagnosis.

How is surgery for breast cancer advancing?

Recent advances in surgery have focused on reducing morbidity. Breast conserving surgery by wide local excision is the preferred option, with mastectomy predominantly reserved for tumours not suitable for wide local excision and for patients who request it. In selected cases where breast conserving surgery is not possible, neoadjuvant chemotherapy or hormone therapy may be used to "downstage" the tumour, thus potentially allowing conservative surgery (fig 2).

Sentinel lymph node biopsy

At surgery the axillary nodes are dissected to provide prognostic information that will guide adjuvant therapy and to achieve local control. Biopsy of the sentinel lymph node is accepted as the standard of care in early breast cancer, with removal of the first lymph node or nodes that drain the tumour. The decision to proceed to a full axillary clearance can potentially be made during surgery with touch imprint cytology, fresh frozen section histology, or with molecular

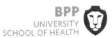

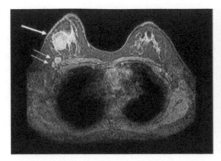
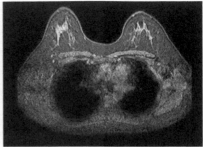

Fig 2 Contrast enhanced magnetic resonance scan of the breast. Left: At presentation from a 39 year old woman with a 3 cm breast cancer in the right upper outer quadrant (large arrow) with two involved lymph nodes (small arrows). Right: Same woman after neoadjuvant chemotherapy. Surgical pathology tests confirmed a pathologically complete remission

polymerase chain reaction assays such as the GeneSearch BLN Assay (Veridex, USA).[21] Sentinel lymph node biopsy is safe, with a false negative rate of less than 10% and reduced arm morbidity and hospital stay compared with full axillary clearance.[22] Current research is evaluating the role of complete axillary clearance versus radiotherapy after a positive sentinel lymph node biopsy. In addition, uncertainty remains over the correct management of micrometastases (metastases less than 2 mm) and isolated tumour cells in the biopsy, which by themselves do not alter prognosis.

Endoscopic assisted surgery

Endoscopic removal of axillary nodes and endoscopic mastectomy have been examined in small series with encouraging reports of improved morbidity.[23] Currently the evidence is insufficiently robust to advocate widespread use of these techniques outside clinical trials or specialist centres. Nipple endoscopy is finding a role in the investigation of nipple discharge.

Minimally invasive techniques

Percutaneous ablation of small (generally less than 3 cm) breast tumours has been examined with radiofrequency ablation, laser therapy, and cryotherapy. Insufficient evidence exists of the effectiveness of these techniques for use outside a research setting.

Oncoplastic surgery

Reconstruction of the breast with better implants and reconstructive surgical techniques continues to improve the cosmetic results of mastectomy. Immediate reconstruction is often feasible, although many centres prefer to delay reconstruction until after adjuvant radiotherapy if that is required. The overlying skin and nipple can be spared in selected cases of ductal carcinoma in situ and small cancers.[24] In addition, there are several new approaches to performing oncoplastic procedures after breast conserving surgery.

Improvements in adjuvant radiotherapy

After breast conserving surgery all women require breast radiotherapy, which reduces local recurrence rates from 26% to 7%.[25] Until recently, radiotherapy was given over five weeks, but long term follow-up of randomised trials has shown that accelerated hypofractionated radiotherapy (for example, 40 Gy in 15 fractions over three weeks) produces equivalent low rates of local recurrence[26] [27] without prejudicing cosmesis or late effects. Accelerated radiotherapy requires fewer visits for the patient and has substantial cost savings.

Meta-analysis of randomised trials has shown that radiotherapy after mastectomy improves survival in women with axillary node metastases,[28] and it is generally accepted that women with four or more involved nodes benefit from radiotherapy. However, since many of these trials were conducted, the risk of local recurrence has improved substantially, owing to better surgery and systemic adjuvant therapy, as well as to stage migration. The relevance, therefore, of the meta-analysis to women with one to three node involvement is less clear and is subject to ongoing randomised trials.

Current radiotherapy research is examining techniques to decrease toxicity and further accelerate treatment, with partial breast irradiation after wide local excision. Examples include:

- Intraoperative radiotherapy. Delivery of a single dose of radiotherapy during surgery to the breast cavity. Early results suggest encouragingly low recurrence rates, and large randomised studies are examining this further[29]
- Brachytherapy, most commonly with MammoSite (Hologic, USA). Delivery of a radioactive seed directly into the breast cavity via a catheter placed at surgery, typically with five to 10 days of brachytherapy. Recurrence rates are low in early clinical trials[30]
- Three dimensional conformal radiotherapy.

The evidence base for partial breast irradiation is not as strong as for conventional external beam radiotherapy and should, in general, be given in the context of a clinical trial.

We thank Katharine Piggott and Mo Keshtgar for critically reading this manuscript and the reviewers for their helpful suggestions.

Contributors: Both authors planned and wrote this review and act as guarantors.

Competing interests: ALJ has received consultancy and lecturing fees from AstraZeneca, Bristol-Myers Squibb, GlaxoSmithKline, Roche, and Sanofi-Aventis.

Provenance and peer review: Commissioned; externally peer reviewed

Patient consent obtained.

1   Peto R, Boreham J, Clarke M, Davies C, Beral V. UK and USA breast cancer deaths down 25% in year 2000 at ages 20-69 years. Lancet2000;355:1822.
2   Michels KB, Mohllajee AP, Roset-Bahmanyar E, Beehler GP, Moysich KB. Diet and breast cancer: a review of the prospective observational studies. Cancer2007;109(suppl):2712-49.
3   Chlebowski RT, Blackburn GL, Thomson CA, Nixon DW, Shapiro A, Hoy MK, et al. Dietary fat reduction and breast cancer outcome: interim efficacy results from the women's intervention nutrition study. J Natl Cancer Inst2006;98:1767-76.
4   Pierce JP, Natarajan L, Caan BJ, Parker BA, Greenberg ER, Flatt SW, et al. Influence of a diet very high in vegetables, fruit, and fiber and low in fat on prognosis following treatment for breast cancer: the women's healthy eating and living (WHEL) randomized trial. JAMA2007;298:289-98.
5   Beral V. Breast cancer and hormone-replacement therapy in the million women study. Lancet2003;362:419-27.

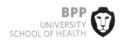

BMJ | BPP UNIVERSITY SCHOOL OF HEALTH

<table>
<tr><td>

TIPS FOR NON-SPECIALISTS

- All patients with a possible presentation of breast cancer should be referred urgently for rapid assessment in a specialist clinic. In the UK all patients referred with a breast problem should be seen by a specialist within two weeks

- Patients with a strong family history of breast and/or ovarian cancer should be referred to specialist clinics for risk and cancer genetics assessment. Local guidelines will determine referral practice

</td></tr>
</table>

<table>
<tr><td>

ADDITIONAL EDUCATIONAL RESOURCES

Resources for healthcare professionals

- See *Journal of Oncology* 2008;26:5 (http://jco.ascopubs.org/content/vol26/issue5/). A review issue devoted to in-depth discussions on the current issues of breast cancer

Resources for patients

- Breakthrough (www.breakthrough.org.uk)—Charity tackling breast cancer through research, campaigning, and education

- CancerHelp UK (www.cancerhelp.org.uk/)—The patient information website of Cancer Research UK. It provides a free information service about cancer and cancer care for people with cancer and their families

- US National Cancer Institute (www.cancer.gov/)—Provides comprehensive information about cancer for patients

</td></tr>
</table>

<table>
<tr><td>

ONGOING RESEARCH

- Large cohort studies are recruiting participants to identify new risk factors for breast cancer and to examine links between environmental factors and genetics

- Aromatase inhibitors and other agents in the prevention of breast cancer

- Appropriate management of patients after biopsy of the sentinel lymph node

- Safety and side effects of techniques for partial breast irradiation

</td></tr>
</table>

6   Heiss G, Wallace R, Anderson GL, Aragaki A, Beresford SA, Brzyski R, et al. Health risks and benefits 3 years after stopping randomized treatment with estrogen and progestin. *JAMA* 2008;299:1036-45.

7   Brohet RM, Goldgar DE, Easton DF, Antoniou AC, Andrieu N, Chang-Claude J, et al. Oral contraceptives and breast cancer risk in the international BRCA1/2 carrier cohort study: a report from EMBRACE, GENEPSO, GEO-HEBON, and the IBCCS Collaborating Group. *J Clin Oncol* 2007;25:3831-6.

8   Cuzick J, Powles T, Veronesi U, Forbes J, Edwards R, Ashley S, et al. Overview of the main outcomes in breast-cancer prevention trials. *Lancet* 2003;361:296-300.

9   Ettinger B, Black DM, Mitlak BH, Knickerbocker RK, Nickelsen T, Genant HK, et al. Reduction of vertebral fracture risk in postmenopausal women with osteoporosis treated with raloxifene: results from a 3-year randomized clinical trial. Multiple Outcomes of Raloxifene Evaluation (MORE) Investigators. *JAMA* 1999;282:637-45.

10 Vogel VG, Costantino JP, Wickerham DL, Cronin WM, Cecchini RS, Atkins JN, et al. Effects of tamoxifen vs raloxifene on the risk of developing invasive breast cancer and other disease outcomes: the NSABP study of tamoxifen and raloxifene (STAR) P-2 trial. *JAMA* 2006;295:2727-41.

11 Stratton MR, Rahman N. The emerging landscape of breast cancer susceptibility. *Nat Genet* 2008;40(1):17-22.

12 Travis LB, Hill D, Dores GM, Gospodarowicz M, van Leeuwen FE, Holowaty E, et al. Cumulative absolute breast cancer risk for young women treated for Hodgkin lymphoma. *J Natl Cancer Inst* 2005;97:1428-37.

13 King MC, Wieand S, Hale K, Lee M, Walsh T, Owens K, et al. Tamoxifen and breast cancer incidence among women with inherited mutations in BRCA1 and BRCA2: national surgical adjuvant breast and bowel project (NSABP-P1) breast cancer prevention trial. *JAMA* 2001;286:2251-6.

14 Robson M, Offit K. Clinical practice. Management of an inherited predisposition to breast cancer. *N Engl J Med* 2007;357:154-62.

15 Meijers-Heijboer H, van Geel B, van Putten WL, Henzen-Logmans SC, Seynaeve C, Menke-Pluymers MB, et al. Breast cancer after prophylactic bilateral mastectomy in women with a BRCA1 or BRCA2 mutation. *N Engl J Med* 2001;345:159-64.

16 Metcalfe KA, Birenbaum-Carmeli D, Lubinski J, Gronwald J, Lynch H, Moller P, et al. International variation in rates of uptake of preventive options in BRCA1 and BRCA2 mutation carriers. *Int J Cancer* 2008;122:2017-22.

17 Gotzsche PC, Nielsen M. Screening for breast cancer with mammography. *Cochrane Database Syst Rev* 2006(4):CD001877.

18 International Agency for Research on Cancer. *IARC Handbook of cancer prevention. Volume 7. Breast cancer screening.* Lyon, IARC, 2002.

19 Leach MO, Boggis CR, Dixon AK, Easton DF, Eeles RA, Evans DG, et al. Screening with magnetic resonance imaging and mammography of a UK population at high familial risk of breast cancer: a prospective multicentre cohort study (MARIBS). *Lancet* 2005;365:1769-78.

20 Kuhl CK, Schrading S, Bieling HB, Wardelmann E, Leutner CC, Koenig R, et al. MRI for diagnosis of pure ductal carcinoma in situ: a prospective observational study. *Lancet* 2007;370:485-92.

21 Blumencranz P, Whitworth PW, Deck K, Rosenberg A, Reintgen D, Beitsch P, et al. Scientific impact recognition award. Sentinel node staging for breast cancer: intraoperative molecular pathology overcomes conventional histologic sampling errors. *Am J Surg* 2007;194:426-32.

22 Mansel RE, Fallowfield L, Kissin M, Goyal A, Newcombe RG, Dixon JM, et al. Randomized multicenter trial of sentinel node biopsy versus standard axillary treatment in operable breast cancer: the ALMANAC trial. *J Natl Cancer Inst* 2006;98:599-609.

23 Lim SM, Lam FL. Laparoscopic-assisted axillary dissection in breast cancer surgery. *Am J Surg* 2005;190:641-3.

24 Cunnick GH, Mokbel K. Skin-sparing mastectomy. *Am J Surg* 2004;188:78-84.

25 Clarke M, Collins R, Darby S, Davies C, Elphinstone P, Evans E, et al. Effects of radiotherapy and of differences in the extent of surgery for early breast cancer on local recurrence and 15-year survival: an overview of the randomised trials. *Lancet* 2005;366:2087-106.

26 Whelan T, MacKenzie R, Julian J, Levine M, Shelley W, Grimard L, et al. Randomized trial of breast irradiation schedules after lumpectomy for women with lymph node-negative breast cancer. *J Natl Cancer Inst* 2002;94:1143-50.

27 The UK standardisation of breast radiotherapy (START) trial B of radiotherapy hypofractionation for treatment of early breast cancer: a randomised trial. *Lancet* 2008;371:1098-107.

28 Gebski V, Lagleva M, Keech A, Simes J, Langlands AO. Survival effects of postmastectomy adjuvant radiation therapy using biologically equivalent doses: a clinical perspective. *J Natl Cancer Inst* 2006;98:26-38.

29 Vaidya JS, Tobias JS, Baum M, Keshtgar M, Joseph D, Wenz F, et al. Intraoperative radiotherapy for breast cancer. *Lancet Oncol* 2004;5:165-73.

30 Benitez PR, Keisch ME, Vicini F, Stolier A, Scroggins T, Walker A, et al. Five-year results: the initial clinical trial of MammoSite balloon brachytherapy for partial breast irradiation in early-stage breast cancer. *Am J Surg* 2007;194:456-62.

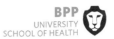

An update on the medical management of breast cancer

Belinda Yeo breast unit research fellow[1], Nicholas C Turner consultant medical oncologist[12], Alison Jones consultant medical oncologist[3]

[1]Breast Unit, Royal Marsden Hospital, London SW3 6JJ, UK

[2]Breakthrough Breast Cancer Research Centre, Institute of Cancer Research, London SW3 6JB, UK

[3]Royal Free Hospital, London NW3 2QG, UK

Corresponding authors: A Jones (Alisonjones6@nhs.net) N C Turner (nicholas.turner@icr.ac.uk)

Cite this as: BMJ 2014;348:g3608

‹DOI› 10.1136/bmj.g3608
http://www.bmj.com/content/348/bmj.g3608

Breast cancer remained the most common cancer in women in 2013 and its incidence continues to rise.[1] Nonetheless, mortality is falling, partly as a result of earlier diagnosis through mammographic screening,[2] improved surgical techniques and attention to margins, improved delivery of radiotherapy, and better adjuvant medical therapies (fig 1). Despite these improvements, breast cancer remains the second most common cause of death from cancer in women.

This review focuses on the medical treatment of breast cancer in the adjuvant and metastatic settings, with particular attention to recent advances and changes in practice since our last review in 2008.[3] [4] We discuss how targeted therapies can be used to individualise and tailor the management of breast cancer according to tumour biology and molecular subtype.

Early breast cancer

Diagnosis

Guidelines on the diagnosis of early breast cancer have changed little since our last review. Population based mammography screening for asymptomatic women is currently offered in the United Kingdom by the NHS Breast Screening Programme from age 47 to 73 years, with self referral encouraged thereafter.[2] Women or men with breast symptoms are referred urgently to local specialist breast units (under the two week rule in the UK) for rapid assessment, including clinical assessment with mammography or ultrasound (or both) and biopsy as needed (triple assessment).

Local therapy

The breast

Surgical management aims to excise invasive and non-invasive cancer with clear margins. Breast conserving surgery followed by radiotherapy has equivalent survival to mastectomy.[5] It should be offered if complete cancer

excision can be achieved with adequate margins (>1 mm) and an acceptable cosmetic outcome.[6] Mastectomy may be recommended when breast conserving surgery is not possible owing to tumour size, multifocal disease, aesthetically unfavourable ratio of breast size to tumour volume, or at the patient's request. Primary medical (neoadjuvant) therapies are increasingly given before surgery to reduce tumour size and facilitate breast conservation.

The axilla

At the time that breast cancer is diagnosed, clinical staging of the ipsilateral axilla is achieved with axillary ultrasound and cytology or core biopsy of any suspicious lymph nodes. If the axilla is clinically negative, pathological axillary staging can be achieved with sentinel lymph node biopsy (SLNB), which is usually performed at the same time as breast surgery. In the past, axillary lymph node dissection (ALND) was recommended in patients with clinically positive nodes preoperatively and those who were positive at SLNB after a negative clinical assessment. The aim of ALND was to clear additional disease, maintain effective local disease control, and assess the total nodal disease burden as a way to accurately determine prognosis and the need for adjuvant therapies.

However, these two node positive groups of patients are very different with regard to disease burden; half of patients with a positive SLNB will have no further involved axillary lymph nodes on completion ALND performed after assessment of the sentinel lymph node.[7] The Zoo11 trial has questioned whether all SLN positive axillae require completion ALND.[8] In this trial, more than 800 patients were randomised after breast conserving surgery and a positive SLNB (27% of whom had further involved lymph nodes) to either completion ALND or no further axillary surgery.[8] Adjuvant therapies were offered according to pathological staging and local protocols. No significant difference was found in the risk of local or distant relapse at 6.3 years' median follow-up between the SLNB only arm (about 27% of whom should have had further axillary disease) and the completion ALND arm.[8] It was postulated that adjuvant therapy (especially breast radiotherapy, which reaches the lower axillae) eradicates residual axillary disease.

There is no international consensus as to which patients require ALND after a positive SLNB, and recent guidelines suggest that most women with one or two positive SLNBs who are having breast conservation surgery followed by breast radiotherapy may not need ALND.[9] In addition, a recent trial that compared completion ALND with axillary radiotherapy for SLN positive axillae found that radiotherapy provided similar disease control to ALND, with less toxicity.[10]

Pathology and molecular subtyping: deciding on appropriate adjuvant therapy

The planning of adjuvant postsurgical therapy in breast cancer is dictated by the pathology report, in which tumour burden is reported by tumour and axillary nodal

---

SOURCES AND SELECTION CRITERIA

We used PubMed to identify recent published updates on the medical management of breast cancer. We also referenced presentations from international conferences and consulted with other experts in the breast cancer field.

SUMMARY POINTS

- Despite the increasing incidence of breast cancer, death rates are falling owing to earlier diagnosis, better surgical and radiotherapy techniques, and improved systemic therapies
- The best management of the axilla in clinically node negative disease is unclear
- Adjuvant decision making is driven by tumour biology, with particular attention to the distinct molecular subtypes of breast cancer
- There is substantial evidence for extended hormone therapy in premenopausal and postmenopausal women with hormone receptor positive early breast cancer
- In metastatic HER2 positive breast cancer there are now multiple lines of HER2 targeted therapies

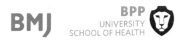

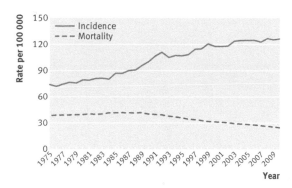

Fig 1 Incidence of breast cancer in women and mortality rates in the United Kingdom over the past 30 years. Data from Cancer Research UK[1]

status. Tumour biology is reported as histological grade, expression of the hormone receptors (oestrogen receptor and progesterone receptor), and amplification status of the *HER2* gene. These factors are combined to estimate the prognosis and hence likely benefit from adjuvant therapies, often using online web based tools, such as Adjuvant Online! or the PREDICT tool, which incorporates the proliferation marker, Ki67, in its algorithm.

Additional molecular tests can be performed to give more information on tumour biology and improve the prediction of prognosis. These tests have been driven by the recognition of distinct molecular subtypes of breast cancer (fig 2).[11] In particular, these tests can help differentiate between the two major groups of oestrogen receptor positive breast cancer—high proliferation cancers with a poor prognosis (luminal B tumours) and low proliferation cancers with a good prognosis (luminal A tumours).

The most widely used prognostic test is the Oncotype DX assay. This 21 gene assay on paraffin blocks is used to calculate a recurrence score and is currently validated in women with oestrogen receptor positive, lymph node negative cancers (fig 3). Mammaprint is another gene assay that uses 70 genes to estimate prognosis but is currently performed only on frozen material. In the UK, the National Institute for Health and Care Excellence recommends Oncotype DX to aid decisions about chemotherapy after surgery in some patients with oestrogen receptor positive, lymph node negative early breast cancer. Although these tests do not directly differentiate between luminal A and luminal B subtypes, they do assay the differences in biology that underlie these two subtypes.

Adjuvant systemic therapy in early breast cancer
Hormone treatment in the first five years
The aim of adjuvant therapy is to increase the chance of cure by eradicating micrometastatic disease. About 80% of breast cancers are oestrogen receptor positive. For these cancers, five years of adjuvant tamoxifen, a selective oestrogen receptor modulator, reduces the relative risk of relapse by 41% and death from breast cancer by 31%.[13] Tamoxifen remains the standard of care for premenopausal women.

For postmenopausal women, aromatase inhibitors have been shown to be superior to tamoxifen. Two large trials (ATAC and BIG1-98) of nearly 10 000 women compared five years of an aromatase inhibitor with five years of tamoxifen with a mean follow-up of 5.8 years. They showed a 2.9% absolute decrease in recurrence (9.6% v 12.6%; P <0.001) favouring the aromatase inhibitor arm,[14] although the absolute improvement in overall survival was small. Adverse

effects that are more common with aromatase inhibitors than with tamoxifen include hot flushes, arthralgias, and bone thinning. For patients taking aromatase inhibitors, it is important to monitor bone mineral density at baseline and every two years in the setting of osteopenia or osteoporosis, with calcium and vitamin D replacement considered in those with osteopenia, and the addition of a bisphosphonate or denosumab in those with osteoporosis.[15] Women who are premenopausal at diagnosis but later become postmenopausal (naturally or as a result of chemotherapy), benefit from switching to an aromatase inhibitor after two to three years of tamoxifen.[14]

Adjuvant hormonal therapy extended beyond five years
In oestrogen receptor positive breast cancer, as many recurrences occur after five years' follow-up as in the first five years.[16] For women who complete five years of tamoxifen and are postmenopausal, there is a 42% relative risk reduction (hazard ratio 0.57; P<0.001) with a further five years of the non-steroidal aromatase inhibitor letrozole.[17]

For women who remain premenopausal after five years of tamoxifen, or who are intolerant of aromatase inhibitors, recent evidence suggests benefit of continuing tamoxifen beyond five years. The ATLAS trial of nearly 7000 women with oestrogen receptor positive early breast cancer reported a further reduction in recurrence (617 recurrences v 711; P=0.002) and breast cancer mortality (331 deaths v 397 deaths; P=0.01) for women who continue tamoxifen to 10 years, rather than stopping at five years.[18] In a recent meta-analysis of five trials of extended adjuvant tamoxifen (>20 000 women), the absolute risk reduction was 2.1% in lymph node negative (number needed to treat 49) and 4.1% in lymph node positive (25) patients.[19] The risk of endometrial cancer was increased during years 5-14 in women who continued tamoxifen compared with those who stopped after five years (3.1% v 1.6%).[18]

Similar results were seen in the ATTom trial of 6953 women.[20] Pooled data from the ATLAS and ATTom trials confirm that, compared with no endocrine therapy, 10 years of adjuvant tamoxifen reduces death from breast cancer by one third in the first 10 years of follow-up, with a continued benefit beyond 10 years.[20] Continued adjuvant endocrine therapy for 10 years has become a standard option, especially for women who originally had node positive breast cancer.

Chemotherapy
Combination adjuvant chemotherapy reduces the relative risk of death from breast cancer by about a third,[21] with the absolute risk reduction depending on the risk of relapse. However, in many patients who receive adjuvant chemotherapy, the improvement in survival is small, because their chance of being cured by surgery and hormone therapy alone is high. Selection of which patients actually need chemotherapy is a major area of research. Molecular tests such as Oncotype DX improve the prediction of prognosis and can help identify which patients are likely to be cured by hormone therapy and surgery alone. However, many patients achieve an intermediate result with these molecular tests, and the management of these women is the subject of large trials that have completed accrual but are yet to report (TAILORx (NCT00310180) and MINDACT (NCT00433589)). Recent studies have also examined how morbidity from chemotherapy can be reduced by refining chemotherapy schedules,[22] and such schedules are

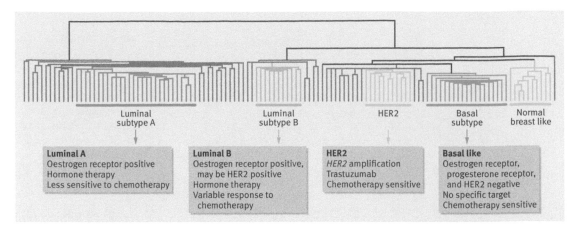

Fig 2 The three major molecular subtypes of breast cancer: luminal-type (subtype A and B), *HER2* amplified, and basal-like. Luminal-type breast cancers express the oestrogen receptor and related genes and can be targeted with hormonal therapies. Subtype A may be less sensitive to chemotherapy and less aggressive than subtype B. HER2 breast cancers are characterised by overexpression of the growth factor receptor HER2, with amplification of the *HER2* gene. They are more aggressive than HER2 negative breast cancers, but can be targeted with the monoclonal antibody trastuzumab and may be highly chemosensitive. About 50% of HER2 positive breast cancers express the oestrogen receptor. Basal-like breast cancers do not usually express oestrogen or progesterone receptors or overexpress *HER2*, a cancer phenotype often referred to as "triple negative." Basal-like breast cancers are highly proliferative and often have a poor prognosis, although they are highly sensitive to chemotherapy. Adapted from Sorlie and colleagues[12]

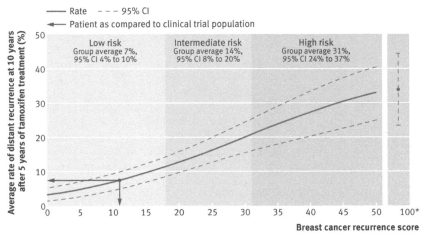

* For recurrence scores >50, group average rate of distant recurrence and 95% CI shown

Fig 3 Example of the molecular prediction of risk recurrence using the Oncotype DX assay. The recurrence score was 11 (low risk), which corresponds to a 7% (95% confidence interval (CI) 5% to 10%) average risk of distant relapse after 10 years of follow-up assuming that the patient took tamoxifen for five years. This risk was considered too low for chemotherapy to have sufficient additional benefit, so the patient was subsequently prescribed adjuvant hormone therapy and no chemotherapy

increasingly being used worldwide. As well as acute side effects, many chemotherapy schedules for breast cancer are associated with a low (<1%) risk of secondary myeloid cancers and cardiomyopathy.

HER2 directed therapy

About 15% of breast cancers have amplification of the *HER2* gene, and these cancers have an intrinsically worse prognosis than other cancers.[23] Trastuzumab is a monoclonal antibody against the extracellular domain of the HER2 receptor, and given every three weeks for a year improves disease-free survival (218 v 321 recurrence events favouring trastuzumab arm; hazard ratio 0.64; P<0.0001) and overall survival (59 v 90 deaths favouring trastuzumab arm; 0.66; P=0.0115).[24] [25] Trastuzumab has few adverse effects, although about 3% of patients experience a drop in left ventricular function,[26] which is usually reversible. After treatment with trastuzumab is interrupted and an angiotensin converting enzyme inhibitor is started, many patients with left ventricular dysfunction can restart and complete the course of trastuzumab.

Bisphosphonates

A recent meta-analysis of 36 randomised controlled trials found that treatment with bisphosphonates is associated with a reduced risk of recurrence of breast cancer in postmenopausal women only.[27] In the analysis of more than 11 000 postmenopausal woman, those treated with bisphosphonates had significantly fewer distant recurrences (18.4% v 21.9%; P<0.001) and fewer bone recurrences (5.9% v 8.8%; P<0.001) than those not taking bisphosphonates. Currently, this evidence has not translated into routine use of bisphosphonates solely for this purpose.

Neoadjuvant therapy and locally advanced breast cancer

Patients with large tumours currently not suitable for conservative surgery can be treated with preoperative chemotherapy, HER2 targeted therapy, or endocrine therapy to downstage the tumour and to facilitate breast conserving surgery.[28] Neoadjuvant therapy in this setting also provides the opportunity to assess sensitivity to systemic therapy by monitoring response during neoadjuvant treatment before surgical excision. Patients who achieve a complete

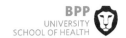

pathological response to chemotherapy, especially those with oestrogen receptor negative breast cancer, have a good prognosis.[29]

Patients with locally advanced breast cancer may start chemotherapy to reduce tumour bulk before mastectomy. Inflammatory breast cancer presents with erythema and oedema of the breast, with or without an underlying mass. This type of cancer is less likely to be oestrogen receptor positive and more likely to be HER2 positive than non-inflammatory breast cancers. Optimal treatment is usually preoperative chemotherapy, followed by surgery or radiotherapy (or both) using a multidisciplinary approach.

Management of advanced breast cancer

The aim of systemic therapy in advanced breast cancer is to palliate symptoms, control disease, and improve overall survival, while minimising the toxicity of treatment. Median survival after distant metastasis varies according to breast cancer subtype. In historical series, median duration of survival after distant metastasis varied from 2.2 years for luminal A subtype cancer to 0.5 years for basal-like breast cancers.[30] Over the past three decades, overall survival has improved substantially, particularly in HER2 positive breast cancer.[31] Metastatic breast cancer remains incurable in all but a few patients, yet many patients continue to live for many years with a good quality of life.

Hormone therapy

For oestrogen receptor positive metastatic disease, hormone treatment is recommended as firstline therapy, in the absence of life threatening visceral disease. The choice of hormone therapy depends on previous treatments and menopausal status.

Resistance to hormone therapy in the metastatic setting is inevitable, and recent research has focused on attempts to restore sensitivity. The enzyme mTOR (mammalian target of rapamycin) is activated in many oestrogen receptor positive cancers that become resistant to hormone therapy.[32] The combination of everolimus, an inhibitor of mTOR, with the hormone therapy exemestane controls disease for substantially longer than exemestane and placebo (median progression-free survival 10.6 v 4.1 months; P<0.001).[33] Everolimus can have serious adverse effects, with stomatitis, rash, diarrhoea, fatigue, and pneumonitis being the most common. These adverse effects must be carefully monitored and treated promptly. Everolimus is licensed in Europe and North America for the treatment of advanced hormone receptor positive, HER2 negative breast cancer, although access to drugs varies. The inhibition of many other pathways similar to mTOR using targeted therapies is being investigated in phase I-III clinical trials.

Chemotherapy

Chemotherapy is used for hormone resistant cancer, hormone receptor negative disease, and rapidly progressive disease, as well as most HER2 positive cancers irrespective of oestrogen receptor status. The choice of which chemotherapy to use depends on patient factors (such as performance status, comorbidities), acceptance of potential toxicity such as alopecia, tumour factors (for example, triple negative v HER2 positive), and duration and response to previous chemotherapy. It is often given for a fixed number of cycles, especially with regimens that incur toxicity, although some regimens may be given long term (for example, paclitaxel and capecitabine). There is no consensus on the optimal duration of chemotherapy.

HER2 amplified breast cancer

In the past HER2 amplified breast cancer had a poor prognosis, but medical treatment has improved this (fig 4). The monoclonal antibody trastuzumab added to taxane chemotherapy significantly improves overall survival (25.1 v 20.3 months; P=0.046) in patients who have not received adjuvant trastuzumab.[34] In patients who progress after trastuzumab, lapatinib—a small molecule kinase inhibitor of HER2—is approved in combination with capecitabine as second line treatment.[35]

Further advances have been made recently through better targeting of HER2. In a phase III study, more than 800 patients were randomised to either docetaxel, trastuzumab, and pertuzumab or docetaxel, trastuzumab, and placebo. Combined inhibition of HER2 with pertuzumab, another monoclonal antibody that inhibits HER2 by blocking dimerisation with HER3, and trastuzumab, improved disease control by 6.1 months (18.5 v 12.4 months; P<0.001),[36] and overall survival (hazard ratio 0.66; P<0.001).[37] The addition of pertuzumab resulted in a modest increase in the side effects of diarrhoea and infections.

Trastuzumab-emtansine is an antibody-drug conjugate that specifically targets chemotherapy to HER2 positive breast cancer cells.[38] In the randomised phase III EMILIA study, this treatment was better tolerated than standard lapatinib and capecitabine chemotherapy and also improved disease control (9.6 v 6.4 months; P<0.001) and overall survival (30.9 v 25.1 months; P<0.001).[39] As a consequence of these steady improvements, the median survival of a woman with HER2 positive metastatic breast cancer diagnosed today is more than three years.[39]

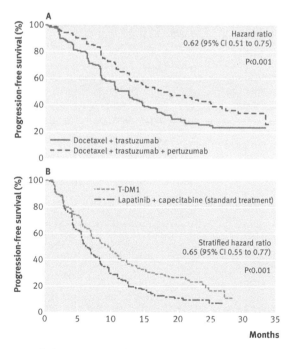

Fig 4 Continuing progress in the management of HER2 positive metastatic breast cancer. In the past, HER2 positive breast cancers had a poor prognosis but the development of trastuzumab (Herceptin) greatly improved prognosis in early and metastatic disease. Recent further advances in targeting HER2 are further improving outcome. (A) Results of the CLEOPATRA randomised trial.[36] The addition of pertuzumab (a second HER2 antibody) resulted in a 48% improvement in progression-free survival. (B) Results of the EMILIA randomised trial that compared lapatinib and capecitabine with T-DM1 (trastuzumab linked to a potent chemotherapeutic agent) in patients who had already been treated with trastuzumab, showing an improvement in progression-free survival in the T-DM1 arm

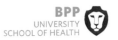

Preventing complications from skeletal metastases in breast cancer

Bone metastases occur in 60-80% of patients with advanced disease.[40][41] Skeletal related events include pain, fractures, and cord compression from extraosseous extension of vertebral metastases. These effects are reduced by the use of bisphosphonates, which inhibit osteoclast mediated bone resorption.[42]

Denosumab is a subcutaneously injected monoclonal antibody that inhibits the membrane protein known as the RANK ligand, and this prevents the activation of osteoclast mediated bone destruction.[43] In a randomised study of denosumab versus zoledronic acid in more than 2000 patients with breast cancer and bone metastases, denosumab was more effective in reducing skeletal related events.[44] Bisphosphonates and denosumab, can cause hypocalcaemia, so calcium and vitamin D supplementation should be considered. The incidence of osteonecrosis of the jaw is around 0.5-1.0% a year in patients taking either of these agents,[45] and patients taking them should maintain good oral hygiene and avoid major invasive dental surgery.

Brain metastases from advanced breast cancer

As the treatment of advanced breast cancer improves, with better control of extracranial disease, the problem of cerebral metastases has become more evident, particularly in HER2 positive patients, because drugs such as trastuzumab cannot cross the blood-brain barrier.[46] Whole brain radiotherapy is the standard treatment for multiple brain metastases. Patients with solitary metastases, or oligometastatic disease, may be considered for surgical debulking, and stereotactic radiotherapy such as the CyberKnife and Gamma Knife systems. Some women with brain metastases have a relatively good prognosis with treatment, and can live for years after these metastases are diagnosed.[47]

Where are we heading in the management of breast cancer?

The somatic genetic events that cause breast cancer have recently been described in detail,[48][49] and it is becoming evident that breast cancer is a highly heterogeneous disease at the genetic level. For cancers with *HER2* amplification, there is substantial cause for optimism that, as new treatments for metastatic HER2 positive disease are brought into the adjuvant setting, we are on the way to curing most women with this form of breast cancer. This illustrates the benefit of identifying, and then targeting, the key genetic event that has driven the development of breast cancer.

Yet many other potentially targetable events occur in just a small proportion of breast cancers, and this presents a major challenge for academic oncology to develop strategies to target these rare genetic events. We are on the brink of an era of diverse molecular stratification of breast cancer, and the development of increasingly personalised medicine. Through such approaches, the survival rates of patients with breast cancer are likely to continue to steadily improve.

We thank Fiona MacNeill for her review and comments on the manuscript. We acknowledge NHS funding to the NIHR Biomedical Research Centre for Cancer. NT is a Cancer Research UK clinician scientist.

Contributors: BY, NT, and AJ conceived, drafted, and approved the manuscript. NT is guarantor.

Competing interests: We have read and understood BMJ policy on declaration of interests and declare the following interests: NT has received advisory board honorariums from AstraZeneca, Roche, Novartis, and Pfizer as well as research funding from AstraZeneca. AJ has received advisory board honorariums and speakers fees from Roche, Novartis, Amgen, and AstraZeneca as well as speaker's fees from Genomic Health. BY: none.

Provenance and peer review: Commissioned; externally peer reviewed.

1. Cancer Research UK. Breast cancer incidence statistics. www.cancerresearchuk.org/cancer-info/cancerstats/types/breast/incidence/uk-breast-cancer-incidence-statistics#trends.
2. Independent UK Panel on Breast Cancer Screening. The benefits and harms of breast cancer screening: an independent review. *Lancet* 2012;380:1778-86.
3. Turner NC, Jones AL. Management of breast cancer—part I. *BMJ* 2008;337:a421.
4. Turner NC, Jones AL. Management of breast cancer—part II. *BMJ* 2008;337:a540.
5. Fisher B, Anderson S, Bryant J, Margolese RG, Deutsch M, Fisher ER, et al. Twenty-year follow-up of a randomized trial comparing total mastectomy, lumpectomy, and lumpectomy plus irradiation for the treatment of invasive breast cancer. *N Engl J Med* 2002;347:1233-41.
6. Moran MS, Schnitt SJ, Giuliano AE, Harris JR, Khan SA, Horton J, et al. Society of Surgical Oncology-American Society for Radiation oncology consensus guideline on margins for breast-conserving surgery with whole-breast irradiation in stages i and ii invasive breast cancer. *J Clin Oncol* 2014;32:1507-15.
7. Kim T, Giuliano AE, Lyman GH. Lymphatic mapping and sentinel lymph node biopsy in early-stage breast carcinoma: a metaanalysis. *Cancer* 2006;106:4-16.
8. Giuliano AE, McCall L, Beitsch P, Whitworth PW, Blumencranz P, Leitch AM, et al. Locoregional recurrence after sentinel lymph node dissection with or without axillary dissection in patients with sentinel lymph node metastases: the American College of Surgeons Oncology Group Z0011 randomized trial. *Ann Surg* 2010;252:426-32; discussion 32-3.
9. Lyman GH, Temin S, Edge SB, Newman LA, Turner RR, Weaver DL, et al. Sentinel lymph node biopsy for patients with early-stage breast cancer: American Society of Clinical Oncology clinical practice guideline update. *J Clin Oncol* 2014;32:1365-83.
10. Rutgers EJ, Donker M, Straver ME, Meijnen P, Van De Velde CJH, Mansel RE, et al. Radiotherapy or surgery of the axilla after a positive sentinel node in breast cancer patients: final analysis of the EORTC AMAROS trial (10981/22023). *J Clin Oncol* 2013;31(suppl):abstract LBA1001.
11. Perou CM, Sorlie T, Eisen MB, van de Rijn M, Jeffrey SS, Rees CA, et al. Molecular portraits of human breast tumours. *Nature* 2000;406:747-52.
12. Sorlie T, Tibshirani R, Parker J, Hastie T, Marron JS, Nobel A, et al. Repeated observation of breast tumor subtypes in independent gene expression data sets. *Proc Natl Acad Sci U S A* 2003;100:8418-23.
13. Early Breast Cancer Trialists' Collaborative Group. Effects of chemotherapy and hormonal therapy for early breast cancer on recurrence and 15-year survival: an overview of the randomised trials. *Lancet* 2005;365:1687-717.
14. Dowsett M, Cuzick J, Ingle J, Coates A, Forbes J, Bliss J, et al. Meta-analysis of breast cancer outcomes in adjuvant trials of aromatase inhibitors versus tamoxifen. *J Clin Oncol* 2010;28:509-18.
15. Kanis JA, McCloskey EV, Johansson H, Cooper C, Rizzoli R, Reginster JY. European guidance for the diagnosis and management of osteoporosis in postmenopausal women. *Osteoporos Int* 2013;24:23-57.

ADDITIONAL EDUCATIONAL RESOURCES

Resources for healthcare professionals

- ESMO clinical practice guidelines for early breast cancer: Senkus E, Kyriakides S, Penault-Llorca F, Poormans P, Thompson A, Thompson A, et al. Primary breast cancer: ESMO clinical practice guidelines for diagnosis, treatment and follow-up. *Ann Oncol* 2013;24(suppl 6):vi7-23
- Advanced breast cancer guidelines: Cardoso F, Costa A, Norton L, Cameron D, Cufer T, Fallowfield L, et al. 1st International consensus guidelines for advanced breast cancer (ABC 1). *Breast* 2012;21:242-52
- UK guidelines on the management of metastatic disease: Coleman RE, Bertelli G, Beaumont T, Kunkler I, Miles D, Simmonds PD, et al. UK guidance document: treatment of metastatic breast cancer. *Clin Oncol* 2012;24:169-76
- National Institute for Health and Care Excellence guidelines on early and locally advanced breast cancer (www.nice.org.uk/CG80) and advanced breast cancer (www.nice.org.uk/CG81)

Resources for patients

- Cancer Research UK www.cancerresearchuk.org/cancer-help/type/breast-cancer/)—Comprehensive information for patients on breast cancer and its treatment
- Breakthrough Breast Cancer (www.breakthrough.org.uk/)—Dedicated to saving lives through improving early diagnosis, developing new treatments, and preventing all types of breast cancer
- Breast Cancer Care (www.breastcancercare.org.uk/)—Provides information and support for women with breast cancer and campaigns for improved standards of care

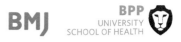

16   Davies C, Godwin J, Gray R, Clarke M, Cutter D, Darby S, et al. Relevance of breast cancer hormone receptors and other factors to the efficacy of adjuvant tamoxifen: patient-level meta-analysis of randomised trials. *Lancet*2011;378:771-84.

17   Goss PE, Ingle JN, Martino S, Robert NJ, Muss HB, Piccart MJ, et al. Randomized trial of letrozole following tamoxifen as extended adjuvant therapy in receptor-positive breast cancer: updated findings from NCIC CTG MA.17. *J Natl Cancer Inst*2005;97:1262-71.

18   Davies C, Pan H, Godwin J, Gray R, Arriagada R, Raina V, et al. Long-term effects of continuing adjuvant tamoxifen to 10 years versus stopping at 5 years after diagnosis of oestrogen receptor-positive breast cancer: ATLAS, a randomised trial. *Lancet* 2013;381:805-16.

19   Al-Mubarak M, Tibau A, Templeton AJ, Cescon DW, Ocana A, Seruga B, et al. Extended adjuvant tamoxifen for early breast cancer: a meta-analysis. *PloS One*2014;9:e88238.

20   Gray RG, Rea D, Handley K, Bowden SJ, Perry P, Helena ME, et al. ATTom: long-term effects of continuing adjuvant tamoxifen to 10 years versus stopping at 5 years in 6953 women with early breast cancer. *J Clin Oncol*2013;31(suppl):abstract 5.

21   Early Breast Cancer Trialists' Collaborative Group, Clarke M, Coates AS, Darby SC, Davies C, Gelber RD, et al. Adjuvant chemotherapy in oestrogen-receptor-poor breast cancer: patient-level meta-analysis of randomised trials. *Lancet*2008;371:29-40.

22   Goldstein LJ, O'Neill A, Sparano JA, Perez EA, Shulman LN, Martino S, et al. Concurrent doxorubicin plus docetaxel is not more effective than concurrent doxorubicin plus cyclophosphamide in operable breast cancer with 0 to 3 positive axillary nodes: North American Breast Cancer Intergroup Trial E 2197. *J Clin Oncol*2008;26:4092-9.

23   Slamon DJ, Clark GM, Wong SG, Levin WJ, Ullrich A, McGuire WL. Human breast cancer: correlation of relapse and survival with amplification of the HER-2/neu oncogene. *Science*1987;235:177-82.

24   Piccart-Gebhart MJ, Procter M, Leyland-Jones B, Goldhirsch A, Untch M, Smith I, et al. Trastuzumab after adjuvant chemotherapy in HER2-positive breast cancer. *N Engl J Med*2005;353:1659-72.

25   Smith I, Procter M, Gelber RD, Guillaume S, Feyereislova A, Dowsett M, et al. 2 year follow-up of trastuzumab after adjuvant chemotherapy in HER2-positive breast cancer: a randomised controlled trial. *Lancet* 2007;369:29-36.

26   Suter TM, Procter M, van Veldhuisen DJ, Muscholl M, Bergh J, Carlomagno C, et al. Trastuzumab-associated cardiac adverse effects in the herceptin adjuvant trial. *J Clin Oncol*2007;25:3859-65.

27   Coleman R, Gnant M, Paterson A, Powles T, con Minckwitc G, Pritchard K, et al. Effects of bisphosphonate treatment on recurrence and cause-specific mortality in women with early breast cancer: a meta-analysis of individual patient data from randomized trials. 2013 San Antonio Breast Cancer Symposium. December 12, 2013, abstract S4-07.

28   Fisher B, Brown A, Mamounas E, Wieand S, Robidoux A, Margolese RG, et al. Effect of preoperative chemotherapy on local-regional disease in women with operable breast cancer: findings from national surgical adjuvant breast and bowel project B-18. *J Clin Oncol*1997;15:2483-93.

29   von Minckwitz G, Untch M, Blohmer JU, Costa SD, Eidtmann H, Fasching PA, et al. Definition and impact of pathologic complete response on prognosis after neoadjuvant chemotherapy in various intrinsic breast cancer subtypes. *J Clin Oncol*2012;30:1796-804.

30   Kennecke H, Yerushalmi R, Woods R, Cheang MC, Voduc D, Speers CH, et al. Metastatic behavior of breast cancer subtypes. *J Clin Oncol*2010;28:3271-7.

31   Giordano SH, Buzdar AU, Smith TL, Kau SW, Yang Y, Hortobagyi GN.Is breast cancer survival improving? *Cancer*2004;100:44-52.

32   Miller TW, Balko JM, Fox EM, Ghazoui Z, Dunbier A, Anderson H, et al. ERalpha-dependent E2F transcription can mediate resistance to estrogen deprivation in human breast cancer. *Cancer Discov*2011;1:338-51.

33   Baselga J, Campone M, Piccart M, Burris HA, 3rd, Rugo HS, Sahmoud T, et al. Everolimus in postmenopausal hormone-receptor-positive advanced breast cancer. *N Engl J Med*2012;366:520-9.

34   Slamon DJ, Leyland-Jones B, Shak S, Fuchs H, Paton V, Bajamonde A, et al. Use of chemotherapy plus a monoclonal antibody against HER2 for metastatic breast cancer that overexpresses HER2. *N Engl J Med*2001;344:783-92.

35   Geyer CE, Forster J, Lindquist D, Chan S, Romieu CG, Pienkowski T, et al. Lapatinib plus capecitabine for HER2-positive advanced breast cancer. *N Engl J Med*2006;355:2733-43.

36   Baselga J, Cortes J, Kim SB, Im SA, Hegg R, Im YH, et al. Pertuzumab plus trastuzumab plus docetaxel for metastatic breast cancer. *N Engl J Med*2012;366:109-19.

37   Swain SM, Kim SB, Cortes J, Ro J, Semiglazov V, Campone M, et al. Pertuzumab, trastuzumab, and docetaxel for HER2-positive metastatic breast cancer (CLEOPATRA study): overall survival results from a randomised, double-blind, placebo-controlled, phase 3 study. *Lancet Oncol* 2013;14:461-71.

38   Lewis Phillips GD, Li G, Dugger DL, Crocker LM, Parsons KL, Mai E, et al. Targeting HER2-positive breast cancer with trastuzumab-DM1, an antibody-cytotoxic drug conjugate. *Cancer Res*2008;68:9280-90.

39   Verma S, Miles D, Gianni L, Krop IE, Welslau M, Baselga J, et al. Trastuzumab emtansine for HER2-positive advanced breast cancer. *N Engl J Med*2012;367:1783-91.

40   Coleman RE, Rubens RD. The clinical course of bone metastases from breast cancer. *Br J Cancer*1987;55:61-6.

41   Hortobagyi GN. Novel approaches to the management of bone metastases in patients with breast cancer. *Semin Oncol*2002;29(3 suppl 11):134-44.

42   Pavlakis N, Schmidt R, Stockler M. Bisphosphonates for breast cancer. *Cochrane Database Syst Rev*2005;3:CD003474.

43   Baron R, Ferrari S, Russell RG. Denosumab and bisphosphonates: different mechanisms of action and effects. *Bone*2011;48:677-92.

44   Stopeck A. Denosumab findings in metastatic breast cancer. *Clin Adv Hematol Oncol*2010;8:159-60.

45   Saad F, Lattouf JB. Bisphosphonates: prevention of bone metastases in prostate cancer. *Recent Results Cancer Res*2012;192:109-26.

46   Lin NU, Winer EP. Brain metastases: the HER2 paradigm. *Clin Cancer Res*2007;13:1648-55.

47   Sperduto PW, Chao ST, Sneed PK, Luo X, Suh J, Roberge D, et al. Diagnosis-specific prognostic factors, indexes, and treatment outcomes for patients with newly diagnosed brain metastases: a multi-institutional analysis of 4259 patients. *Int J Radiat Oncol Biol Phys*2010;77:655-61.

48   Cancer Genome Atlas Network. Comprehensive molecular portraits of human breast tumours. *Nature*2012;490:61-70.

49   Curtis C, Shah SP, Chin SF, Turashvili G, Rueda OM, Dunning MJ, et al. The genomic and transcriptomic architecture of 2000 breast tumours reveals novel subgroups. *Nature* 2012;486:346-52.

Related links

bmj.com

Previous articles in this series

- Skin disease in pregnancy (BMJ 2014;348:g3489)
- Management of cutaneous viral warts (BMJ 2014;348:g3339)
- Posterior circulation ischaemic stroke (BMJ 2014;348:g3175)
- Managing common breastfeeding problems in the community (BMJ 2014;348:g2954)
- Spontaneous pneumothorax (BMJ 2014;348:g2928)

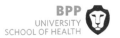

Management of women at high risk of breast cancer

Anne C Armstrong consultant medical oncologist[1], Gareth D Evans professor of medical genetics and cancer epidemiology[23]

[1]Department of Oncology, Christie Hospital Manchester, Manchester, UK

[2]Manchester Centre for Genomic Medicine, Manchester Academic Health Science Centre, University of Manchester, Manchester, UK

[3]Department of Genetic Medicine, St Mary's Hospital, Central Manchester Foundation Trust, Manchester, UK

Correspondence to: A C Armstrong
anne.armstrong@christie.nhs.uk

Cite this as: *BMJ* 2014;348:g2756

<DOI> 10.1136/bmj.g2756
http://www.bmj.com/content/348/bmj.g2756

Breast cancer is the commonest malignancy diagnosed in women worldwide and accounts for over 30% of all cancers diagnosed in women in the United Kingdom.[1] The average lifetime risk of developing breast cancer for women in the United Kingdom and United States is estimated to be 12%,[1] although this may be an overestimate, as it is not clear what age this assumes a woman lives to and whether full adjustment has been made for those who die young from other causes. It is also unclear whether multiple breast cancers in a single woman are counted as several women with breast cancer.

The risk of breast cancer is multifactorial and is an interaction between environmental, lifestyle, hormonal, and genetic factors.[2][3] Some women have a particularly high risk of breast cancer owing to their family history, or, less commonly, after supradiaphragmatic radiotherapy for Hodgkin's lymphoma. This review discusses how to identify women who are at high risk of breast cancer as a result of their family history or irradiation and outlines the management options for such women, including surveillance and risk reducing strategies. A further group of women diagnosed on the basis of a breast biopsy as having atypical ductal or lobular hyperplasia are also at increased risk of breast cancer; these women are not discussed further in this review.

When should a woman be considered at high risk of breast cancer?

A risk assessment for breast cancer is complex and no consistent definition or threshold for high risk has been established. Within UK practice, high risk, as defined by the National Institute for Health and Care Excellence,[4] is a lifetime risk of 30% or greater, which equates to a more than 8% risk of breast cancer at age 40-50 years. The high risk threshold used in the United Kingdom is similar to that in other European countries, although in North America the threshold for screening using magnetic resonance imaging is a lifetime risk of 20-25%.[5] NICE guidelines have algorithms for identifying high risk women, which include two close (first or second degree) relatives with breast cancer with an average age of less than 50, three with breast cancer aged less than 60, or four with breast cancer at any age. These are "catch all" criteria, which will not make all women who meet these criteria fit the lifetime or 10 year risk criterion. Another high risk criterion includes women with a family history of both breast and ovarian cancer, which specifically highlights the possibility of a BRCA1/2 mutation given the increased risk of both cancers associated with mutations in these genes.

In most women with breast cancer the cause is unknown. Those with breast cancer can be considered at high risk if they meet the criteria mentioned above, including their own breast cancer. Each close relative with a diagnosis of breast cancer increases a woman's risk of developing breast cancer, especially with a diagnosis at a young age (<50 years). Such families may have a genetic predisposition to the development of breast cancer, with about 5% of all breast cancers being attributable to inherited mutations in specific genes such as BRCA1, BRCA2, and TP53. In any individual the genetic risk factors will be modified by other risk factors.

In women of Ashkenazi Jewish descent a family history of breast cancer poses a higher risk than in women of non-Jewish descent because of the high prevalence and penetrance of BRCA1 and BRCA2 mutations (2.5%).[6] In this population any breast cancer is associated with a 10% carrier rate of BRCA1/2, with higher rates for women with a diagnosis at a younger age. Furthermore, three specific "founder" mutations (two in BRCA1 and one in BRCA2) have been identified within this population, making genetic testing based on only these mutations a much more sensitive and specific test.

It is also clear that women who received supradiaphragmatic radiotherapy at a young age as treatment for Hodgkin's lymphoma have a high risk of breast cancer, which 20-40 years after treatment is nearly as high as that of carriers of BRCA1/2.[7] The peak risk is around age 14 years, which may be attributable to the accumulation of radiation damage in dividing cells during breast development.

Which genes are implicated in a high risk of breast cancer?

Several genes are associated with a high risk of breast cancer. Of the known high risk genes, mutations in BRCA1 and BRCA2 are the most common and account for about 20% of the familial component. Germline mutations in other high

SOURCES AND SELECTION CRITERIA

We searched PubMed using search terms such as "breast cancer risk" and "hereditary breast cancer." Studies included were those written in English, and included case-control studies, randomised control trials, and meta-analyses. We also consulted relevant national and international guidelines, including those of the National Institute for Health and Care Excellence, and we were part of the NICE Guideline Development Group where all relevant evidence was identified and summarised.

SUMMARY POINTS

- The risk of breast cancer is multifactorial, but some women will have a high risk because of a genetic predisposition or, rarely, as a consequence of radiotherapy at a young age
- Women with a family history suggestive of a genetic predisposition to cancer should be referred to local genetics services for formal assessment
- Annual magnetic resonance imaging and mammography (unless a carrier of the TP53 gene) in high risk women identifies more breast cancers than does mammography alone
- Risk reducing bilateral salpingo-oophorectomy and risk reducing mastectomy reduces the risk of breast cancer by 50% and 90-95%, respectively, in carriers of BRCA1 and BRCA2 mutations
- Chemoprevention with drugs such as tamoxifen for five years reduces the risk of breast cancer by about 30% and can be a useful alternative to risk reducing surgery

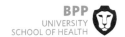

Table 1 Breast cancer associated cancer predisposition syndromes and associated risk of breast cancer[9]

Disease gene	Location	Tumours	Tumour age (years)	Risk (%)		Birth incidence of mutations	Life expectancy
CHEK2	22q	Breast cancer	>25		20	1 in 200	?Normal
ATM	11q	Breast cancer	>25		20	1 in 200	?Normal
BRIP		Breast cancer	>25		20	1 in 1000	?Normal
PALB2		Breast cancer	>25	30-40		<1 in 1000	?Normal
NF1	17q	Neurofibroma, glioma, breast cancer	1st year, 1st year, >25	100, 12, 17		1 in 2600	54-72 years
PTEN Cowden	10q	Breast cancer, thyroid	>25, 30	60, 10		1 in 200 000-250 000	Reduced in women
PJS STK11	19p	Gastrointestinal malignancy, breast	20, >25	60, 40		1 in 25 000	58 years
LFSTP53	17p	Sarcoma, breast cancer (women), gliomas	1st year, >16, 1st year	80, 95, 20		1 in 30 000	Severely reduced
CDH1	16q	Gastric, breast (women)	>16, >35	70-80, 20-40		Rare	Reduced
BRCA2	13q	Breast/ovary (women), prostate (men), pancreas	>18, >30, >30	40-90, 20, 5		1 in 800	68 years
BRCA1	17q	Breast (women), ovary	>18, >20	60-90, 40-60		1 in 1000	62 years

risk genes such as TP53, PTEN, and STK11 are less common and identified in less than 1% of families with breast cancer (table 1).[8]

Carriers of mutations in BRCA1 and BRCA2 have a high lifetime risk of breast cancer (around 65-85% with BRCA1 and 40-85% with BRCA2)[10] [11] [12] as well as a high risk of ovarian cancer (40-60% with BRCA1 and 10-30% with BRCA2). BRCA2 mutations also confer an excess risk of prostate cancer, pancreatic cancer, and melanoma. The frequencies of BRCA1/BRCA2 mutations in breast cancer populations unselected for family history or age of diagnosis are, however, low and account for about 2-3% of breast cancers overall,[13] but they are about 10% in founder populations such as Ashkenazi Jewish.

Most breast cancers that arise in carriers of the BRCA1 mutation are "triple negative"—that is, the cancers lack receptors for oestrogen, progesterone, and human epidermal growth factor receptor 2 (Her2).[13] The immune phenotye of

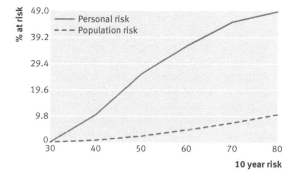

Woman aged 30 years
Age at menarch, 12 years
Age at first birth, 26 years
Person is premenopausal
Height, 5 ft 4 in (1.63 m)
Weight 9 stone (57.2 kg)
Never used hormone replacement therapy
Risk after 10 years, 10.26%
10 year population risk, 0.523%
Lifetime risk, 48.82%
Lifetime population risk, 10.21%
Probability of being a carrier of BRCA1 gene, 20.97%
Probability of being a carrier of BRCA2 gene, 22.55%

Tyrer-Cuzick readout of a woman (arrowed) at high risk of breast cancer. The woman is eligible without genetic testing for annual screening by magnetic resonance imaging aged 30-50 and for genetic testing. Her affected mother and aunt, if alive, can be offered genetic testing for BRCA1/2 as they qualify on all algorithms (Manchester score 30 is well above the 15 threshold for 10%). If they are not alive the proband and her sister could have genetic testing as they have a >10% chance of a BRCA1/2 mutation. The sister, now aged 35, could be offered tamoxifen for five years

cancers associated with BRCA2 mutations reflect that of sporadic cancers, with most cancers expressing receptors for oestrogen and progesterone with only 16% triple negative.[14]

When and how should a family history be taken?

Although 2004 guidelines from NICE did not advocate taking a family history proactively, much has changed in terms of extra available surveillance and preventive options for those women with at least moderate risk.[15] Moderate risk as defined by NICE is a lifetime risk of 17-29% or a 10 year risk at age 40 of 3-7.9%. When risk is being assessed in primary or secondary care, at least a two generation family history, including paternal relatives, should be taken from women seeking advice. A family history of breast cancer should also be sought in women aged more than 30 starting combined oral contraception and women aged more than 50 starting combined hormone replacement therapy. Women meeting at least moderate risk criteria (for instance a mother or sister with breast cancer at age <40 or two close relatives at any age) should be offered a referral to secondary care (the local family history clinic or breast clinic) but for women with a known family gene mutation, direct referral to genetic services is appropriate (table 2). In the United Kingdom, family history clinics are available in most localities, with over 100 countrywide, but models may differ in other countries. None the less, much management of familial breast cancer does take place in secondary care around the world, with surveillance organised by local breast surgeons and gynaecologists.

When referred to a secondary care clinic, women will have a preclinic questionnaire administered to assess eligibility or a family history elicited directly. Other non-genetic risk factors such as pregnancy history and age at menarche and menopause are also taken. The woman's risk is assessed usually by use of a risk algorithm such as Tyrer-Cuzick[16] or BOADICEA.[17] If a woman is in the high risk category (lifetime risk .30%) or she or her affected relative has a 10% or more chance of carrying a BRCA1/2 mutation she will be offered referral to a tertiary care genetics service. Extra surveillance will be offered as appropriate (table 3). An assessment will also be made of others in the family who may benefit from screening or genetic testing. Use of a risk algorithm to assess the 10% threshold can be made in family history clinics using a simple scoring system such as the Manchester score[18] or a computer algorithm such as BOADICEA.[17] Women from founder populations such as Ashkenazi Jewish (carrier frequency 2.5%) and Icelandic

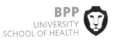

Table 2   Referral criteria for family history and genetics clinics*[4]

Referral to family history clinics/secondary care	Referral to genetics clinics/tertiary care
One first degree relative with breast cancer at age <40 years	Triple negative breast cancer at age <40 years
One first degree male relative with breast cancer at any age	Two first or second degree relatives with breast cancer at age <50 years
Two first or second degree relatives with breast cancer at any age	Three first or second degree relatives at age <60 years with breast cancer
Two close relatives with breast cancer at any age and a close relative with ovarian cancer	Four first degree relatives with breast cancer at any age
Three first or second degree relatives with breast cancer at any age	Ovarian or male breast cancer at any age and on same side of family and any of: one first or second degree relative aged <50 years; two first or second degree relatives aged <60 years; another ovarian cancer at any age
Three first or second degree relatives with breast cancer at any age	Any breast cancer and Jewish ancestry

*For bilateral breast cancer each breast cancer counts as one relative.

Table 3   Screening for women at high risk of breast cancer*[4]

Age (years)	Annual mammographic surveillance	Annual breast magnetic resonance imaging
≤29	No surveillance	TP53 carrier†
30-39	Known or suspected BRCA1/BRCA2 mutation	Known or suspected BRCA1/BRCA2/TP53 mutation
40-49	Known or suspected BRCA1/BRCA2 mutation	Known or suspected BRCA1/BRCA2/TP53 mutation
50-59	Known or suspected BRCA1/BRCA2 mutation	Known TP53 mutation
60-69	Known or suspected BRCA1/BRCA2 mutation	Known TP53 mutation

*For guidance on surveillance for women at moderate risk of breast cancer see National Institute for Health and Care Excellence guidelines.[4]
†Mammographic surveillance is not recommended for TP53 carriers owing to risk of ionising radiation in this patient group.

(0.5%) can be considered for BRCA1/2 testing with much less significant family histories. Several algorithms may be used in tertiary care. The figure shows an example of a risk output from Tyer-Cuzick version 6. Fully comprehensive algorithms such as Tyrer-Cuzick incorporate family history with other known risk factors such as age at menarche and menopause and at first full term pregnancy, overweight or obesity, and breast biopsy information. Newer risk factors such as mammographic density are being incorporated. Efforts are under way internationally to target screening, and preventive measures by proper risk stratification and accurate risk assessments are vital to this aim.

Counselling

Counselling includes advising women about their risk of breast cancer and what they can do about it, as well as the possibility of genetic testing. Although many genes and genetic factors have been identified, currently there is really only good utility in offering testing for women with high risk genes and in particular mutations in BRCA1 and BRCA2. Testing will usually start with the woman who has breast or ovarian cancer to develop a definitive test for that family. Women undergoing testing need to be aware of the likelihood of testing positive for a mutation that causes disease as well as for a variant of uncertain significance (about 5% of BRCA1/2 tests find missense mutations, most of which are thought to be harmless).

The decision to undergo presymptomatic testing for a known BRCA1/2 mutation can involve complex emotions and bring back memories of a relative's diagnosis, treatment, and death. Many women do not choose to have testing, and those that do may leave this for many years, particularly if they are a young adult when first eligible. As such most genetics centres see women at least twice before taking a predictive sample. Women who are considering being tested for a known family mutation or being considered for testing where no living relative is available will need a full discussion of their risks for breast and ovarian cancer, how these can be managed, and any effects on life or health insurance dependent on where they live.

How are high risk women followed up?

Surveillance

Breast screening aims to diagnose cancer earlier to allow timely therapeutic intervention that may consequently be more effective than if left to later. In all women, breast screening with mammography is predicted to reduce breast cancer mortality,[19] although controversy remains about the absolute benefit of screening as well as the impact of overdiagnosis and overtreatment of screen detected low grade and in situ breast cancers. In the United Kingdom, women are offered screening from age 47-50 within the NHS breast screening programme. Many similar screening programmes exist across Europe and worldwide.

Mammographic screening of younger women is generally less effective than of older women because of increased breast density. Digital mammography is more accurate than film mammography in younger women with dense breasts and is therefore recommended for the high risk population. There are, however, concerns about exposing young women to regular doses of ionising radiation. One study modelled the risk of radiation induced cancers against reductions in mortality from mammographic screening in carriers of the BRCA mutation and suggested no net benefit of mammographic screening in women aged less than 30.[20] NICE advocate no mammography in women aged less than 30 with a familial risk.[2] Breast magnetic resonance imaging, with no exposure to radiation, has a sensitivity of about 80% and identifies more cancers in high risk women than does mammography (sensitivity 30-40%).[21] [22] Magnetic resonance imaging is less specific, leading to additional imaging and biopsies. In high risk women, surveillance with both magnetic resonance imaging and mammography is better than either test alone.[22] [23]

National[2] and international guidelines recommend enhanced screening for women with a very high risk of familial breast cancer who have not had risk reducing mastectomies (table 3). This includes annual surveillance with magnetic resonance imaging from age 30-49 years for women who have a known BRCA1, BRCA2, or TP53 mutation or are at a more than 30% probability of such and, for BRCA1/2, annual mammography from the age of 40 to 69. UK guidelines also recommend the use of annual mammography and magnetic resonance imaging in women

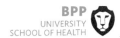

who have received supradiaphragmatic radiotherapy when less than 36, starting eight years after treatment.[24]

Breast cancer surveillance is non-invasive, has few adverse long term effects, and does not interfere with child bearing. The risk of false positive results can lead to additional investigations, including imaging and biopsies, and some women find magnetic resonance imaging unacceptably claustrophobic. Furthermore, magnetic resonance imaging does not prevent breast cancer and there is no evidence as yet that breast screening reduces the risk of breast cancer deaths in high risk women.

When is prophylactic surgery or chemoprevention considered?

Risk reducing mastectomies

Women with high risk of breast cancer may decide to undergo surgery to reduce their risk. Bilateral risk reducing mastectomies remove most but not all breast tissue. Case-control studies in patients with BRCA1/2 mutations found than surgery reduced the risk of breast cancer by 90-95%.[25] Although randomised trials comparing the efficacy of bilateral risk reducing mastectomy with regular surveillance would be an ethical challenge, prospective observational studies have been published, with one study of more than 2000 years of patient observation finding 57 breast cancer cases in the surveillance group compared with none in the surgical group.[26] Overall survival benefits from bilateral risk reducing mastectomy alone have yet to be shown, but one study reported that any form of risk reducing surgery in women with BRCA1 or BRCA2 mutations improved survival,[27] and in two recent studies contralateral mastectomy has been shown to improve survival in women with BRCA1/2 mutations.[28][29]

Bilateral risk reducing mastectomy is a major undertaking for women, who need time to discuss their options and the risks of each procedure, including the potential for ongoing interventions such as surgical revisions and nipple tattooing. There is a small (about 2-5%) possibility of finding an occult malignancy during risk reducing mastectomy, despite preoperative screening investigations.[26] Several studies have evaluated the psychological impact of bilateral risk reducing mastectomies, which in general (but not universally) show good levels of satisfaction and reduced anxiety after the procedure.[30][31]

Bilateral risk reducing salpingo-oophorectomy

Women who have inherited mutations of BRCA1 and BRCA2 may also undergo risk reducing bilateral salpingo-oophorectomy. This reduces the risk of ovarian and breast cancer; a meta-analysis of all case series of the procedure suggesting that bilateral salpingo-oophorectomy performed before natural menopause reduces the risk of breast cancer by up to 50%.[32] This is thought to be due to the reduction in circulating oestrogen. The benefits of risk reducing bilateral salpingo-oophorectomy may be greater in carriers of the BRCA2 mutation compared with BRCA1 mutation, which is likely to relate to the greater frequency of oestrogen receptor positive breast cancer in carriers of the BRCA2 mutation. Nevertheless, ongoing breast surveillance is still recommended in these women and there are some prospective case series that suggest the incidence of breast cancer after risk reducing bilateral salpingo-oophorectomy is still high.[33]

The ideal age for risk reducing bilateral salpingo-oophorectomy remains uncertain, but studies suggesting an earlier age of onset of cancers in carriers of the BRCA1 mutation support earlier intervention compared with carriers of the BRCA2 mutation. A surgical menopause can result in acute symptoms and long term risks of oestrogen deficiency. Although the use of hormone replacement therapy after natural menopause has been in decline since the association between breast cancer and hormone replacement therapy use in the Million Womens Study,[34] the use of hormone replacement therapy for women with BRCA1 and BRCA2 mutations until the age of an expected menopause seems to be safe[35] and is advised.[4] Risk reducing bilateral salpingo-oophorectomy at ages 38-40 for carriers of the BRCA1 mutation and at ages 40-45 for carriers of the BRCA2 mutation would seem to be a reasonable balance.

Chemoprevention

In women with a diagnosis of (an oestrogen receptor positive) cancer, selective oestrogen receptor modulators, such as tamoxifen and raloxifene, and aromatase inhibitors reduce the risk of recurrence of that cancer as well as the risk of a contralateral primary breast cancer. Such drugs have therefore been investigated as preventive agents as an alternative to risk reducing surgery in women with a high risk of breast cancer. Tamoxifen has efficacy in premenopausal and postmenopausal women, whereas aromatase inhibitors are only effective in postmenopausal women. Raloxifene only has efficacy data in postmenopausal women.

A meta-analysis of randomised trials of selective oestrogen receptor modulators for breast cancer prevention, with data on 83 000 women, showed a 38% reduction in incidence of oestrogen receptor positive (but not oestrogen receptor negative) breast cancer with five years of treatment.[36] The absolute benefit of treatment depended on the absolute risk of breast cancer, but overall this equated to a need to treat 42 women to prevent one cancer. Similar to the benefit of adjuvant endocrine treatment for breast cancer, the benefits of chemoprevention extend beyond the five years that the drug is taken, with evidence of risk reduction extending to at least five years after completion.

Other studies have investigated the use of the aromatase inhibitors, exemestane and anastrozole, as chemopreventive agents. The recently published IBIS-II study, in which 3864 postmenopausal women were randomly assigned to anastrozole 1 mg daily or to placebo, showed an enhanced risk reduction with anastrozole treatment for five years compared with the risk reduction seen in the studies using selective oestrogen receptor modulators. After five years of follow-up 40 women in the anastrozole arm had developed breast cancer compared with 85 in the placebo arm (hazard ratio 0.47, 95% confidence interval 0.32 to 0.68).[37] Selective oestrogen receptor modulators and aromatase inhibitors have yet to be compared head to head in the same study.

No study has as yet shown an overall survival advantage from any chemopreventive strategy. Furthermore, from the available evidence the drugs prevent the incidence of oestrogen receptor positive but not oestrogen receptor negative cancers and may not be as effective in BRCA1 carriers where triple negative cancers predominate. Chemoprevention can be associated with potentially serious adverse events—for example, tamoxifen causes a small excess risk of venous thrombosis (around 4-7 events per 1000 women over five years) and endometrial malignancy (around 4 excess cases per 1000, with most of the excess risk in postmenopausal women).[38] Aromatase inhibitors (which are not currently approved for chemoprevention by

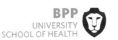

NICE) cause loss of bone mineral density and an increased risk of osteoporosis. All women starting treatment with an aromatase inhibitor should have baseline bone mineral density monitoring according to national guidelines.[39]

The uptake of chemoprevention worldwide is low despite favourable national guidance by NICE (for tamoxifen and raloxifene), the American Society of Clinical Oncology, and other institutions. Possible explanations for this include concerns about side effects of the drugs and a lack of awareness among women and healthcare providers.[40] For women at high risk of an oestrogen receptor positive breast cancer, these drugs can be a useful option if they wish to avoid or delay risk reducing surgery. The drugs are, however, less effective than risk reducing surgery and have the potential for serious adverse events. The potential benefits and risks of these drugs require careful counselling and quantifying, which may best be performed within secondary or tertiary care settings. Decision aids are being developed to help women make a decision regarding treatment with these drugs.

Competing interests: We have read and understood the BMJ Group policy on declaration of interests and declare the following interests: AA was an expert member of the NICE Familial Breast Cancer Guideline Development Group (2013 update). GE was the chair of the same group. GE and AA are coauthors of a manuscript in preparation.

Provenance and peer review: Commissioned; externally peer reviewed.

1   Cancer Research UK. Breast cancer incidence statistics. 2012. www.cancerresearchuk.org/cancer-info/cancerstats/types/breast/incidence/#risk.

2   Parkin DM, Boyd L, Walker LC. The fraction of cancer attributable to lifestyle and environmental factors in the UK in 2010. Summary and conclusions. *Br J Cancer*2011;105(S2):S77-81.

3   Turkoz FP, Solak M, Petekkaya I, Keskin O, Kertmen N, Sarici F, et al. Association between common risk factors and molecular subtypes in breast cancer patients. *Breast*2013;22:344-50.

4   National Institute for Health and Care Excellence. Familial breast cancer: classification and care of people at risk of familial breast cancer and management of breast cancer and related risks in people with a family history of breast cancer. (Clinical guideline 164.) 2013. http://guidance.nice.org.uk/CG164.

5   Saslow D, Boetes C, Burke W, Harms S, Leach MO, Lehman CD, et al. American Cancer Society guidelines for breast screening with MRI as an adjunct to mammography. *CA Cancer J Clin*2007;57:75-89.

6   Rubinstein WS. Hereditary breast cancer in Jews. *Fam Cancer*2004;3:249-57.

7   Swerdlow AJ, Cooke R, Bates A, Cunningham D, Falk SJ, Gilson D, et al. Breast cancer risk after supradiaphragmatic radiotherapy for Hodgkin's lymphoma in England and Wales: a national cohort study. *J Clin Oncol*2012;30:2745-52.

8   Lalloo F, Evans DG. Familial breast cancer. *Clin Genet*2012;82:105-14.

9   Evans DG, Ingham RL. Reduced life expectancy seen in hereditary diseases which predispose to early-onset tumors. *Appl Clin Genet*2013;6:53-61.

10   Antoniou A, Pharoah PD, Narod S, Risch HA, Eyfjord JE, Hopper JL, et al. Average risks of breast and ovarian cancer associated with BRCA1 or BRCA2 mutations detected in case series unselected for family history: a combined analysis of 22 studies. *Am J Hum Genet*2002;72:1117-30.

11   Chen S, Parmigiani G. Meta-analysis of BRCA1 and BRCA2 penetrance. *J Clin Oncol*2007;25:1329-33.

12   Evans DG, Shenton A, Woodward E, Lalloo F, Howell A, Maher ER. Penetrance estimates for BRCA1 and BRCA2 based on genetic testing in a clinical cancer genetics service setting: risks of breast/ovarian cancer quoted should reflect the cancer burden in the family. *BMC Cancer*2008;8:155.

13   Papelard H, de Bock GH, van Eijk R, Vliet Vlieland TP, Cornelisse CJ, Devilee P, et al. Prevalence of BRCA1 in a hospital-based population of Dutch breast cancer patients. *Br J Cancer*2000;83:719-24.

14   Mavaddat N, Barrowdale D, Andrulis IL, Domchek SM, Eccles D, Navanlinna H, et al. Pathology of breast and ovarian cancers among BRCA1 and BRCA2 mutation carriers: results from the Consortium of Investigators of Modifiers of BRCA1/2 (CIMBA). *Cancer Epidemiol Biomarkers Prev*2012;21:134-47.

15   Harris H, Nippert I, Julian-Reynier C, Schmidtke J, van Asperen C, Gadzicki D, et al. Familial breast cancer: is it time to move from a reactive to a proactive role? *Fam Cancer*2011;10:501-3.

16   Tyrer J, Duffy SW, Cuzick J. A breast cancer prediction model incorporating familial and personal risk factors. *Stat Med*2005;23:1111-30.

17   Antoniou AC, Hardy R, Walker L, Evans DG, Shenton A, Eeles R, et al. Predicting the likelihood of carrying a BRCA1 or BRCA2 mutation: validation of BOADICEA, BRCAPRO, IBIS, Myriad and the Manchester scoring system using data from UK genetics clinics. *J Med Genet*2008;45:425-31.

18   Evans DG, Lalloo F, Cramer A, Jones E, Knox F, Amir E, et al. Addition of pathology and biomarker information significantly improves the performance of the Manchester scoring system for BRCA1 and BRCA2 testing. *J Med Genet*2009;46:811-7.

19   Independent UK Panel on Breast Cancer Screening. The benefits and harms of breast cancer screening: an independent review. *Lancet*2012;380:1778-86.

20   Berrington de Gonzalez A, Berg CD, Visvanathan K, Robson M. Estimated risk of radiation-induced breast cancer from mammographic screening for young BRCA mutation carriers. *J Natl Cancer Inst*2009;101:205-9.

21   Kriege M, Brekelmans CT, Boetes C, Besnard PE, Zonderland HM, Obdeijn IM, et al. Efficacy of MRI and mammography for breast-cancer screening in women with a familial or genetic predisposition. *N Engl J Med*2004;351:427-37.

22   Leach MO, Boggis CR, Dixon AK, Easton DF, Eeles RA, Evans DG, et al. MARIBS study group. Screening with magnetic resonance imaging and mammography of a UK population at high familial risk of breast cancer: a prospective multicentre cohort study (MARIBS). *Lancet*2005;365:1769-78.

23   Warner E, Messersmith H, Causer P, Eisen A, Shumak R, Plewes D. Systematic review: using magnetic resonance imaging to screen women at high risk for breast cancer. *Ann Intern Med*2008;148:671-9.

24   Ralleigh G, Given-Wilson R. Breast cancer risk and possible screening strategies for young women following supradiaphragmatic irradiation for Hodgkin's disease. *Clin Radiol*2004;59:647-50.

25   Rebbeck TR, Friebel T, Lynch HT, Neuhausen SL, van't Veer L, Garber JE, et al. Bilateral prophylactic mastectomy reduces breast cancer in BRCA1 and BRCA2 mutation carriers: the PROSE Study Group. *J Clin Oncol*2004;22:1055-62.

26   Heemskerk-Gerritsen BA, Menke-Pluijmers MB, Jager A, Tilanus-Linthorst MM, Koppert LB, Obdeijn IM, et al. Substantial breast cancer risk reduction and potential survival benefit after bilateral mastectomy when compared with surveillance in healthy BRCA1 and BRCA2 mutation carriers: a prospective analysis. *Ann Oncol*2013;24:2029-35.

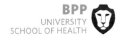

27 Ingham SL, Sperrin M, Baildam A, Ross GL, Clayton R, Lallo F, et al. Risk-reducing surgery increases survival in BRCA1/2 mutation carriers unaffected at time of family referral. *Breast Cancer Res Treat*2013;142:611-8.

28 Evans DG, Ingham SL, Baildam A, Ross GL, Lalloo F, Buchan I, et al. Contralateral mastectomy improves survival in women with BRCA1/2-associated breast cancer. *Breast Cancer Res Treat*2013;140:135-42.

29 Metcalfe K, Gershman S, Ghadirian P, Lynch HT, Snyder C, Tung N, et al. Contralateral mastectomy and survival after breast cancer in carriers of BRCA1 and BRCA2 mutations: retrospective analysis. *BMJ*2014;348:g226.

30 Hallowell N, Baylock B, Heiniger L, Butow PN, Patel D, Meiser B, et al. Looking different, feeling different women's reactions to risk-reducing breast and ovarian surgery. *Fam Cancer*2012;11:215-24.

31 Montgomery LL, Tran KN, Heelan MC, Van Zee KJ, Massie MJ, Payne DK, et al. Issues of regret in women with contralateral prophylactic mastectomies. *Ann Surg Oncol*1999;6:546-52.

32 Rebbeck TR, Kauff ND, Domchek SM. Meta-analysis of risk reduction estimates associated with risk-reducing salpingo-oophorectomy in BRCA1 or BRCA2 mutation carriers. *J Natl Cancer Inst*2009;101:80-7.

33 Fakkert IE, Mourits MJ, Jansen L, van der Kolk DM, Meijer K, et al. Breast cancer incidence after risk-reducing salpingo-oophorectomy in BRCA1 and BRCA2 mutation carriers. *Cancer Prev Res (Phila)*2012;5:1291-7.

34 Beral V; Million Women Study Collaborators. Breast cancer and hormone-replacement therapy in the Million Women Study. *Lancet*2003;362:419-27.

35 Rebbeck TR, Friebel T, Wagner T, Lynch HT, Garber JE, Daly MB, et al. Effect of short-term hormone replacement therapy on breast cancer risk reduction after bilateral prophylactic oophorectomy in BRCA1 and BRCA2 mutation carriers: the PROSE Study Group. *J Clin Oncol*2005;23:7804-10.

36 Cuzick J, Sestak I, Bonanni B, Costantino JP, Cummings S, et al. Selective oestrogen receptor modulators in prevention of breast cancer: an updated meta-analysis of individual participant data. *Lancet*2013;381:1827-34.

37 Cuzick J, Sestak I, Forbes JF, Dowsett M, Knox J, Cawthorn S, et al. Anastrozole for prevention of breast cancer in high-risk postmenopausal women (IBIS-II): an international, double-blind, randomised placebo-controlled trial. *Lancet*2013;383:1041-8.

38 Moyer VA. Medications for risk reduction of primary breast cancer in women: US Preventative Services Task Force recommendation statement. *Ann Intern Med*2013;159:698-708.

39 Reid DM, Doughty J, Eastell R, Heys SD, Howell A, et al. Guidance for the management of breast cancer treatment-induced bone loss: a consensus position statement from a UK Expert Group. *Cancer Treat Rev*2008;34(Suppl 1):S3-18.

40 Waters EA, McNeel TS, Stevens WM, Freedman AN. Use of tamoxifen and raloxifene for breast cancer chemoprevention in 2010. *Breast Cancer Res Treat*2012;134:875-80.

Related links

bmj.com
Previous articles in this series
- Gallstones (BMJ 2014;348: g2669)
- First seizures in adults (BMJ 2014;348:g2470)
- Obsessive-compulsive disorder (BMJ 2014;348:g2183)
- Modern management of splenic trauma (BMJ 2014;348:g1864)
- Fungal nail infection: diagnosis and management (BMJ 2014;348:g1800)

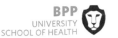

Gynaecomastia and breast cancer in men

Catherine B Niewoehner professor of medicine[1], Anna E Schorer associate professor of medicine[2]

[1]Metabolism Section, VA Medical Center 111G, One Veterans Drive, Minneapolis, MN 55417, USA

[2]Hematology/Oncology Section, VA Medical Center 111E, Minneapolis, USA

Correspondence to: C B Niewoehner niewo002@umn.edu

Cite this as: BMJ 2008;336:709-13

‹DOI› 10.1136/bmj.39511.493391.BE http://www.bmj.com/ content/336/7646/709

Breast disorders in males can be distressing for both patients and examining doctors. Patients often feel embarrassed and anxious. Although cancers are diagnosed in only about 1% of cases of male breast enlargement, practitioners may feel uncertain about how to differentiate gynaecomastia (benign breast enlargement) from malignancy and how to manage these disorders. This review covers the causes, evaluation, and treatment of gynaecomastia and the risk factors for and evaluation and treatment of breast cancer in males.

What is gynaecomastia?

Gynaecomastia is the benign enlargement of male breast tissue (>2 cm palpable, firm, subareolar gland and ductal tissue) resulting from a relative decrease in androgen effect or increase in oestrogen effect. Breast enlargement due to adipose tissue is called pseudogynaecomastia.

How do hormones affect the breast?

Male breast tissue contains receptors for androgen, oestrogen, and progesterone. Oestrogen stimulates duct development and progesterone stimulates alveolar development in the presence of the permissive anterior pituitary hormones luteinising hormone, follicle stimulating hormone, and growth hormone. Androgens antagonise the effects of oestrogen. A high prolactin level does not stimulate breast tissue growth but alters the production of luteinising hormone by suppressing production of gonadotrophin hormone releasing hormone.

What are the hormone sources in men?

Testicular Leydig cells produce 95% of testosterone. The adrenal cortex produces the rest. About 50% of circulating testosterone is bound to sex hormone binding globulin.

Much of the remainder is weakly bound to albumin. Only the free hormone is active. Oestrogen is less bound to sex hormone binding globulin than testosterone, so increases in sex hormone binding globulin reduce the ratio of active testosterone to oestrogen.

Testosterone can be converted to another potent androgen, dihydrotestosterone, by the enzyme 5 α reductase in peripheral tissues. Testosterone also can be converted to oestradiol by the enzyme aromatase, found especially in adipose tissue. The weak adrenal androgen androstenedione can be converted by aromatase to oestrone, a weak oestrogen. Oestradiol and oestrone can be interconverted in peripheral tissues (fig 1).

When is gynaecomastia physiological?

Overall, 65-90% of neonates have breast tissue, which results from the transfer of maternal and placental oestrogen and progesterone and persists up to several months.

By age 14 up to 60% of boys have gynaecomastia. This usually resolves within one or two years (table 1). At puberty, surges of luteinising hormone and follicle stimulating hormone in conjunction with growth hormone and insulin-like growth factor-1 stimulate testosterone production in Leydig cells. Oestrogen concentrations increase threefold, peaking earlier than testosterone concentrations that eventually increase up to 30-fold. Whether gynaecomastia results from the relative delay in full testosterone production, a temporary increase in aromatase activity, varying sensitivity to oestrogen, or all of these is uncertain.

Gynaecomastia increases with age as free testosterone levels decline and obesity becomes more common (table 1).[1] In an unselected group of men admitted to hospital, the prevalence and diameter of breast enlargement was highly correlated with increasing body mass index.[2] Autopsy studies have found gynaecomastia in 40-55% of unselected cases.[3]

Table 1 Prevalence of gynaecomastia

Age group	Percentage with gynaecomastia
Neonates	65-90
Puberty (age 14)	60
16-20 years	19
25-45 years	33-41
>50 years	55-60

What disorders or drugs enlarge the breast?

Non-physiological gynaecomastia develops with disorders or drugs associated with low testosterone levels, high testosterone conversion to oestrogen, high oestrogen levels, and high sex hormone binding globulin levels resulting in low free testosterone (see boxes).

Drugs, creams, cosmetics, and lotions

Body builders who use high doses of androgen frequently develop significant gynaecomastia, often with breast tenderness, because of androgen conversion to oestrogen.[4] At the opposite end of the spectrum, men prescribed

SOURCES AND SELECTION CRITERIA

We searched Medline for English language papers with the key words "gynaecomastia", "gynecomastia", and "male breast cancer"; the Cochrane database for clinical trials; our personal archives of references; and websites with those terms. We also referred to our institutional experience with gynaecomastia and male breast cancer.

SUMMARY POINTS

- Most breast enlargement in males is due to the benign enlargement of breast tissue (gynaecomastia)
- Physiological gynaecomastia occurs in neonates, at puberty, and with obesity and ageing
- Gynaecomastia is due to an increased oestrogen to testosterone ratio; possible causes are many
- Treatments for painful or embarrassing gynaecomastia include an anti-oestrogen, such as tamoxifen, or surgery (liposuction or mammoplasty)
- One per cent of breast cancers occur in men, with higher rates in men with a family history of breast cancer or previous chest radiation
- Irregular, eccentric, hard or fixed breast tissue, ulceration, nipple abnormalities, or associated adenopathy suggest breast cancer
- Men typically have more advanced breast cancer at diagnosis than women; management is similar

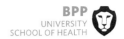

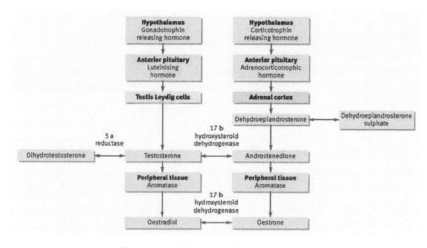

Fig 1 Sources of hormones affecting breast tissue

DISEASES ASSOCIATED WITH GYNAECOMASTIA

Low androgen levels

Hypogonadotrophic hypogonadism (Kallmann's syndrome); high prolactin states; pituitary disease; primary hypogonadism—infection (viral orchitis), trauma, infiltration (haemachromatosis), chemotherapy, neurological disease (spinal cord injury, myotonic dystrophy); Klinefelter's syndrome; true hermaphrodism; congenital defects in testosterone synthesis

High androgen and high oestrogen levels

Testicular feminisation, Leydig cell tumour, human chorionic gonadotrophin producing tumour, congenital adrenal hyperplasia

High oestrogen levels

Abnormal aromatase (activating mutation), tumour aromatase, feminising adrenal carcinoma, Sertoli cell tumour, starvation and refeeding

High sex hormone binding globulin levels leading to low free testosterone levels

High oestrogen states, genetic high sex hormone binding globulin level, hyperthyroidism

Other or multifactorial

Cirrhosis, renal failure, idiopathic

DRUGS ASSOCIATED WITH GYNAECOMASTIA

Low androgen levels: inhibition of testosterone synthesis

Ketoconazole; metronidazole; gonadotrophin releasing hormone agonists (chronic) and antagonists; spironolactone; chemotherapy (cytotoxic drugs)

Low androgen levels: inhibition of testosterone action

Androgen receptor blockers—bicalutamide, flutamide, nilutamide, spironolactone, eplerinone, cyproterone; 5 α reductase inhibitors—finasteride, dutasteride; H2 blockers and proton pump inhibitors—cimetidine, ranitidine, proton pump inhibitors; marijuana

High androgen levels resulting in high oestrogen levels

Androgen administration—excessive testosterone replacement, anabolic steroids, androgen containing contraceptives; human chorionic gonadotrophin

High oestrogen levels or oestrogen action

Oestrogen administration; occupational exposure to oestrogen; oestrogen containing creams or cosmetics; isoflavones; phytoestrogens—cosmetics, soy products, beer, tea tree oil, lavender oil; oestrogen action—diethylstilbesterol, clomiphene, phenytoin, digitalis

Other or multifactorial

Angiotensin converting enzyme inhibitors, alcohol, amiloride, amiodarone, amphetamines, calcium channel blockers, ciclosporin, diazepam, growth hormone, highly active antiretroviral therapy, heroin, methyldopa, isoniazid, reserpine, risperidone, theophylline, tricyclic antidepressants (increase prolactin levels)

---

combined gonadotrophin releasing hormone agonist-androgen receptor antagonist therapy or androgen receptor antagonist monotherapy for prostate cancer develop gynaecomastia 10-20% and 50-60% of the time, respectively.[5] Gynaecomastia is much less common in men taking 5

α reductase inhibitors for benign prostatic hypertrophy (0.3-1.1%).

Patients treated with highly active antiretroviral therapy for HIV report gynaecomastia, but the prevalence and mechanisms are uncertain.[6] Pseudogynaecomastia can occur in patients with HIV associated lipodystrophy. HIV does not increase the risk for breast cancer, but HIV associated lymphoma can present as a lymphomatous breast mass.

Cosmetics, creams, and lotions may contain oestrogens or compounds with oestrogen effects. Children are particularly vulnerable to these sources. Three healthy prepubertal boys developed gynaecomastia, which was traced to repeated application of a "healing balm" containing lavender oil (*Lavandula augustifolia*), lavender scented soap and skin lotions, and shampoo and styling gel containing lavender and tea tree oil (*Melaleuca alternifolia*), respectively. Antiandrogenic effects of lavender and tea tree oil were confirmed using human breast cancer cell lines.[7] Gynaecomastia resolved within a few months of stopping these applications.

Starvation and refeeding
Children and adults refed after starvation or who have been treated with growth hormone can develop transient gynaecomastia. The mechanisms are thought to be similar to those governing gynaecomastia during puberty.

Illness
Multiple mechanisms may operate in systemic diseases. Thyrotoxicosis increases production of androstenedione, increases oestrogen production in peripheral tissue, and increases sex hormone binding globulin levels. Androgen catabolism is reduced in liver disease, making more available for conversion to oestrogen in peripheral tissue. Renal failure has many effects on hormone and drug metabolism.

Tumours
All types of testicular tumours have increased aromatase activity.[8] Leydig and Sertoli cell tumours produce androgen and oestrogen. Germ cell tumours produce intratesticular human chorionic gonadotrophin, which can cause dysfunction of Leydig cells and reduced testosterone production. Lung and hepatic tumours can produce enough systemic human chorionic gonadotrophin to increase Leydig cell testosterone secretion, which is readily converted to oestrogen through increased aromatase activity. Gynaecomastia may follow cancer treatment if chemotherapy or radiation damages Leydig cells.

Genetic causes
Several families (fathers and sons) have been described with oestrogen excess due to mutations activating the aromatase gene.[9] They developed prepubertal gynaecomastia and accelerated prepubertal growth.

Who is at higher risk for breast cancer?
Table 2 lists the conditions associated with breast cancer in males.

Male breast cancer represents about 1% of all cases of breast cancer, but in sub-Saharan Africa 7-14% of breast cancer cases occur in men. Population based US tumour registries show that rates are highest in African-American men, intermediate in non-Hispanic Caucasian men and Asian-Pacific Islanders, and lowest in Hispanic men.[10] Male

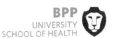

Table 2 Risk factors for male breast cancer

Category	High risk established	High risk suggested
Oestrogen excess	Klinefelter's syndrome, exogenous oestrogen	Cirrhosis
Androgen deficiency	Cryptorchidism, orchitis, orchiectomy	
Ethnic and familial	Family with history of breast cancer; sub-Saharan African	Ashkenazi Jew
Specific genes	BRCA2, BRCA1	Androgen receptor mutation, CHEK2* mutation, CYP17† mutation, PTEN‡ mutation
Exposures	Radiation	Electromagnetic fields, occupational, polycyclic aromatic hydrocarbons

*Cell cycle checkpoint kinase regulating responses to DNA damage.
†Cytochrome P450c17a gene coding enzyme involved in oestrogen and androgen synthesis.
‡Tumour suppressor gene associated with Cowden syndrome, an autosomal dominant susceptibility to multiple hamartomas.

Table 3 Physical examination in male breast enlargement

Gynaecomastia	Malignancy
Bilateral (usually) or unilateral	Unilateral (usually) or bilateral
Painless or painful (occasionally)	Painless or painful (uncommon)
Central (subareolar)	Central (70-90%) or eccentric*
Smooth	Irregular*
Firm	Rubbery or hard*
Mobile	Fixed†
Normal nipple	Nipple deformity (17-30%) or discharge (<10%)*
Normal skin	Thickened, red, or ulcerated skin*
Normal axilla	Axillary adenopathy†

*Mandates surgical evaluation.
†May be associated with locally advanced malignancy.

breast cancer can occur at any age but mean age is 65 years.

The risk of gynaecomastia and breast cancer coexists in high oestrogen states. Men with Klinefelter's syndrome, who have testicular failure shortly after puberty, have a 58-fold higher risk than normal males for breast cancer, with an absolute risk that approaches 3%.[11] Breast cancer has been reported in male to female transsexuals who were castrated and given high dose oestrogen. In one nested case-control study of 41 Swedish men who developed breast cancer after treatment for prostate cancer, the risk was higher in men treated with oestrogen than in other survivors of prostate cancer.[12]

A family history of breast cancer increases the risk of breast cancer in males. In some families this is linked to the breast cancer risk gene BRCA2, which is also associated with excess risk for prostate cancer. Ashkenazi Jews have a higher prevalence of BRCA1 and BRCA2 and an increased risk of male breast cancer than the general population.[13] Male carriers of BRCA2 have a cumulative risk for breast cancer of 7% by age 80. The excess risk in male carriers of BRCA1 is much less. Table 2 shows other genetic markers considered possible risk factors for male breast cancer.

Exposure to ionising radiation may also increase the risk of breast cancer. The incidence of breast cancer is higher in male survivors of cancer who have received therapeutic chest irradiation, particularly at a young age. The rate of breast cancer in Japanese men exposed to nuclear fallout was threefold greater than in non-exposed men.[14]

How should male breast tissue be evaluated?

Examination
Table 3 lists differences in the presentation of gynaecomastia and malignancy. If breast tissue enlargement is unilateral, a diagnosis other than gynaecomastia must be considered. In the absence of exogenous androgen or other drugs,

rapid development of breast enlargement outside puberty suggests a tumour producing luteinising hormone or human chorionic gonadotrophin. Almost no lobular tissue exists in normal adult male breast tissue. Gynaecomastia is characterised by proliferation of ductules and loose connective tissue. Increasing glandular tissue in adult men increases the concern for malignancy.

Other important physical findings include adiposity, signs of hyperthyroidism, liver disease, hypogonadism (gynoid body habitus, decreased body hair, small testes consistent with Klinefelter's syndrome), excessive musculature indicating exogenous androgen administration, or a testicular mass.

Initial laboratory evaluation
If the cause of breast enlargement is not obvious, laboratory evaluation is needed (fig 2). Such evaluation is unnecessary for boys at puberty, for typical asymptomatic senile changes, for enlargement consisting mostly of adipose tissue, for men taking drugs known to cause gynaecomastia, or for physical findings strongly suggesting breast cancer.

Imaging
Imaging is not necessary if cancer is not suspected. Ultrasonography and mammography can, however, differentiate adipose tissue from gynaecomastia and can be useful if surgical intervention is planned. Mammography is about 90% sensitive and 90% specific for malignant compared with benign masses in men.[15] Invasive cancers are solid on ultrasonography. A complex cystic mass also is suspicious.

Biopsy
Biopsy is the only way to make a definitive diagnosis. Patients with a hard, irregular or asymmetrical mass, nipple discharge (bloody or non-bloody), axillary adenopathy, or a mass fixed to skin or the chest wall must have a biopsy (table 3). Core biopsy is recommended over fine needle or excisional biopsy.

Most primary breast carcinomas in men are ductal, either invasive or non-invasive (ductal carcinoma in situ).[16] Papillary histology is more common and lobular histology is rare in men (fig 3). Ninety per cent of breast cancers in men have oestrogen and progesterone receptors.

Metastatic and non-malignant breast masses
Rare causes of male breast masses include metastatic carcinoma from lung, prostate, and liver; haematological malignancies, including lymphoma, Hodgkin's disease, and plasmacytoma; and benign conditions, including myofibroblastoma, papillary hyperplasia, lupus mastitis, haemangioma, hamartoma, and granulomatous mastitis.

When and how should gynaecomastia be treated?

Non-surgical treatment
Physiological gynaecomastia requires no treatment unless accompanied by pain or significant embarrassment. Withdrawing an offending drug or treating an underlying disorder may be sufficient, especially if gynaecomastia is relatively recent.

Testosterone replacement for hypogonadal men can be beneficial, but longstanding fibrotic gynaecomastia is unlikely to respond. One small study showed more stable testosterone levels and more resolution of gynaecomastia with transdermal testosterone than with biweekly

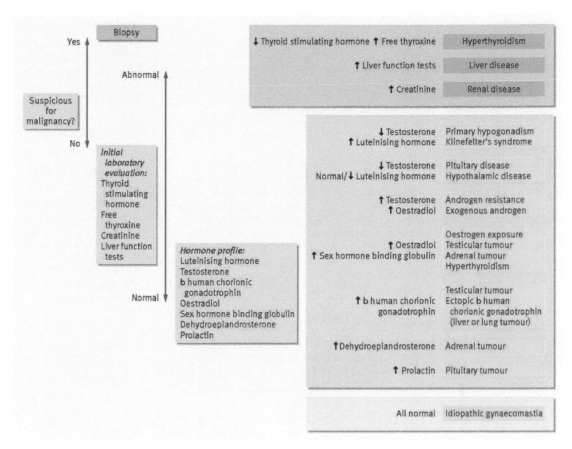

Fig 2 Evaluation of non-physiological breast enlargement in men when cause is not obvious

intramuscular testosterone injections that resulted in high initial testosterone levels with potential to cause high oestrogen levels.[17] Danazol, a weak androgen, is less effective.

Anti-oestrogen treatment with tamoxifen 10-20 mg/day significantly reduced pain and breast volume in 40-80% of boys with persistent pubertal gynaecomastia[18] and men with prostate cancer treated with an androgen receptor blocker (bicalutamide).[19] Trials of raloxifene and clomiphene are too small or results too mixed to be conclusive. The aromatase inhibitor anastrazole was no better than placebo for reducing breast volume during puberty[20] and was less effective than tamoxifen in men treated with bicalutamide.[19]

Local irradiation (10-12 Gy) prevented gynaecomastia in men with prostate cancer treated with bicalutamide,[20] but tamoxifen achieved significantly better results.[21]

Surgical treatment
Men with findings suspicious for malignancy or gynaecomastia causing persistent pain or embarrassment should be referred to a surgeon. Goals of surgery include removing abnormal breast tissue, restoring the normal male breast contour, and reducing pain.

Liposuction is effective if breast enlargement is mostly caused by adipose tissue and the overlying skin is fairly taut. Subcutaneous mastectomy is required for removal of glandular tissue and redundant skin (visible inframammary skinfolds) and pain relief. Complications include haematoma, seroma, infection, sensory changes, pain, breast asymmetry, skin redundancy, and scarring.[22] [23] The most common complication is a poor cosmetic outcome. Final results of surgery may not be apparent for a year.

How is male breast cancer treated?
No prospective studies have been done of male breast cancer. Management is extrapolated from female breast cancer and from case series in single institutions. Local surgical management is modified radical mastectomy (simple mastectomy plus axillary dissection or sentinel node biopsy), with postoperative radiation for bulky tumour, involved or close margins, clinically positive nodes, or inflammatory carcinoma.

Men usually are offered adjuvant hormone therapy with tamoxifen 20 mg/day for five years, as several retrospective studies have shown improved survival.[24] If the tumour has adverse features, adjuvant systemic therapy (chemotherapy or HER2 antibody trastuzumab, or both) should be offered. Experience of using adjuvant aromatase inhibitors in men is limited. The management of metastatic and recurrent disease is similar to that in women.

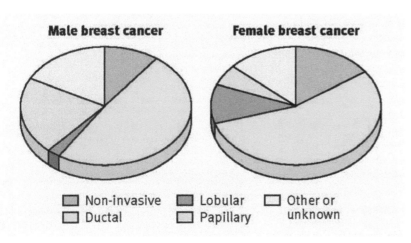

Fig 3 Histology of breast cancers in men and women

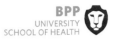

PATIENT VIGNETTE

A 33 year old man mentioned fatigue; headaches; painful, enlarged breasts; and impotence. He had been a heavy user of androgen containing substances for muscle enhancement until three months previously. Examination revealed moderate obesity; normal visual fields; 7 cm tender, firm palpable subareolar breast tissue on the left and 4 cm non-tender tissue on the right; and soft 5 ml testes bilaterally. Levels of follicle stimulating hormone, luteinising hormone, and testosterone were low. His prolactin level was mildly elevated. Magnetic resonance imaging showed a 5 mm pituitary mass. Levels of thyroid stimulating hormone, free thyroxine, morning cortisol, and adrenocorticotrophic hormone were normal. A mammogram showed noticeably increased glandular tissue, especially on the left.

Gynaecomastia was thought primarily to be due to conversion of previous high dose androgen to oestrogen in adipose tissue. Suppression of the hypothalamic-pituitary-gonadal axis can persist for months to years after prolonged exposure to exogenous androgen. Prolactin induced suppression of the gonadotrophin releasing hormone pulse generator may have contributed. The patient was given a dopamine agonist (cabergoline) to suppress prolactin. Levels of follicle stimulating hormone, luteinising hormone, and testosterone remained low. Transdermal testosterone caused skin irritation. Biweekly intramuscular testosterone reduced fatigue, but the high peak testosterone levels increased oestrogen levels, which, in turn, increased prolactin levels. He developed more gynaecomastia (to 6 cm) and pain in his right breast. He refused tamoxifen. He has been referred to a surgeon because of ongoing breast pain.

ADDITIONAL EDUCATIONAL RESOURCES

- Giordano SH, Buzdar AU, Hortobagyi GN. Breast cancer in men. *Ann Intern Med* 2002;137:678-87
- Braunstein GD. Aromatase and gynecomastia. *Endocr Relat Cancer* 1999; 6:315-324
- Chin HW, Nguyen T, Kumar G, Durning J, Crowell C. Male breast cancer. *Fed Pract* Apr;2006:40-7
- Gynecomastia: etiology, diagnosis, and treatment (www.endotext.org/male/male14/male14.htm)—An extensive discussion of male breast development and a brief summary of diagnosis and treatment
- Gynecomastia (www.emedicine.com/med/topic934.htm)—A concise description of the causes, clinical evaluation, and treatment of gynaecomastia
- Sports shorts (www.aap.org/family/sportsshorts12.pdf)—Quick guides to performance enhancing substances, for paediatricians, parents, coaches, and athletes
- Gynaecomastia: its features and when and how to treat it (www.ccjm.org/PDFFILES/BEMB0604.pdf)—A description of the causes, clinical features, diagnosis, and treatment of gynaecomastia
- Mastectomy for gynaecomastia (medpolicy.unicare.com/policies/SURG/gynecomastia.html)—Indications for when mastectomy is considered medically necessary, with links for additional information
- Detailed guide to breast cancer in men (www.cancer.org/docroot/CRI/CRI_2_3x.asp?dt=28)—A clear, concise reference covering risk factors, diagnosis, and staging and treatment of male breast cancer
- Male breast cancer treatment (www.cancer.gov/cancertopics/pdq/treatment/malebreast)—A review of risk factors, prognostic factors, and treatment options for breast cancer in men
- No registration is needed for these websites

Information resources for patients

- Welcome to Gynecomastia.org (www.gynecomastia.org)—Addresses questions about causes and treatments for gynaecomastia with some information about breast cancer
- Male breast cancer (www.psaweb.med.navy.mil/BREASTHEALTH/malecancer.html)—A concise description of many facets of male breast cancer, with clear illustrations
- General information about breast cancer (www.cancer.gov/cancertopics/pdq/treatment/malebreast)—A review of risk factors, prognosis, and treatments for male patients with breast cancer
- No registration is needed for these websites

TIPS FOR NON-SPECIALISTS

- Breast tissue is a common finding in males and is almost always benign in newborns, at puberty, and in otherwise healthy older men, especially if they are obese
- If the physical examination is suspicious for cancer (see table 3) then refer for biopsy

Men are less likely to be diagnosed as having breast cancer at an early stage, but diagnosis at the preinvasive (in situ) stage has increased since the 1980s,[18] perhaps owing to the heightened awareness of patients and clinicians.

QUESTIONS FOR FUTURE RESEARCH

- What is the best treatment for painful gynaecomastia?
- Should breast cancer in men be treated differently from that in women?
- Which hormone therapy is most appropriate for male breast cancer in the adjuvant setting?
- What is the role for immunotherapy or anti-angiogenesis therapy in men with aggressive or refractory breast cancer?

When men and women are matched for tumour stage and histology, no sex difference is found in tumour specific survival. Overall survival is shorter in men, possibly because they tend to be older and have more comorbid conditions.

Contributors: CBN did the literature review, wrote the section on gynaecomastia and the patient vignette, and prepared figure 1. AES did the literature review, wrote the section on breast cancer, and prepared figures 2 and 3. Both authors are guarantors.

Competing interests: None declared.

Provenance and peer review: commissioned; externally peer reviewed.

Patient consent: provided.

1 Nuttall FQ. Gynecomastia as a physical finding in normal men. *J Clin Endocrinol Metab*1979;48:338-40.
2 Niewoehner CB, Nuttall FQ. Gynecomastia in a hospitalized male population. *Am J Med*1984;77:633-7.
3 Andersen JA, Gram JB. Male breast at autopsy. *Acta Path Microbiol Immunol Scand*1982;90:191-7.
4 Friedl KE, Yesalis, CE. Self-treatment of gynecomastia in bodybuilders who use anabolic steroids. case reports. *Physician Sports Med*1989;17:67-79.
5 Dobs B, Darkes MJM. Incidence and management of gynecomastia in men treated for prostate cancer. *J Urol*2005;174:1737-42.
6 Allen EA, Parwant AV, Siddiqui MT, Clark DP, Ali SZ. Cytopathologic findings in breast tissues in men with HIV infection. *Acta Cytologica*2003;47:183-7.
7 Henley DV, Lipson N, Korach KS, Bloch CA. Pubertal gynecomastia linked to lavender and tea tree oils. *N Engl J Med*2007;356:479-85.
8 Tseng A, Horning SJ, Freiha FS, Resser KJ, Hannigan JF, Torti FM. Gynecomastia in testicular cancer patients. *Cancer*1985;56:2534-8.
9 Shozu M, Sebastian S, Takayama K, Hsu W-T, Schultz RA, Neely K, et al. Estrogen excess associated with novel gain-of-function mutations affecting the aromatase gene. *N Engl J Med*2003;348:1855-65.
10 Sasco AJ, Lowenfels AB, Pasker-de Jong P. Review article: epidemiology of male breast cancer. A meta-analysis of published case-control studies and discussion of selected aetiological factors. *Int J Cancer*1993;53:538-49.
11 Swerdlow AJ, Schoemaker MJ, Higgins CD, Wright AF, Jacobs PA. Cancer incidence and mortality in men with Klinefelter syndrome: a cohort study. *J Natl Cancer Inst*2005;97(16):1204-10
12 Karlsson CT, Malmer B, Wiklund F, Gronberg H. Breast cancer as a second primary in patients with prostate cancer—estrogen treatment or association with family history of cancer? *J Urol*2006 Aug;176(2):538-43.
13 Struewing JP, Hartge P, Wacholder S, Baker SM, Berlin M, McAdams M, et al. The risk of cancer associated with specific mutations of BRCA1 and BRCA2 among Ashkenazi Jews. *N Engl J Med*1997;336:1401-8.
14 Weiss JR, Moysich KB, Swede H. Epidemiology of male breast cancer. *Cancer Epidemiol Biomarkers Prev*2005;14:20-6.
15 Evans GFF, Anthony T, Appelbaum AH, Schumpert TD, Levy KR, Amirkhan RH, et al. The diagnostic accuracy of mammography in the evaluation of male breast disease. *Am J of Surg*2001;181:96-100.
16 Anderson WF, Devesa SS. In situ breast carcinoma in the surveillance, epidemiology, and end results database of the National Cancer Institute. *Cancer*2005;104:1733-41.
17 Dobs AS, Meikle AW, Arver S, Sanders SW, Carmelli KE, Mazer NA. Pharmacokinetics, efficacy, and safety of a permeation-enhanced testosterone transdermal system in comparison with bi-weekly injections of testosterone enanthate for the treatment of hypogonadal men. *J Clin Endocrinol Metab*1999;84:3469-78.
18 Lawrence SE, Faught KA, Vethamuthu J, Lawson ML. Beneficial effects of raloxifene and tamoxifen in the treatment of pubertal gynecomastia. *J Pediatrics*2004;145:71-6.
19 Boccardo F, Rubagotti A, Battaglia M, Di Tonno P, Selvaggi FP, Conti G, et al. Evaluation of tamoxifen and anastrazole in the prevention of gynecomastia and breast pain induced by bicalutamide monotherapy of prostate cancer. *J Clin Oncol*2005;23:808-15.
20 Plourde PV, Reite FQ, Jou HC, Desrochers PE, Rubin SD, Bercu BB, et al. Safety and efficacy of anastrazole for the treatment of pubertal gynecomastia: a randomized, double-blind, placebo-controlled trial. *J Clin Endocrinol Metab*2004;89:4428-33.
21 Perdonna S, Autorino R, De Placido S, D'Armiento M, Gallo A, Damiano R, et al. Efficacy of tamoxifen and radiotherapy for prevention

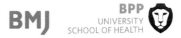

and treatment of gynaecomastia and breast pain caused by bicalutamide in prostate cancer: a randomized, controlled trial. *Lancet Oncol*2005;6:295-300.

22   Fruhstorfer BH, Malata CM. A systematic approach to the surgical treatment of gynecomastia. *Br J Plast Surg*2003;56:237-46.

23   Goes JC, Landecker A. Ultrasound-assisted lipoplasty (UASL) in breast surgery. *Aesthetic Plast Surg*2002;26:1-9.

24   Ribeiro GG, Swindell R, Harris M, Banerjee S, Cramer A. A review of the management of male breast carcinoma based on an analysis of 420 treated cases. *Breast*1996;5:141-6.

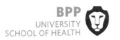

Pancreatic adenocarcinoma

Giles Bond-Smith general and hepatopancreatic-biliary surgical registrar[1], Neal Banga general and transplant surgical registrar[1], Toby M Hammond general and colorectal surgical registrar[2], Charles J Imber consultant hepatopancreatic-biliary and liver transplant surgeon[1]

[1]Hepatopancreatic-biliary Surgery and Liver Transplant Unit, Royal Free Hospital, London NW3 2QG, UK

[2]Department of Surgery, St Mark's Hospital, Harrow, Middlesex

Correspondence to: G Bond-Smith gelsmith@yahoo.co.uk

Cite this as: BMJ 2012;344:e2476

‹DOI› 10.1136/bmj.e2476
http://www.bmj.com/content/344/bmj.e2476

In 2008, an estimated 217 000 new cases of pancreatic cancer were diagnosed worldwide, and in the UK 8000 new cases of pancreatic cancer are reported every year.[4] [5] [6] Worldwide, pancreatic cancer is 13th in incidence but 8th in terms of cancer death.[4] In the UK, pancreatic cancer is the 5th most common cause of cancer death in both sexes, despite being only the 11th most common cancer overall.[7] This is largely due to red flag symptoms usually appearing only once the disease has progressed to involve other structures. Consequently, only 10-20% of patients will have resectable pancreatic cancer at presentation.[7]

The term pancreatic cancer encompasses both exocrine and endocrine tumours (see box 1), of which over 80% are adenocarcinomas. The aim of this review is to update the non-specialist clinician on the cause, clinical presentation, and current management of so called curable and incurable pancreatic adenocarcinomas. The main surgical options available to the patient are discussed, including the decision making process involved in considering patients for curative surgery. The potential complications and morbidity of current treatment regimes, and their management, is covered.

How does pancreatic cancer present?

Almost 50% of cases of pancreatic cancer are diagnosed on attending an emergency department for non-specific abdominal pain or jaundice or both. Only 13% are diagnosed via the two week wait pathway utilised by general practitioners in the UK.[8]

The peak incidence for pancreatic cancer is in the seventh and eighth decades of life. There is no difference in incidence between the sexes.[2] Courvoisier's sign, described as a palpable gallbladder in the presence of painless jaundice, occurs in less than 25% of patients. The majority of patients present with non-specific symptoms. Those presenting late frequently have symptoms secondary to metastatic spread. Approximately 80% of patients have unresectable disease at the time of diagnosis.[2]

Abdominal pain and jaundice are the most common presenting complaints. Abdominal pain predominantly features in up to two thirds of patients, and is typically located in the epigastric region, radiating through to the back, but can present as simple back pain. This can usually be attributed to direct invasion of the celiac plexus or secondary to pancreatitis. Thirteen per cent of patients will present with painless jaundice, and 46% will present with both pain and jaundice.[9] It is reported that those patients presenting with painless jaundice have a better prognosis than those patients that present with pain alone.[10] Pancreatic cancer should be considered in the differential diagnosis of any elderly patient presenting for the first time with acute pancreatitis, particularly in the absence of known precipitating factors such as gallstones or alcohol abuse.

Unexplained weight loss may occur as a result of anorexia, or malabsorption due to pancreatic exocrine insufficiency. This is usually secondary to a blocked pancreatic duct, and often manifests as steatorrhoea. Patients describe foul smelling, oily stools that are difficult to flush away. Peripancreatic oedema or a large tumour may compress the duodenum or the stomach, causing gastric outlet obstruction or delayed gastric emptying, with associated nausea and early satiety.

Development of any of the above symptoms in the presence of late onset diabetes should strongly alert the physician to the possibility of pancreatic cancer. Patients over the age of 50 years with late onset diabetes have an eightfold increased risk of developing pancreatic cancer within three years of the diagnosis compared to the general population (see box 2 for other risk factors).[11]

The clinician should be alert to a potential diagnosis of pancreatic cancer with patients over 50 years old who present with unexplained weight loss, persistent abdominal or back pain, dyspepsia, vomiting, or change of bowel function. Currently there is no specific diagnostic algorithm for pancreatic cancer within the National Institute for Health and Clinical Excellence guidelines for cancer referral. If pancreatic cancer is suspected, patients should be referred to a high volume specialist pancreatic centre. In the UK, this can be performed via the suspected upper gastrointestinal cancer two week wait referral pathway.

What is the pathology of pancreatic cancer?

Ninety five per cent of pancreatic cancers originate from the exocrine portion of the gland. A proposed mechanism for the development of invasive pancreatic adenocarcinoma is a stepwise progression through genetically and histologically well defined non-invasive precursor lesions, called pancreatic intraepithelial neoplasias (PanINs). They are microscopic lesions in small (less than 5 mm) pancreatic ducts, and are classified into three grades (see box 3). The understanding of molecular alterations in PanINs has provided rational candidates for the development of early detection biomarkers and therapeutic targets.[12]

SOURCES AND SELECTION CRITERIA

We searched PubMed to identify peer reviewed original research articles, meta-analyses, and reviews. Search terms were pancreatic cancer, pancreatic adenocarcinoma, pancreatic neoplasia or neoplasm. Only papers written in English were considered.

SUMMARY POINTS

- Pancreatic cancer can present with non-specific symptoms, such as abdominal or back pain, dyspepsia, and unexplained weight loss, as well as the classic presentation of painless jaundice
- The majority of pancreatic cancer is incurable at presentation[1] [2]
- Whether or not pancreatic cancer is deemed curable, current surgical, endoscopic, and oncological management regimes can significantly improve quality of life
- Trials are currently ongoing to improve outcomes in pancreatic cancer[3]

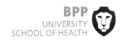

BOX 1 TYPES OF PANCREATIC CANCER

Pancreatic exocrine cancers

- Adenocarcinoma
- Acinar cell carcinoma
- Adenosquamous carcinoma
- Giant cell tumour
- Intraductal papillary mucinous neoplasm (IPMN)
- Mucinous cystadenocarcinoma
- Pancreatoblastoma
- Serous cystadenocarcinoma
- Solid and pseudopapillary tumours

Pancreatic endocrine cancers (pancreatic neuroendocrine tumours)

- Gastrinoma
- Glucagonoma
- Insulinoma
- Nonfunctional islet cell tumour
- Somatostatinoma
- Vasoactive intestinal peptide releasing tumour (VIPoma)

BOX 2 RISK FACTORS FOR PANCREATIC CANCER

Risk factors

- Smoking
- Alcohol
- Increased BMI
- Diabetes mellitus
- Chronic pancreatitis
- Family history of pancreatic cancer

Familial cancer syndromes

- BRCA1, BRCA2
- Familial adenomatous polyposis (FAP)
- Peutz-Jeghers syndrome
- Familial atypical multiple mole melanoma syndrome (FAMMM)
- Lynch syndrome
- von Hippel-Lindau syndrome
- Multiple endocrine neoplasia type 1
- Gardner syndrome

Other medical conditions

- Inflammatory bowel disease
- Periodontal disease
- Peptic ulcer disease

BOX 3 TYPES OF PANCREATIC INTRAEPITHELIAL NEOPLASIA (PANIN)

PanIN 1 (low grade)

- Minimal degree of atypia
- Subclassified into PanIN 1A: absence of micropapillary infoldings of the epithelium; and 1B, presence of micropapillary infoldings of the epithelium

PanIN 2 (intermediate grade)

- Moderate degree of atypia, including loss of polarity, nuclear crowding, enlarged nuclei, pseudostratification, and hyperchromatism
- Mitoses are rarely seen

PanIN 3 (high grade/carcinoma in situ)

- Severe atypia, with varying degrees of cribriforming, luminal necrosis, and atypical mitoses
- Contained within the basement membrane

How do we investigate and diagnose suspected pancreatic cancer?

The most important investigative tool for the diagnosis of pancreatic cancer is computed tomography. However, certain blood tests help guide further management and can be performed while the patient is awaiting specialist review.

Blood tests and tumour markers

A full blood count may reveal a normochromic anaemia or thrombocytosis or both. Those presenting with obstructive jaundice will have significant elevations in serum bilirubin (conjugated and total), alkaline phosphatase, and γ-glutamyltransferase. Serum aspartate aminotransferase (AST) and serum alanine aminotransferase (ALT) may also be raised, but usually to a lesser extent. Liver metastases alone are not frequently associated with clinically evident jaundice, but may result in relatively low grade elevations of serum alkaline phosphatase and transaminase levels.

Carbohydrate 19-9 (CA19-9), also known as sialylated Lewis (a) antigen, was first identified in pancreatic cancer patients in 1981.[13] It is now one of the most widely used serum tumour markers. CA19-9 is normally found in the cells of the biliary tract, and therefore any disease affecting these cells can cause serum elevations, including pancreatitis, cirrhosis, and cholangitis. Five per cent of the population lack the Lewis (a) antigen, and are not able to produce CA19-9, resulting in a sensitivity of 80% and specificity of 73% for pancreatic cancer.[14] As such, it is not currently recommended as a screening tool. CA19-9 does, however, have a role to play in assessing response to surgery and chemoradiotherapy, and as a surveillance tool following treatment.

With the advancement of high throughput techniques (DNA arrays and proteomics), a number of other potential molecular markers for pancreatic cancer have been identified, but to date these have not been found to be any more discriminating than CA19-9.

Imaging

Imaging is not only the most important diagnostic tool for pancreatic cancer, but will also guide the multidisciplinary team in determining whether the disease is surgically curable.

Abdominal ultrasound is safe, non-invasive, and inexpensive. Its main role is in formulating a differential diagnosis among the possible causes of obstructive jaundice. Bile duct dilation (>7 mm, or >10 mm if previous cholecystectomy) with pancreatic duct dilation (>2 mm) can be an indirect sign of pancreatic cancer (the so called double duct sign). Abdominal ultrasound is not as sensitive as computed tomography in imaging the pancreas, and small tumours (less than 3 cm) will frequently be missed.[15] Liver metastases and ascites are important findings in the work-up of a patient with suspected pancreatic cancer and can normally be visualised by ultrasound.

Triple phase computed tomography, preceded by non-contrast computed tomography, is currently the best technique for detecting pancreatic neoplasms and assessing resectability. It is performed in the arterial, pancreatic parenchymal, and portal venous phase (pancreas protocol computed tomography). Multidetector computed tomography is up to 90% effective at predicting the resectability of a pancreatic cancer.[16] There are reports that computed tomography can only reliably detect lesions larger than 3 cm.[14]

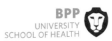
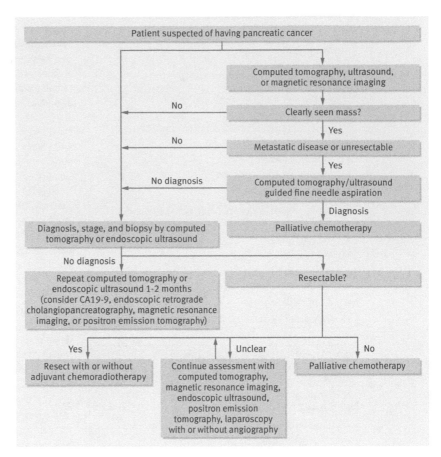

Fig 1 Clinical management pathway

Endoscopic ultrasound (EUS) is becoming an increasingly important imaging modality. A recent meta-analysis showed that it had a sensitivity of 96% (range 85-100%) for diagnosing pancreatic cancer.[17] In comparison to computed tomography, diagnostic sensitivities were significantly in favour of endoscopic ultrasound, especially for small (<3cm) tumours.[12] Endoscopic ultrasound can also accurately detect the involvement of loco-regional lymph nodes.[18] It is further employed to guide fine needle aspiration (FNA) for cytological evaluation of lesions in which there is diagnostic uncertainty. The sensitivity of endoscopic ultrasound guided FNA ranges from 85% to 90% with a false negative rate of up to 15%.[19] Routine endoscopic ultrasound guided FNA of all pancreatic masses is therefore controversial. In a patient with resectable disease who is deemed physiologically fit for surgery, it is arguable whether an FNA is required, as a negative result would not rule out neoplasia, and could delay a potentially curable procedure. The benefit of FNA is mainly in those patients with unresectable disease, as the results may guide further oncological management, or in those patients with significant comorbidities in whom the risk to benefit ratio of surgical intervention is less clear.

The role of MRI (magnetic resonance imaging) remains uncertain at present. Its use in detecting small lesions and determining resectability is increasing as new, faster MRI techniques enable imaging of the pancreas with higher resolution. In a comparative study to determine the diagnostic role of endoscopic ultrasound, computed tomography, and MRI in patients suspected of having pancreatic cancer, the respective sensitivities were 94%, 69%, and 83%.[20]

Positron emission tomography (PET) scanning uses ^{18}F-fluorodeoxyglucose (FDG) to image the primary tumour and establish the presence of metastatic disease. When combined with simultaneous computed tomography scanning (PET-CT), it is more sensitive than conventional imaging for the detection of pancreatic cancer and extra-hepatic metastases. Its role in the staging of disease is, however, yet to be fully ascertained.

Similar to endoscopic ultrasound, endoscopic retrograde cholangiopancreatography with brush cytology or forceps biopsy is an effective way (90-95% sensitivity) to confirm the diagnosis of pancreatic adenocarcinoma. Endoscopic retrograde cholangiopancreatography is, however, an invasive procedure that carries a 5-10% risk of significant complications including pancreatitis, and gastrointestinal or biliary perforation, and is therefore usually reserved as a therapeutic procedure for biliary obstruction or for the diagnosis of unusual pancreatic neoplasms.

Staging and treatment of pancreatic adenocarcinoma

The classification of pancreatic adenocarcinoma is shown in table 1, and how it relates to disease stage and prognosis are shown in table 2.[21][22] At present, surgical resection is the only curative treatment for pancreatic adenocarcinoma. Surgery with curative intent has a five year survival of 10-15%, and median survival of 11 to 18 months. For patients unwilling or not medically fit enough to undergo major pancreatic surgery, alternatives include systemic chemotherapy, chemoradiotherapy, image guided stereotactic radiosurgical systems (such as CyberKnife), surgical bypass, ablative therapies, and endoscopic biliary and gastrointestinal stenting. These are palliative procedures that can improve patients' quality of life by alleviating tumour related symptoms (such as pain and pruritus).

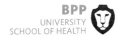

Table 1 TNM classification of pancreatic adenocarcinoma

Tumour (T)	
TX	Primary tumour cannot be assessed
T0	No evidence of primary tumour
Tis	Carcinoma in situ
T1	Tumour limited to the pancreas, 2 cm or smaller in greatest dimension
T2	Tumour limited to the pancreas, larger than 2 cm in greatest diameter
T3	Tumour extension beyond the pancreas but not involving the coeliac axis or superior mesenteric artery
T4	Tumour involves the coeliac axis or superior mesenteric artery
Regional lymph nodes (N)	
NX	Regional lymph nodes cannot be assessed
N0	No regional lymph node metastasis
N1	Regional lymph node metastasis
Distant metastasis (M)	
MX	Distant metastasis cannot be assessed
M0	No distant metastasis
M1	Distant metastasis

Table 2 Staging and TNM (tumour, lymph node, metastasis) classification related to incidence, treatment, and prognosis

Stage	TNM classification	Clinical classification	Incidence at diagnosis (%)	5-year survival rate (%)
0	Tis, N0, M0	Resectable	7.5	15.2
IA	T1, N0, M0	—	—	—
IB	T2, N0, M0	—	—	—
IIA	T3, N0, M0	—	—	—
IIB	T1-3, N1, M0	Locally advanced	29.3	6.3
III	T4, any N, M0	—	—	—
IV	Any T, any N, M1	Metastatic	47.2	1.6

Table 3 Mortality following pancreatic resection in high, medium, and low volume centres[21]

Centre	No. of resections per year	30 day mortality (%)
High volume	>18	2.4
Medium volume	5-18	5.9
Low volume	<5	9.2

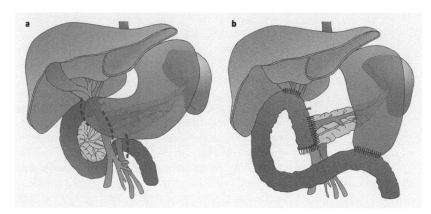

Fig 2 A: Normal anatomy of liver, stomach, duodenum, and pancreas. Dotted lines indicate resection margins at pancreaticoduodenectomy. B: Surgical anastomoses to restore gastrointestinal continuity following a pancreaticoduodenectomy, include a gastrojejunostomy, choledochojejunostomy, and pancreaticojejunostomy (diagram not to scale)

The role of the multidisciplinary team is to determine which patients are suitable to undergo curative surgery, if there is a role for preoperative (neoadjuvant) or postoperative (adjuvant) therapy, or to decide on the most appropriate mode of palliation.

What is resectable and unresectable pancreatic cancer?
The absolute contraindications to pancreatic resection are liver, peritoneal, or distant lymph node metastases, or the patient being deemed medically unfit for major surgery. The age of the patient, size of the tumour, local lymph node metastases, and continuous invasion of the stomach or duodenum are not contraindications to resection.

Advances in surgical techniques and perioperative care mean that tumour involvement of the major vessels around the pancreas is no longer an absolute contraindication to curative resection,[23] although encasement of the hepatic artery, superior mesenteric artery, and coeliac axis means surgery is unlikely to confer any survival benefit. Pancreaticoduodenectomy with resection of the portal and/ or superior mesenteric vein is safe and feasible, with a similar mortality and morbidity to pancreaticoduodenectomy without vascular resection.[24] It should, however, only be performed if a disease-free (R0) resection margin can be achieved. If an R0 resection can be obtained, median survival is vastly improved compared to resections with tumour positive margins (13 versus 6 months; p=0.0002).[25]

Neoadjuvant chemotherapy and chemoradiation
The rationale for neoadjuvant therapy is to increase the incidence of R0 resections, downstage borderline resectable disease to allow resection, and reduce loco-regional recurrence. However, there are no large multicentre randomised controlled trials of neoadjuvant therapy for pancreatic cancer. Meta-analysis of the available data shows that one third of patients with locally advanced disease without distant metastases can achieve a significant oncological response to neoadjuvant treatment increasing the chances of a achieving a R0 resection,[26] thereby reducing local recurrence and potentially improving disease-free survival.

Curative resection
Pancreaticoduodenectomy
The majority of pancreatic adenocarcinomas (78%) are associated with the head, neck, and uncinate process of the pancreas, and require a pancreaticoduodenectomy.[27] First described in the 1930s, it involves resection of the proximal pancreas, along with the distal stomach, duodenum, distal bile duct, and gallbladder as an en bloc specimen.[28] Intestinal continuity is restored via a gastrojejunostomy, choledochojejunostomy, pancreaticojejunostomy (figs 2A and B), or pancreaticogastrostomy.

Morbidity following pancreaticoduodenectomy can be as high as 40%; the most common complications being delayed gastric emptying, pancreatic fistula formation, and pancreatic insufficiency.[29] The operation has wide ranging, 30 day mortality, partly dependent on the surgical volume of the centre where the procedure is performed (see table 3).[30]

Distal pancreatectomy
This procedure is performed for tumours of the body and tail of the pancreas, and carries a morbidity and mortality of 28.1% and 1.2% respectively.[31] The most common major complication is pancreatic fistula formation, due to leakage of pancreatic fluid from the pancreatic duct at the resection margin.[32] Laparoscopic distal pancreatectomy can be safely performed in high volume centres with experience in laparoscopic and pancreatic surgery, and results in less intra-operative blood loss, a shorter time to oral intake, and a shorter postoperative hospital stay than open surgery.[33] Centres that have developed expertise in laparoscopic distal pancreatectomy are now also performing laparoscopic pancreaticoduodenectomy, although this remains rare.

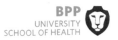

Adjuvant chemotherapy and chemoradiation after curative resection

Treatment regimes have previously employed 5-fluorouracil and radiotherapy.[34] The ESPAC-1 trial in 2004 showed a clear advantage for adjuvant chemotherapy in patients with resected pancreatic cancer over chemoradiotherapy, which had a deleterious impact on survival.[35] ESPAC-3 showed there was no difference between 5-flurouracil/folinic acid and gemcitabine, which is now the most commonly used chemotherapy agent.[36] The ESPAC-4 trial is currently in phase 3, and compares gemcitabine alone against combination therapy of gemcitabine plus capecitabine in patients within one year of a potentially curative resection.

Palliative treatment

Biliary tract or duodenal obstruction can be relieved by surgical, endoscopic, or radiological techniques. Palliative chemotherapy usually involves gemcitabine based regimes. Monoclonal antibodies and the telomerase vaccine GV1001 (the TeloVac trial) are currently under investigation to prolong survival in patients with unresectable or metastatic pancreatic cancer.[3]

How are common postoperative and palliative problems managed?

Locally advanced disease and pancreatic surgery can lead to exocrine insufficiency causing fat malabsorption, which tends to present as excess flatulence, diarrhoea, fatty and offensive smelling stools, or progressive weight loss. These symptoms can be significantly improved by prescribing supplemental pancreatic enzymes (pancreatin). Pancreatin is inactivated by gastric acid and therefore works best when taken with food. There is no linear relationship between the dose of pancreatic enzymes and the symptoms of exocrine insufficiency, so there is no definitive starting dose. Normally the pancreatin preparation is started at a dose of 25 000 to 40 000 units per meal and titrated according to effect on the individual patient.[15]

Delayed gastric emptying is common, causes considerable discomfort, and can prolong the patient's hospital stay. General treatment measures include long term nasogastric drainage, correction of fluid and electrolyte abnormalities, commencement of a proton pump inhibitor or an H2 antagonist, and nutritional supplementation. Prokinetic medications (such as metoclopramide) to improve gastric emptying can also be considered.[15] The onset of delayed gastric emptying shortly after surgery (or an episode of pancreatitis), can indicate an intra-abdominal fluid collection and should be investigated by either ultrasound or computed tomography.

Pancreatic fistulas can result following an anastomotic leak. This is a difficult problem to resolve, with a reported incidence of 0-25%.[37] Early recognition is crucial as a pancreatic fistula may be associated with intra-abdominal sepsis, pseudoaneurysm formation, and possible haemorrhage. If haemorrhage occurs, often preceded by a so called herald bleed, then urgent angiographic imaging is needed to identify and control the source of bleeding, via coil embolisation. The management of simple pancreatic fistulation is still debated. Some advocate conservative management, which includes treatment of sepsis, drainage of intra-abdominal collections, nasogastric suction, total parenteral nutrition, and reducing pancreatic secretions, whereas others favour reoperation.

Contributors: GB-S and NB performed the literature search and wrote the initial draft of the manuscript. TMH and CJI edited and rewrote the manuscript. The original concept for the article was devised by TMH. CJI is guarantor.

Competing interests: All authors have completed the ICMJE uniform disclosure form at www.icmje.org/coi_disclosure.pdf (available on request from the corresponding author) and declare: no support from any organisation for the submitted work; no financial relationships with any organisations that might have an interest in the submitted work in the previous three years; and no other relationships or activities that could appear to have influenced the submitted work.

Provenance and peer review: Not commissioned; externally peer reviewed.

ADDITIONAL EDUCATIONAL RESOURCES

Resources for healthcare professionals

- Hruban RH, Adsay NV, Albores-Saavedra J, Compton C, Garrett ES, Goodman SN, et al. Pancreatic intraepithelial neoplasia: a new nomenclature and classification system for pancreatic duct lesions. *Am J Surg Pathol* 2001;25:579-86—describes a new classification system for pancreatic cancer

- Safi F, Roscher R, Beger HG. Tumour markers in pancreatic cancer. Sensitivity and specificity of CA 19-9. *Hepatogastroenterology* 1989;36:419-23—summarises the role of CA19-9 in pancreatic cancer

- Yeo CJ, Cameron JL, Lillemoe KD, Sohn TA, Campbell KA, Sauter PK, et al. Panctreaticoduodenectomy with or without distal gastrectomy and extended retroperitoneal lymphadenectomy for periampullary adenocarcinoma, part 2: randomized controlled trial evaluating survival, morbidity and mortality. *Ann Surg* 2002;236:355-66—report of a trial showing no benefit for extended lymphadenectomy at the time of pancreaticoduodenectomy for pancreatic cancer

- Zavoral M, Minarikova P, Zavada F, Salek C, Minarik M. Molecular biology of pancreatic cancer. *World J Gastroenterol* 2011;17:2897-908—review of molecular biology of pancreatic cancer

- Hruban RH, Canto MI, Goggins M, Schulick R, Klein AP. Update on familial pancreatic cancer. *Adv Surg* 2010;44:293-311—introduction to familial pancreatic cancer

- Dieterich S, Gibbs IC. The CyberKnife in clinical use: current roles, future expectations. *Front Radiat Ther Oncol* 2011;43:181-94.

Resources for patients

- Pancreatic Cancer UK (www.pancreaticcancer.org.uk)
- Cancer Research UK (www.cancerresearchuk.org)
- Pancreatic Cancer Action (www.pancreaticcanceraction.org)
- Macmillan Cancer Support (www.macmillan.org.uk)
- Patient.co.uk (www.patient.co.uk)
- HPB London (www.hpblondon.com)

TIPS FOR NON-SPECIALISTS

- Patients in the UK with suspected pancreatic cancer should be referred to a specialist pancreatic centre via the two week wait pathway
- Pancreatic cancer should always be considered in the differential diagnosis of an elderly patient with unexplained weight loss, even in the absence of abdominal pain or jaundice
- Multidetector computed tomography is the initial investigation of choice
- All patients with pancreatic cancer should be assessed and managed in a high volume specialist pancreatic centre

---

ONGOING RESEARCH

- **ESPAC 4 trial:** Phase III trial to investigate whether combination adjuvant chemotherapy (gemcitabine and capecitabine) in patients who have undergone resection of pancreatic cancer improves survival when compared to adjuvant chemotherapy (gemcitabine) alone

- **PanGen-EU study:** A large European case control study involving the collection of epidemiological, clinical, and biological information on pancreatic cancer, which aims to validate previous findings as well as explore developmental and progression mechanisms for pancreatic cancer

- **TeloVac trial:** Phase III trial comparing combination chemotherapy (gemcitabine and capecitabine) with concurrent and sequential immunotherapy using the telomerase vaccine (GV1001) in locally advanced and metastatic pancreatic cancer. It is closed to recruitment and the results are expected soon

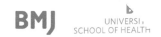

1   Singh SM, Longmire WP Jr, Reber HA. Surgical palliation for pancreatic cancer. The UCLA experience. *Ann Surg*1990;212:132-9.

2   Singh SM, Reber HA. Surgical palliation for pancreatic cancer. *Surg Clin North Am*1989;69:599-611.

3   Bernhardt SL, Gjertsen MK, Trachsel S, Møller M, Eriksen JA, Meo M, et al. Telomerase peptide vaccination of patients with non-resectable pancreatic cancer: a dose escalating phase I/II study. *Br J Cancer*2006;95:1474-82.

4   Anderson K, Mack TM, Silverman DT. Cancer of the pancreas. In: Schottenfeld D, Fraumeni JF Jr, eds. Cancer epidemiology and prevention. 3rd ed. Oxford University Press, 2006.

5   Cancer Research UK. Cancer mortality: UK statistics. 2009. http://info.cancerresearchuk.org/cancerstats/mortality.

6   Hariharan D, Saied A, Kocher HM. Analysis of mortality rates for pancreatic cancer across the world. *HPB (Oxford)*2008;10:58-62.

7   Cancer Research UK. Pancreatic cancer: UK incidence statistics. 2011. http://info.cancerresearchuk.org/cancerstats/types/pancreas/incidence.

8   Elliss-Brookes L. Routes to diagnosis. National Cancer Intelligence Network, 2010. www.ncin.org.uk/publications/data_briefings/routes_to_diagnosis.aspx.

9   Gullo L, Tomassetti P, Migliori M, Casadei R, Marrano D. Do early symptoms of pancreatic cancer exist that can allow an earlier diagnosis? *Pancreas*2001;22:210-3.

10   Watanabe I, Sasaki S, Konishi M, Nakagohri T, Inoue K, Oda T, et al. Onset symptoms and tumor locations as prognostic factors of pancreatic cancer. *Pancreas*2004;28:160-5.

11   Chari ST, Leibson CL, Rabe KG, Ransom J, de Andrade M, Petersen GM. Probability of pancreatic cancer following diabetes: a population-based study. *Gastroenterology*2005;129:504-11.

12   Maitra A, Adsay NV, Argani P, Iacobuzio-Donahue C, De Marzo A, Cameron JL, et al. Multicomponent analysis of the pancreatic adenocarcinoma progression model using a pancreatic intraepithelial neoplasia tissue microarray. *Mod Pathol*2003;16:902-12.

13   Koprowski H, Herlyn M, Steplewski Z, Sears HF. Specific antigen in serum of patients with colon carcinoma. *Science*1981;212:53-5.

14   Valls C, Andía E, Sanchez A, Fabregat J, Pozuelo O, Quintero JC, et al. Dual-phase helical CT of pancreatic adenocarcinoma: assessment of resectability before surgery. *AJR Am J Roentgenol*2002;178:821-6.

15   Shrikhande, S, Freiss H, Buchler M, eds. Surgery of pancreatic tumors. BI Publications Pvt Ltd, 2008.

16   Tabuchi T, Itoh K, Ohshio G, Kojima N, Maetani Y, Shibata T, et al. Tumor staging of pancreatic adenocarcinoma using early- and late-phase helical CT. *AJR Am J Roentgenol*1999;173:375-80.

17   Iglesias Garcia J, Lariño Noia J, Domínguez Muñoz JE. Endoscopic ultrasound in the diagnosis and staging of pancreatic cancer. *Rev Esp Enferm Dig*2009;101:631-8.

18   Kahl S, Malfertheiner P. Role of endoscopic ultrasound in the diagnosis of patients with solid pancreatic masses. *Dig Dis*2004;22:26-31.

19   Chang KJ, Nguyen P, Erickson RA, Durbin TE, Katz KD. The clinical utility of endoscopic ultrasound-guided fine needle aspiration in the diagnosis and staging of pancreatic adenocarcinoma. *Gastrointest Endosc*1997;45:387-93.

20   Müller MF, Meyenberger C, Bertschinger P, Schaer R, Marincek B. Pancreatic tumors: evaluation with endoscopic US, CT, and MR imaging. *Radiology*1994;190:745-51.

21   American Joint Committee on Cancer. AJCC cancer staging manual. 6th ed. Springer, 2002.

22   Jemal A, Clegg LX, Ward E, Ries LA, Wu X, Jamison PM, et al. Annual report to the nation on the status of cancer 1975-2001, with a special feature regarding survival. *Cancer*2004;101:3-27.

23   Reddy SK, Tyler DS, Pappas TN, Clary BM. Extended resection for pancreatic adenocarcinoma. *Oncologist*2007;12:654-63.

24   Ramacciato G, Mercantini P, Petrucciani N, Giaccaglia V, Nigri G, Ravaioli M, et al. Does portal-superior mesenteric vein invasion still indicate irresectability for pancreatic carcinoma? *Ann Surg Oncol*2009;16:817-25.

25   Evans DB, Farnell MB, Lillemoe KD, Vollmer C Jr, Strasberg SM, Schulick RD. Surgical treatment of resectable and borderline resectable pancreas cancer: expert consensus statement. *Ann Surg Oncol*2009;16:1736-44.

26   Chua T, Saxena A. Extended pancreaticoduodenectomy with vascular resection for pancreatic cancer: a systematic review. *J Gastrointest Surg*2010;14:1442-52.

27   Gillen S, Schuster T, Meyer Zum Büschenfelde C, Friess H, Kleeff J. Preoperative/neoadjuvant therapy in pancreatic cancer: a systematic review and meta-analysis of response and resection percentages. *PLoS Med*2010;7:e1000267.

28   Whipple AO, Parsons WB, Mullins CR. Treatment of carcinoma of the ampulla of vater. *Ann Surg*1935;102:763-79.

29   Yeo CJ, Cameron JL, Sohn TA, Lillemoe KD, Pitt HA, Talamini MA, et al. Six hundred fifty consecutive pancreaticoduodenectomies in the 1990s: pathology, complications, and outcomes. *Ann Surg*1997;226:248-60.

30   McPhee JT, Hill JS, Whalen GF, Zayaruzny M, Litwin DE, Sullivan ME, et al. Perioperative mortality for pancreatectomy: a national perspective. *Ann Surg*2007;246:246-53.

31   Kelly KJ, Greenblatt DY, Wan Y, Rettammel RJ, Winslow E, Cho CS, et al. Risk stratification for distal pancreatectomy utilizing ACS-NSQIP: preoperative factors predict morbidity and mortality. *J Gastrointest Surg*2011;15:250-61.

32   Zhou W, Lv R, Wang X, Mou Y, Cai X, Herr I. Stapler vs suture closure of pancreatic remnant after distal pancreatectomy: a meta-analysis. *Am J Surg*2010;200:529-36.

33   Briggs CD, Mann CD, Irving GR, Neal CP, Peterson M, Cameron IC, et al. Systematic review of minimally invasive pancreatic resection. *J Gastrointest Surg*2009;13:1129-37.

34   Kalser MH, Ellenberg SS. Pancreatic cancer. Adjuvant combined radiation and chemotherapy following curative resection. *Arch Surg*1985;120:899-903.

35   Neoptolemos JP, Stocken DD, Friess H, Bassi C, Dunn JA, Hickey H, et al. A randomized trial of chemoradiotherapy and chemotherapy after resection of pancreatic cancer. *N Engl J Med*2004;350:1200-10.

36   Neoptolemos JP, Stocken DD, Bassi C, Ghaneh P, Cunningham D, Goldstein D, et al. Adjuvant chemotherapy with fluorouracil plus folinic acid vs gemcitabine following pancreatic cancer resection: a randomized controlled trial. *JAMA*2010;304:1073-81.

37   Yang YM, Tian XD, Zhuang Y, Wang WM, Wan YL, Huang YT. Risk factors of pancreatic leakage after pancreaticoduodenectomy. *World J Gastroenterol*2005;11:2456-61.

Related links

bmj.com
● Get CME credits for this article

bmj.com/archive
Previous articles in this series
● The modern management of incisional hernias (2012;344:e2843)
● Diagnosis and management of bone stress injuries of the lower limb in athletes (2012;344:e2511)
● The management of overactive bladder syndrome (2012;344:e2365)
● Cluster headache (2012;344:e2407)

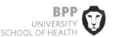

Hepatocellular carcinoma for the non-specialist

T Kumagi lecturer [1], Y Hiasa lecturer[1], G M Hirsch field assistant professor of medicine[2]

[1]Gastroenterology and Metabology, Ehime University, School of Medicine, Ehime, 791-0295, Japan

[2]Liver Centre, Toronto Western Hospital, Toronto, M5T 2S8, Canada

Correspondence to: G M Hirschfield, Toronto Western Hospital, Toronto, ON, M5T 2S8, Canada gideon. hirschfield@uhn.on.ca

Cite this as: BMJ 2009;339:b5039

‹DOI› 10.1136/bmj.b5039
http://www.bmj.com/content/339/
bmj.b5039

Hepatocellular carcinoma is the third most common cause of cancer related mortality worldwide, and in the United Kingdom population data show that age standardised incidence rose from 1.4 to 3.9 per 100000 people between 1975 and 2006 (http://info.cancerresearchuk. org/cancerstats/types/liver). Cirrhosis of the liver is the strongest predisposing factor—80-90% of cases arise from chronic liver disease. Furthermore, in cohort studies of patients with cirrhosis, hepatocellular carcinoma is the leading cause of liver related death.[1] [2]

What predisposes people to hepatocellular carcinoma?

Worldwide rates of hepatocellular carcinoma (fig 1) correlate with widespread infection with hepatitis B in Asia and Africa and hepatitis C in Western countries and Japan. These viral infections are the most common underlying causes of liver disease that predispose to hepatocellular carcinoma (box 1).

Chronic hepatitis B carriers (those seropositive for hepatitis B surface antigen) have a 100-fold higher risk of developing hepatocellular carcinoma than healthy people. In those who also have cirrhosis, the annual incidence of hepatocellular carcinoma is more than 2%,[3] [w1] and risk correlates with viral load.[w2] Aflatoxin B1 is a mycotoxin produced by *Aspergillus* that contaminates grain, particularly in West Africa and China. When ingested it acts as an additive risk factor, as shown by case-control studies using biochemical markers of exposure.[w3] One study found the odds ratio for developing hepatocellular carcinoma was 5.13 (95% confidence interval 7.83 to 29.25) in carriers of hepatitis B surface antigen who had above average concentrations of urinary aflatoxin B1 metabolites compared with those who did not.[w3]

In Western countries and Japan, hepatitis C infection is the most common risk factor: 20-30% of people with chronic hepatitis C develop cirrhosis, with a 3-5% annual incidence of hepatocellular carcinoma.[4] [w4] Sustained alcohol misuse superimposed on chronic viral hepatitis C infection increases the incidence of cancer two to four times.[w5] [w6] Co-viral infections (such as hepatitis B and D, or hepatitis B and C) increase risk further, and in treated patients with HIV—in whom hepatitis C underlies most liver disease—

hepatocellular carcinoma causes 25% of liver related deaths.[w7]

Accurate risk estimates for all other causes of cirrhosis are not available, but alcoholic liver disease, haemochromatosis, and non-alcoholic fatty liver disease—which is becoming increasingly prevalent—are important.[w8-w11] Risk factors for cancer independent of liver disease include age, male sex, and notably metabolic syndrome related to obesity and diabetes.[5] [6] In population based studies,[w12] [w13] diabetes is associated with a two to three times higher risk of developing hepatocellular carcinoma, and a large US prospective cohort study found that liver cancer was one of the cancers in which mortality is higher in obese people.[w14]

How does it present and what is the prognosis?

Patients may remain asymptomatic until malignancy is advanced and symptoms of liver disease—such as right upper quandrant pain, jaundice, ascites, variceal haemorrhage, portal vein thrombosis, or encephalopathy—become evident. Hepatocellular carcinoma should be suspected in patients with chronic liver disease and unexpected decompensation.

Outcomes vary but are poor. One study of 28 asymptomatic patients (tumours ,5 cm) identified by screening found that tumour size doubled in one month to one year (median 117 days).[7] An observational study showed a median survival of 17 months in 102 patients with cirrhosis and unresectable carcinoma managed with treatment of symptoms.[8] Within this group, the best predictors of prognosis were the presence of cancer related symptoms and vascular invasion or extrahepatic spread. For asymptomatic patients without an invasive phenotype, survival at one, two, and three years was 80%, 65%, and 50%, respectively. Overall, the literature supports the following statements[9] [10] [11]:

- The best outcome reported in untreated patients with Child-Pugh class A (table) liver disease and single cancers is 20% survival at five years.

- The prognosis of patients with unresectable hepatocellular carcinoma is poor. In a systematic review, one and two year survival of untreated patients assigned to the control arm in 25 randomised controlled trials ranged from 10% to 72% and from 8% to 50%, respectively.

SOURCES AND SELECTION CRITERIA

We based this review on the available evidence presented in international consensus guidelines and cited in PubMed after searching with the terms "hepatocellular carcinoma", "natural history", "surveillance", "screening", "outcome", "treatment", and "prevention".

SUMMARY POINTS

- Hepatocellular carcinoma is a leading cause of death worldwide, and cirrhosis is the main risk factor
- Infection with hepatitis B and hepatitis C is the main cause of underlying liver disease
- Prevention of chronic liver disease would greatly reduce incidence
- Early tumour diagnosis through screening of at risk groups is cost effective
- New treatments, such as sorafenib, are exciting potential adjuncts to patient care

BOX 1 IMPORTANT RISK FACTORS FOR HEPATOCELLULAR CARCINOMA

- Cirrhosis (any cause)
- Chronic hepatitis B and C infection
- Sustained added excess alcohol consumption
- Non-alcoholic steatohepatitis (both independently and as a cofactor)
- Diabetes
- Aflatoxin exposure
- Older age
- Male sex
- Family history of hepatocellular carcinoma

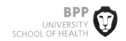

Components of the Child-Pugh score for assessing cirrhosis			
	Score (points)		
Factor	1	2	3
Total bilirubin (µmol/l)	<34	34-50	>50
Serum albumin (g/l)	>35	28-35	<28
International normalised ratio	<1.7	1.71-2.2	>2.2
Ascites	None	Mild (controlled medically)	Severe (poorly controlled)
Encephalopathy	None	Grade I-II	Grade III-IV

This scoring system, although it has been replaced by others for transplantation in particular, is useful for evaluating treatment options in hepatocellular carcinoma. Child-Pugh class A: 5-6 points; Child-Pugh class B: 7-9 points; Child-Pugh class C: 10-15 points.

- People with multinodular asymptomatic tumours without vascular invasion or extrahepatic spread have a median survival of around 16 months.
- Patients with end stage disease and a high tumour burden have a median survival of three months.

Staging systems vary. Most are based on tumour characteristics, the patient's health status, and liver function and are used to help guide management.[12] The Okuda system considers tumour factors (size) and liver function (ascites, albumin, bilirubin) and is used in advanced disease. In contrast, the Cancer of the Liver Italian Program scoring system considers five independent prognostic variables: Child-Pugh class of cirrhosis, tumour size, number of lesions, presence or absence of portal vein thrombosis, and serum concentrations of α fetoprotein. The Barcelona clinic liver cancer staging system found that in early stage disease, survival was negatively correlated with portal hypertension and bilirubin concentrations over 27 µmol/l; for intermediate stages the significant variable was a large multinodular tumour; and for advanced disease, deterioration of performance status (symptoms and functions with respect to ambulatory status and need for care) and the presence of vascular infiltration were important.

Should patients be screened?
Surveillance with ultrasound every six months in patients with cirrhosis, as well as other high risk groups (box 2), is recommended by the American Association for the Study of Liver Diseases,[13] the European Association for the Study of the Liver,[14] and the Japanese Society of Hepatology.[15] The UK hepatocellular carcinoma expert guideline advisory board publish their recommendations imminently. All favour screening, with the aim of decreasing cancer related mortality, despite the potential for generating anxiety and the imperfections of radiology, especially for small tumours.

What evidence supports screening?
A controlled trial in China randomly assigned 18 816 hepatitis B positive patients, aged 35-59, to screening (α fetoprotein and ultrasound every six months) or usual care.[16] Death from hepatocellular carcinoma was lower in the screened group (83.2 v 131.5 per 100 000; mortality rate ratio 0.63, 0.41 to 0.98). However, compliance was less than 60%, the study lacked an intention to treat analysis, outcome was unblinded, and the study's generalisability was questionable. Modelling has also been used to identify patients who might benefit from surveillance.[w15 w16] In the UK, surveillance of people with cirrhosis with six monthly ultrasound and α fetoprotein measurements was cost effective using a decision analysis model.[w17] Modelling data suggest that at an annual individual risk of about 1.5% for developing hepatocellular carcinoma, surveillance becomes effective in terms of life years saved and cost effective if costs are less than $50 000 (£30 150; €33 400) per life year saved.[w18]

Descriptive data support the idea that screening improves survival in patients at risk of hepatocellular carcinoma,[w19] and that cancer is diagnosed earlier and access to treatment is better in these patients.[w20] In a Japanese outpatient surveillance cohort, only 1.4% of the 243 hepatocellular carcinomas detected by screening in 1431 patients with chronic hepatitis C exceeded 3 cm.[w21]

What evidence supports the screening modalities?
A systematic review found six studies evaluating the accuracy of ultrasound for hepatocellular carcinoma at any stage and 13 studies specific to early disease. Surveillance ultrasound detected most tumours, with a pooled sensitivity of 94%, but a lower sensitivity of 63% for early disease.[17] When ultrasound is readily available, α fetoprotein is not routinely measured because it does not identify extra cases and chronic hepatitis may affect concentrations. The reported cut-off point is 20 µg/l, although a large case-control study found that at this value sensitivity was 60% and specificity was 90.6%.[18]

Confirming the diagnosis
To confirm malignancy in a cirrhotic liver, typical radiological features on a variable combination of contrast enhanced computed tomography, magnetic resonance imaging, and ultrasound is needed (fig 2).[13 19] Multidisciplinary teams often coordinate this process, an approach that is validated by observational data.[w22] Advice from the American Association for the Study of Liver Diseases on confirmatory imaging is based on the nodule's size.

Nodules greater than 2 cm
Imaging can confidently establish the diagnosis with no need for biopsy. Characteristic features identified by at least two techniques—ultrasound, computed tomography, or magnetic resonance imaging—is sufficient. Alternatively, if the α fetoprotein is over 200 µg/l, biopsy is not needed when the radiological appearance of the mass is suggestive of hepatocellular carcinoma, such as a large nodule or multifocal disease with arterial hypervascularity.[w23 w24]

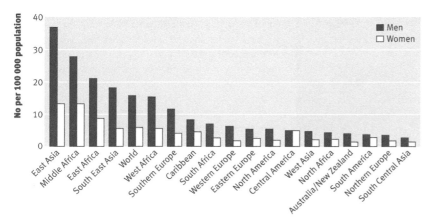

Fig 1 2002 estimates of age standardised incidence of hepatocellular carcinoma. Incidence varies 14-fold across the world for men and 10-fold for women. The disease is still rare in the UK—140th of the 172 countries worldwide for men and 136th for women. Adapted, with permission, from Cancer Research UK

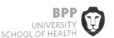

Nodules 1-2 cm

If the appearances are typical of hepatocellular carcinoma—hypervascularity with washout in the portal-venous phase—using two dynamic techniques, the lesion is treated as such. If the findings are not characteristic or the different radiological evaluations of blood supply to the focal lesion are inconsistent, biopsy may be needed. The risks of tumour biopsy include bleeding and needle track seeding—a meta-analysis found that tumour seeding occurred after 2.7% of biopsies.[w25] One study prospectively evaluated the accuracy of contrast enhanced ultrasound and dynamic magnetic resonance imaging for the diagnosis of nodules less than 2 cm detected during ultrasound surveillance. It reported that a diagnosis could be established without a biopsy if both tests were conclusive, but that the sensitivity of these non-invasive criteria was only 33%.[19]

Nodules less than 1 cm

Such nodules need to be followed with ultrasound at three to six month intervals. If no interval change occurs over two years, a return to routine surveillance is advised.

What are the treatment options?

Treatment with curative intent comprises surgery or local tumour ablation. Chemoembolisation and oral chemotherapy aim to prolong survival, but without cure. The stage at diagnosis, the severity of the underlying liver disease, and the risk for future development of hepatocellular cancer are important. Figure 3 shows one recognised but not universally validated treatment algorithm. Despite numerous publications an expert panel found only 80 randomised controlled trials of treatment, of which two thirds had suboptimal study design or methodology.[10 11 20 21]

When is surgery appropriate?

Treatment is most successful after resection or transplantation with curative intent. Case series and multicentre databases show that resection is associated with a five year survival of 50% but a recurrence rate of 70%.[w26 w27] Tumour size is not important for patients without cirrhosis, but in the presence of cirrhosis, outcome is better for those without portal hypertension and very early stage

tumours (<2 cm) and certain patients with tumours less than 5 cm.

Liver transplantation treats not only the cancer but also the underlying liver disease. A pivotal observational study showed that transplantation can successfully treat hepatocellular carcinoma.[w28] It introduced the Milan criteria for transplantation—a single tumour 5.0 cm or less, or two to three tumours of 3.0 cm or less.[w28] Patients outside these criteria may still be good candidates for transplantation, and alternative treatments could possibly be used first as a "bridge" to transplantation.[w29]

What are the alternatives to surgery?

When surgery is not appropriate, or early cancer is identified, locally destructive treatment may be the best option. Radiofrequency ablation using high frequency alternating current or direct percutaneous ethanol injection may be curative. Randomised controlled studies and a systematic review have shown radiofrequency ablation to be superior to percutaneous ethanol ablation, with a four year survival of 74% in patients with small tumours.[22 23 24]

Transarterial chemoembolisation, in which multifocal cancer is treated by angiographically delivered chemotherapy combined with arterial embolisation of tumour feeding vessels, is not curative. It affords median survival of 19-20 months in randomised controlled trials.[25 26] A meta-analysis of these trials showed an improved two year survival with an odds ratio of 0.53 (0.32 to 0.89; P=0.017) when treatment was compared with best supportive care, which translates to a median increase in survival from 16 months to 20 months.[10] This approach is an option for patients who are not candidates for resection, transplantation, or radiofrequency ablation, and it may be useful as a bridge to transplantation. Relative contraindications include portal vein thrombosis, thrombocytopenia, or overt hepatic insufficiency.

What new treatments are available?

New chemotherapeutic agents are emerging, as are adjunctive treatment regimens with radiotherapy. Sorafenib is a multikinase inhibitor with antiproliferative and antiangiogenic activity.[27 w30] The SHARP multicenter phase

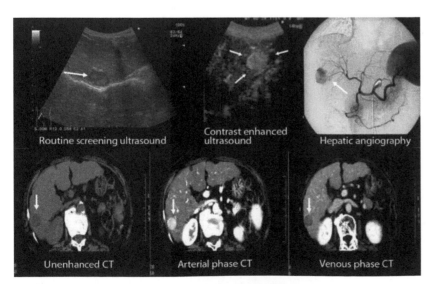

Fig 2 Representative imaging of hepatocellular carcinoma. Selected images obtained of a single hepatocellular carcinoma on screening ultrasound, contrast ultrasound, and computed tomography as well as traditional hepatic angiography. Note the enhancement in the arterial phase of the computed tomogram and washout in the portal venous phase (arrows)

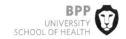

III double blind placebo controlled study randomised 602 patients with advanced hepatocellular carcinoma to either sorafenib or placebo. Patients were not eligible for locoregional treatment and had well preserved liver function (Child-Pugh class A). Median overall survival was 10.7 months in the sorafenib group and 7.9 months in the placebo group (hazard ratio in the sorafenib group, 0.69, 0.55 to 0.87; P<0.001). At present, however, the National Institute for Health and Clinical Excellence (www.nice.org.uk/Guidance/TA/Wave17/8) has not found sorafenib to be a cost effective use of resources.

How is recurrence managed?

Recurrence of hepatocellular carcinoma after resection or local ablation is classified as early (weeks to months) or late (>2 years). Early recurrence is usually the result of incomplete initial treatment or micrometastases, whereas late recurrence is attributed to new cancers. Markers of early recurrence include microvascular or macrovascular tumour invasion and, to a lesser extent, tumour size. No well defined predictors of late recurrence exist, although one report showed the potential for gene expression from surrounding non-tumorous liver tissue to predict risk of recurrence.[w31] The best interventions in such cases are unknown, and multimodal treatment is usually offered on the basis of the timing, size, and site of recurrence, as well as local expertise.

Can this disease be prevented?

As generalists identify more patients with chronic liver disease at an early stage, treatment of the underlying liver disease, especially hepatitis B or C infection, may prevent the development of cancer.

The efficacy of preventing this disease through hepatitis B vaccination is being studied,[w32] and a reduced incidence of hepatocellular carcinoma has been reported in Taiwan in association with universal neonatal vaccination against hepatitis B.[28] Another study randomised 651 patients with compensated hepatitis B cirrhosis to receive lamivudine or placebo. After a median follow-up of 32 months, hepatocellular carcinoma was diagnosed in 3.9% of the lamivudine group and in 7.4% of the controls (P=0.047).[29] In a pooled analysis of 20 hepatitis C treatment studies (4700 patients), analysis of 14 studies (n=3310) reporting sustained virological response rates with antiviral treatment found a reduced risk of hepatocellular carcinoma in patients with viral eradication compared with non-responders (0.35, 0.26 to 0.46; P<0.00001).[30]

Contributors: TG and GMH contributed equally to this article and both act as guarantors; YH contributed to the diagnosis and treatment section, including provision of patient images.

Competing interests: None declared.

Provenance and peer review: Commissioned; externally peer reviewed.

Patient consent obtained.

1　Parkin DM, Bray F, Ferlay J, Pisani P. Global cancer statistics, 2002. *CA Cancer J Clin* 2005;55:74-108.
2　Sangiovanni A, Del Ninno E, Fasani P, De Fazio C, Ronchi G, Romeo R, et al. Increased survival of cirrhotic patients with a hepatocellular carcinoma detected during surveillance. *Gastroenterology* 2004;126:1005-14.
3　Beasley RP, Hwang LY, Lin CC, Chien CS. Hepatocellular carcinoma and hepatitis B virus. A prospective study of 22707 men in Taiwan. *Lancet* 1981;2:1129-33.
4　Lok AS, Seeff LB, Morgan TR, di Bisceglie AM, Sterling RK, Curto TM, et al. Incidence of hepatocellular carcinoma and associated risk factors in hepatitis C-related advanced liver disease. *Gastroenterology* 2009;136:138-48.
5　Naugler WE, Sakurai T, Kim S, Maeda S, Kim K, Elsharkawy AM, et al. Gender disparity in liver cancer due to sex differences in MyD88-dependent IL-6 production. *Science* 2007;317:121-4.

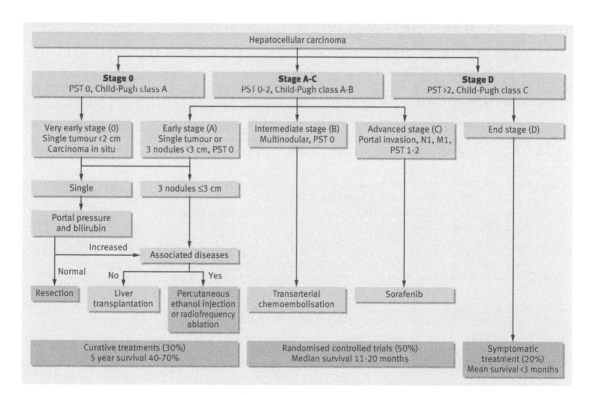

Fig 3 The Barcelona clinic liver cancer staging classification and treatment of hepatocellular carcinoma. Adapted with permission from Llovet et al.[11] This system classifies the disease on the basis of the size of the lesion at presentation and the underlying severity of liver disease. It is widely used, although further independent validation is needed. N1=lymph node involvement; M1=metastatic spread; PST=performance status. PST describes symptoms and functions with respect to ambulatory status and need for care. PST 0=normal activity; PST 1=some symptoms, but still almost fully ambulatory; PST 2=less than 50% ambulatory; PST 3=more than 50% of day spent in bed; PST 4=completely bedridden

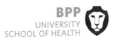

A PATIENT'S PERSPECTIVE

I was diagnosed with liver cancer in October 2008 with no symptoms—just a shadow on a scan taken before a trial to treat my chronic hepatitis C infection. It meant that I could not enter the trial, but instead needed treatment to burn the tumour I didn't even know I had.

To me it not only meant I could not undergo treatment for the virus, but that I was now dealing with a bigger problem. I remember leaving the hospital after hearing the news in a fog. I became quite emotional, and as a man who hadn't cried in 40 years it was a shock to have such strong overwhelming emotions. I became very antisocial and did not want to talk about it except with health professionals. My key support came from my daughter, who was in her first year of university.

It took a few days to process the information, but I decided to beat the cancer at all costs, and after six months of being clear started further treatment for hepatitis. The cancer treatment hurt, but the pain subsided quickly. So for now I have been clear for 11 months, and with the exception of a recent scare, I am relaxed. Life goes on.David, *Toronto*

SELECTED EXAMPLES OF ONGOING RESEARCH

Improvements in screening technology

- Determining the usefulness of non-classic tumour markers, such as lens culinaris agglutinin reactive α fetoprotein (AFP-L3) and des-carboxy prothrombin
- Identification of entirely new tumour markers by serum proteomic evaluation

Histological methods to improve diagnosis and prediction of outcome

- Molecular markers of very early hepatocellular carcinoma and tumour biology
- Tumour and adjacent liver gene expression profiles and prediction of treatment response and recurrence

Improved treatments

- Locally delivered brachytherapy—for example, radioembolisation with yttrium-90 microspheres
- Immunotherapy—for example, tumour vaccine therapy

TIPS FOR GENERAL PRACTITIONERS

- Identifying patients at risk of cirrhosis enables liver disease to be treated and patients to be screened for hepatocellular carcinoma
- Early diagnosis of hepatocellular carcinoma offers a chance for cure, whereas treatment for advanced disease is extremely limited
- Ultrasound—performed at six monthly intervals in at risk groups—is the first line screening tool for hepatocellular carcinoma
- Treatment is usually at tertiary centres, because of its specialist nature, and may involve local or systemic treatments as well as resection or liver transplantation

ADDITIONAL EDUCATIONAL RESOURCES

Resources for healthcare professionals

- US National Cancer Institute (www.nci.nih.gov/cancertopics/pdq/screening/hepatocellular/HealthProfessional/page4)—Detailed information on hepatocellular carcinoma for health professionals
- US National Institutes of Health (http://clinicaltrials.gov/ct2/results?term=Hepatocellular+carcinoma)—Currently registered clinical trials in hepatocellular carcinoma
- Cancer Research UK (http://info.cancerresearchuk.org/cancerstats/types/liver)—Data on the incidence of liver cancer

Information resources for patients

- British Liver Trust (www.britishlivertrust.org.uk/home/the-liver/liver-diseases/liver-cancer.aspx)—Information for patients on liver cancer
- Cancer Research UK (www.cancerhelp.org.uk/help/default.asp?page=4892)—Information about the different types of primary liver cancer
- US National Cancer Institute (www.cancer.gov/cancertopics/types/liver)—Information for patients on liver cancer and current clinical trials
- Mayo Clinic (www.mayoclinic.com/health/liver-cancer/DS00399)—Educational website on liver cancer provided by a private medical organisation

6   Hussain K, El-Serag HB. Epidemiology, screening, diagnosis and treatment of hepatocellular carcinoma. *Minerva Gastroenterol Dietol*2009;55:123-38.

7   Sheu JC, Sung JL, Chen DS, Yang PM, Lai MY, Lee CS, et al. Growth rate of asymptomatic hepatocellular carcinoma and its clinical implications. *Gastroenterology*1985;89:259-66.

8   Llovet JM, Bustamante J, Castells A, Vilana R, Ayuso Mdel C, Sala M, et al. Natural history of untreated nonsurgical hepatocellular carcinoma: rationale for the design and evaluation of therapeutic trials. *Hepatology*1999;29:62-7.

9   Villa E, Moles A, Ferretti I, Buttafoco P, Grottola A, Del Buono M, et al. Natural history of inoperable hepatocellular carcinoma: estrogen receptors' status in the tumor is the strongest prognostic factor for survival. *Hepatology*2000;32:233-8.

10   Llovet JM, Bruix J. Systematic review of randomized trials for unresectable hepatocellular carcinoma: chemoembolization improves survival. *Hepatology*2003;37:429-42.

11   Llovet JM, Di Bisceglie AM, Bruix J, Kramer BS, Lencioni R, Zhu AX, et al. Design and endpoints of clinical trials in hepatocellular carcinoma. *J Natl Cancer Inst*2008;100:698-711.

12   Chen CH, Hu FC, Huang GT, Lee PH, Tsang YM, Cheng AL, et al. Applicability of staging systems for patients with hepatocellular carcinoma is dependent on treatment method—analysis of 2010 Taiwanese patients. *Eur J Cancer*2009;45:1630-9.

13   Bruix J, Sherman M. Management of hepatocellular carcinoma. *Hepatology*2005;42:1208-36.

14   Bruix J, Sherman M, Llovet JM, Beaugrand M, Lencioni R, Burroughs AK, et al. Clinical management of hepatocellular carcinoma. Conclusions of the Barcelona-2000 EASL conference. European Association for the Study of the Liver. *J Hepatol*2001;35:421-30.

15   Makuuchi M, Kokudo N, Arii S, Futagawa S, Kaneko S, Kawasaki S, et al. Development of evidence-based clinical guidelines for the diagnosis and treatment of hepatocellular carcinoma in Japan. *Hepatol Res*2008;38:37-51.

16   Zhang BH, Yang BH, Tang ZY. Randomized controlled trial of screening for hepatocellular carcinoma. *J Cancer Res Clin Oncol*2004;130:417-22.

17   Singal A, Volk ML, Waljee A, Salgia R, Higgins P, Rogers MA, et al. Meta-analysis: surveillance with ultrasound for early-stage hepatocellular carcinoma in patients with cirrhosis. *Aliment Pharmacol Ther*2009;30:37-47.

18   Trevisani F, D'Intino PE, Morselli-Labate AM, Mazzella G, Accogli E, Caraceni P, et al. Serum alpha-fetoprotein for diagnosis of hepatocellular carcinoma in patients with chronic liver disease: influence of HBsAg and anti-HCV status. *J Hepatol*2001;34:570-5.

19   Forner A, Vilana R, Ayuso C, Bianchi L, Sole M, Ayuso JR, et al. Diagnosis of hepatic nodules 20 mm or smaller in cirrhosis: prospective validation of the noninvasive diagnostic criteria for hepatocellular carcinoma. *Hepatology*2008;47:97-104.

20   Lopez PM, Villanueva A, Llovet JM. Systematic review: evidence-based management of hepatocellular carcinoma—an updated analysis of randomized controlled trials. *Aliment Pharmacol Ther*2006;23:1535-47.

21   Llovet JM, Bruix J. Novel advancements in the management of hepatocellular carcinoma in 2008. *J Hepatol*2008;48(suppl 1):S20-37.

22   Shiina S, Teratani T, Obi S, Sato S, Tateishi R, Fujishima T, et al. A randomized controlled trial of radiofrequency ablation with ethanol injection for small hepatocellular carcinoma. *Gastroenterology*2005;129:122-30.

23   Lin SM, Lin CJ, Lin CC, Hsu CW, Chen YC. Randomised controlled trial comparing percutaneous radiofrequency thermal ablation, percutaneous ethanol injection, and percutaneous acetic acid injection to treat hepatocellular carcinoma of 3 cm or less. *Gut*2005;54:1151-6.

24   Cho YK, Kim JK, Kim MY, Rhim H, Han JK. Systematic review of randomized trials for hepatocellular carcinoma treated with percutaneous ablation therapies. *Hepatology*2009;49:453-9.

25   Llovet JM, Real MI, Montana X, Planas R, Coll S, Aponte J, et al. Arterial embolisation or chemoembolisation versus symptomatic treatment in patients with unresectable hepatocellular carcinoma: a randomised controlled trial. *Lancet*2002;359:1734-9.

26   Lo CM, Ngan H, Tso WK, Liu CL, Lam CM, Poon RT, et al. Randomized controlled trial of transarterial lipiodol chemoembolization for unresectable hepatocellular carcinoma. *Hepatology*2002;35:1164-71.

27   Llovet JM, Ricci S, Mazzaferro V, Hilgard P, Gane E, Blanc JF, et al. Sorafenib in advanced hepatocellular carcinoma. *N Engl J Med*2008;359:378-90.

28   Chang MH, Chen CJ, Lai MS, Hsu HM, Wu TC, Kong MS, et al. Universal hepatitis B vaccination in Taiwan and the incidence of hepatocellular carcinoma in children. Taiwan Childhood Hepatoma Study Group. *N Engl J Med*1997;336:1855-9.

29   Liaw YF, Sung JJ, Chow WC, Farrell G, Lee CZ, Yuen H, et al. Lamivudine for patients with chronic hepatitis B and advanced liver disease. *N Engl J Med*2004;351:1521-31.

30   Singal AK, Singh A, Jaganmohan S, Guturu P, Mummadi R, Kuo YF, et al. Antiviral therapy reduces risk of hepatocellular carcinoma in patients with hepatitis C virus-related cirrhosis. *Clin Gastroenterol Hepatol*2009; published online 29 October.

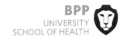

Diagnosis and management of anal intraepithelial neoplasia and anal cancer

J A D Simpson academic surgical registrar, J H Scholefield professor of surgery

¹Division of Gastrointestinal Surgery, Queens Medical Centre Campus, Nottingham University Hospital, Nottingham NG7 2UH, UK

Correspondence to: J A Simpson alastairsimpson@hotmail.com

Cite this as: BMJ 2011;343:d6818

<DOI> 10.1136/bmj.d6818
http://www.bmj.com/content/343/bmj.d6818

Anal cancer accounts for about 4% of large bowel malignancies, but data from the Surveillance Epidemiology and End Results programme show a considerable rise in incidence since 1975[1] from 0.8 to 1.7 per 100 000. The World Health Organization recently estimated that between 350 and 500 new cases of anal squamous cell carcinoma are detected each year in England and Wales.[2]

Observational studies have shown that individuals with genital human papillomavirus (HPV) infection and those who are immunosuppressed, including HIV positive patients, are at increased risk of developing anal cancer.[3][4] A history of cervical or vulval HPV infection and premalignant changes also increases the risk of developing anal cancer, with a reported incidence rate ratio of between 3.97 and 31.09, dependent on age at diagnosis, compared with controls.[5] General practitioners and practice nurses who screen women as part of national programmes for detecting cervical malignancy should be aware of the association between HPV infection and anal cancer.

The majority of anal cancers are of squamous cell origin and 80% are preceded by relatively innocuous skin changes. Early identification is important because anal cancer can often be prevented or treated with conservative management strategies, whereas late presentation often necessitates radical surgery associated with substantial morbidity. We discuss causes, diagnosis, and management of anal cancer, focusing particularly on recent changes in management strategies. We draw on the findings of systematic reviews and cite recognised guidelines where possible.

Who is most at risk?

Observational evidence from the UK has shown that in the past three decades, the greatest increase in incidence of anal cancer has occurred in women.[6][7] Figure 1 illustrates this trend as seen in south east England from the late 1800s through to 1964. The average age for diagnosis in both men and women is 57 years.

Population based case-control studies from Denmark and Sweden[w1] showed that anal cancer is associated with HPV infection in 90% of patients,[1] and a large case-control study found positive associations between incidence of anal cancer and various health and lifestyle factors.[8] This study identified cigarette smoking as a substantial risk factor in both men and women (relative risks 9.4 and 7.7, respectively, compared with non-smoking controls);[8] 28% of patients with anal cancer gave a history of genital warts as a result of HPV infection, compared with only 1-2% of controls, and a history of receptive anal intercourse in men increased the relative risk of developing anal cancer by 33 times compared with controls with colon cancer. HIV infection in men who have sex with men was associated with approximately double the risk of developing anal cancer compared with men who have sex with men who were HIV negative.[8][9]

How do patients with anal cancer present?

Common presenting symptoms include anal pain, bleeding, discharge, pruritus, and ulceration (fig 2). If the anal sphincters are infiltrated by tumour patients may report faecal incontinence and tenesmus. Locally advanced disease may present with perianal infection and fistula formation. It is important to identify palpable inguinal lymphadenopathy at presentation because worse outcomes, higher local failure, and decreased survival have been reported if nodal spread has occurred.[10] Radiological assessment is required to detect distant metastases. Although metastases are not common, occurring in less than 10% of patients with anal cancer, the ACT 1 trial indicated that 40% of this patient subgroup died as a consequence of metastatic spread.[11] Invasive anal cancer is occasionally an unexpected finding after excision of anal tags or haemorrhoids.

Red flag symptoms that should raise suspicion of anal cancer and for which a patient must be promptly referred for investigation are perianal bleeding, a palpable anal mass, and perianal ulceration.

SOURCES AND SELECTION CRITERIA

We searched PubMed for clinically relevant studies, and the Cochrane library, using the search terms anal cancer and anal intraepithelial neoplasia. We consulted the National Institute for Health and Clinical Excellence guidelines and the Association of Coloproctology position statements.

SUMMARY POINTS

- Human papillomavirus infection increases an individual's risk of developing squamous cell carcinoma of the anus; cigarette smoking, high number of previous sexual partners, and previous pre-cancerous lesions of the cervix or vulva (in women) are also associated with increased risk

- Although anal cancer is not an AIDS defining cancer, its incidence is increased in HIV positive individuals and in those who are immunosuppressed

- Anal intraepithelial neoplasia usually precedes development of invasive squamous anal carcinoma and can present in various forms.

- The management of anal cancer has changed in recent years; chemo-irradiation rather than surgery is the first choice treatment for most lesions.

- Surgery may be the primary treatment modality for small perianal lesions which can be locally excised, but is now usually reserved for tumours that fail to respond to chemo-irradiation or for recurrent disease.

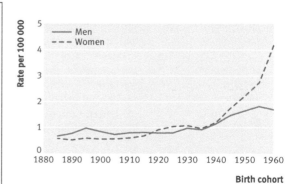

Fig 1 Age standardised rates of anal cancer by birth cohort. Adapted from Robinson et al (Br J Cancer 2009)[7]

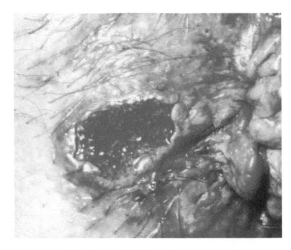

Fig 2 Perianal ulceration, typical of invasive anal cancer, often associated with symptoms of bleeding, pain, and pruritus.

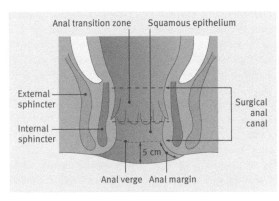

Fig 3 Cross sectional anatomy of the anal canal. Adapted from Renehan et al[12]

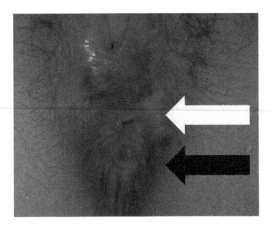

Fig 4 Perianal pigmented anal intraepithelial neoplasia III lesion (black arrow) and associated white plaque (white arrow)

Understanding anal anatomy

Definitions of anal anatomy are not consistent and surgeons, radiologists, and pathologists differ in how they classify structures. The following description is a pragmatic definition taken from the 2011 position statement for management of anal cancer from the Association of Coloproctology of Great Britain and Ireland[12] and relates directly to figure 3.

The anus can be divided into the anal canal and the anal margin; the former is 3.5-4 cm long in men and shorter in women. The anal canal begins where the rectum enters the puborectalis sling at the apex of the anal sphincter complex, and ends with the squamous mucosa blending with the perianal skin, which roughly coincides with the palpable intersphincteric groove. Immediately proximal to the dentate line, a narrow zone of transitional mucosa is variably present—the anal transition zone. Distal to this, the mucosa consists of squamous epithelium devoid of hairs and glands. The anal margin extends distal to the anal verge (the junction of the hair bearing skin) to a 5 cm circumferential area from it. Lymphatic drainage of the anal canal depends on location: below the dentate line drainage is to the inguinal group of nodes; above, lymph drains to the mesorectal, lateral pelvic and inferior mesenteric nodes.[12]

What is anal intraepithelial neoplasia and how do I recognise it?

Anal intraepithelial neoplasia usually precedes the development of invasive squamous anal carcinoma. It can involve both the perianal skin and anal canal. A population based, case-control study has shown that anal intraepithelial neoplasia is strongly associated with HPV infection.[3] It can present as part of a multifocal disease process involving any or all sites of anogenital cancer.[13] There are aetiological and clinical parallels between anal intraepithelial neoplasia, vulval intraepithelial neoplasia, and cervical intraepithelial neoplasia. A recent Association of Coloproctology Position statement suggests that the progression of anal intraepithelial neoplasia to invasive anal cancer more closely resembles the natural history of vulval intraepithelial neoplasia, with expected malignant transformation in about 10% of immunocompetent patients over five years.[14]

Patients may present with pruritus or anal discharge. Suspicious lesions may be raised, scaly, white plaques, erythematous, pigmented, fissured, or eczematous (fig 4). [15] Anal intraepithelial neoplasia is present in 28-35% of excised anal condylomata.[16w2]

How are suspicious lesions investigated?

Evaluation in primary care

Ask the patient about risk factors for anal cancer. Obtaining a careful medical history (including asking about chronic diseases) will help to evaluate a patient's fitness for any future surgery and other treatment. Age over 75 years is associated with reduced tolerance to chemoradiotherapy and increased risk of local disease relapse.[17 18] In view of the association with HPV it is also prudent for a thorough sexual history to be taken.

Although anal cancer is not an AIDS defining cancer (meaning that diagnosis of anal cancer does not indicate the conversion of HIV to AIDS), it is 30 times more common in HIV positive individuals. Therefore HIV status should be considered, and for known HIV positive patients it is sensible to obtain up to date results for viral load and CD4 count.[12]

Patients who describe perianal symptoms consistent with anal intraepithelial neoplasia or anal cancer require examination of the perineum, digital rectal examination, and examination of the inguinal area for palpable nodes. Consider vaginal examination in women because of the multifocal nature of the disease, specifically with a view to identifying lesions on the vulval skin or vaginal mucosa. Suspicious lesions may suggest the presence of vulval intraepithelial neoplasia and should trigger referral to a gynaecological specialist.

Note any changes in pigmentation of the perianal region, as well as ulceration and the presence of skin tags or condylomata. As part of the digital rectal examination it is

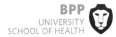

important to document any palpable mass lesion, if possible indicating the distance from the anal verge at which the mass is felt and the proportion of the anal circumference that it occupies. Inspect the glove for blood from the anal canal.

Before referral to a specialist it is helpful to request a full blood count, serum urea and electrolytes, and, in HIV positive patients, an assessment of current CD4 status.

Diagnosing anal intraepithelial neoplasia

Diagnosis of anal intraepithelial neoplasia requires primary care practitioners to maintain a high index of suspicion particularly in patients with known risk factors who present with new symptoms. For a definitive diagnosis a biopsy of the suspicious area is needed. This will normally be performed by a specialist following referral.

Referral of patients with suspected anal cancer

Guidelines from the UK National Institute of Health and Clinical Excellence recommend that patients presenting with bleeding from the anus that has lasted longer than six weeks, a palpable mass on rectal examination, or anaemia without a known cause should be referred for urgent investigation for cancer. Pragmatically this means that they will be included in the two week wait rule and receive a diagnostic investigation within 14 days of referral, because urgent consultation with a specialist has been recognised as a priority.

Investigations undertaken in specialist care

After referral to a specialist, the patient is likely to undergo biopsy of the suspect lesion in order to establish a histological diagnosis. Biopsy often takes place as part of a formal examination under anaesthesia, which can also provide information about the size of the lesion and involvement of adjacent structures, and may be supplemented by sigmoidoscopy.

Imaging is used to inform tumour staging. Distant metastatic spread can be determined by computed tomography of the thorax, abdomen, and pelvis. Magnetic resonance imaging of the pelvis allows assessment of tumour size and local invasion and the involvement of local lymph nodes. Endoanal ultrasound provides a 360° image of the anal canal and is useful for assessing tumour depth, particularly if there is concern that the anal sphincters may be involved. It is useful for assessing local response to treatment but is limited by its restricted field of view and may miss lymph nodes in the mesorectum.

How is anal intraepithelial neoplasia treated?

The priorities of managing anal intraepithelial neoplasia are to minimise symptoms and prevent the development of anal cancer. A number of different strategies can be employed to achieve these end points.

Observation only

Conservative management derives from a combination of single centre studies that have shown low rates of malignant transformation in immunocompetent patients with anal intraepithelial neoplasia[19W3] and high recurrence rates after aggressive surgery. Recurrences after surgery are thought to occur because of the inability to completely eradicate local HPV. Therefore patients with low grade anal dysplasia are followed up every six to 12 months.[w4]

Chemoradiotherapy

No supporting evidence has been established for the use of chemoradiotherapy in anal intraepithelial neoplasia, but anecdotal reports have described success in vulval intraepithelial neoplasia. However the use of radiotherapy in particular may lead to the development of anal stenosis.

Surgery

Local excision of small lesions preserves tissue histology, which can help to guide future management. Local excision is suitable for lesions that cover less than a third of the anal circumference. Before excision the surgeon will usually perform anal mapping to determine the extent of the disease. Mapping involves taking eight to 12 biopsies from around the anal margin and canal. It is useful to record the procedure on an operative mapping sheet or with digital photography.

Brown et al performed preoperative mapping and local excision on 34 patients with high grade anal intraepithelial neoplasia. On review 56% had margin involvement and 63% recurred within 12 months.[w5] No patient developed carcinoma but five developed anal stenosis or faecal incontinence.

Wide local excision has also been considered for larger anal lesions, but these techniques present an even greater risk of postoperative complications and are probably overly aggressive for a disease process in which the natural history is still not fully understood. If the worst areas are excised then the remaining lesions can be managed expectantly.

Immunomodulation therapy

Imiquimod is a nucleoside analogue of the imidazoquinoline family and has pro-inflammatory, anti-tumour, and anti-viral activity. It is prescribed as a 5% cream, and applied topically it can induce regression of anal intraepithelial neoplasia and eradication of HPV. A double blind randomised controlled trial showed sustained regression of high grade intraepithelial neoplasia in 61% of patients, with a median follow-up of 36 months.[w6] In a separate review of cohort studies and case reports, imiquimod was associated with a complete regression in 48% of anal intraepithelial neoplasia lesions and a partial response in 34%. This was associated with a recurrence rate of 36% over 11-39 months of follow-up.[w7] Most studies of imiquimod have assessed its use in HIV positive populations with short follow-up, and the drug has rarely been compared with other treatment strategies. Despite the relative success of this treatment, caution should be used when extrapolating this evidence to other populations of patients with anal intraepithelial neoplasia.

HPV immunotherapy

Vaccination against HPV was first approved in the United States in 2006. The evidence for its use in preventing cervical intraepithelial neoplasia and cervical malignancies as part of a population based immunisation programme is well established.[w8] The quadrivalent vaccine has also shown efficacy against anogenital warts in phase II/III trials. However, clarification of some uncertainties—notably vaccine efficacy in men and HIV infected individuals, and the feasibility to offer vaccination programmes to both sexes—is required to establish the benefits of HPV vaccines for the prevention of malignant and premalignant anal lesions.

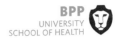

Photodynamic therapy

Case reports and small uncontrolled trials have supported the use of photodynamic therapy in anal intraepithelial neoplasia.[w9] However this type of therapy is painful and often requires multiple treatments.[w10] Larger series with long term follow up are required before it could be recommended as standard therapy.

Ablation

Goldstone et al[w11] retrospectively reviewed 75 cases of high grade anal intraepithelial neoplasia in which patients had received infrared coagulator ablative therapy. They quoted the probability of success as 81% after a single treatment, rising with repeated treatment and with no evidence of serious complications. However, the follow-up period was limited (one to two years) and the outcomes were not as good if the patient was HIV positive before treatment. Other reviews point to a high recurrence rate and substantial postoperative pain, also questioning the ability of ablation to clear HPV.[14] Ablative therapies can include laser ablation, cryotherapy, and electrocautery, but none of these provide histology, which can be useful when planning a patient's long term management.

Anal intraepithelial neoplasia is a complex disease process, the natural history of which remains unclear. Low grade dysplasia (anal intraepithelial neoplasia I and II) represents a much more indolent disease than high grade dysplasia (anal intraepithelial neoplasia III). Progression of disease and therefore associated treatment is more aggressive in HIV positive populations. With this in mind we have reproduced the treatment algorithm from the 2011 Association of Coloproctology guidelines (fig 5).[14]

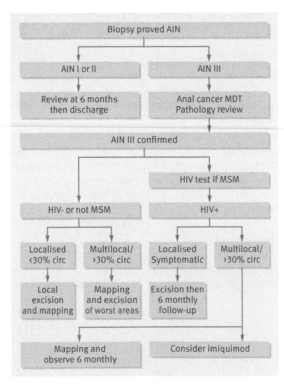

Fig 5 Treatment algorithm for the management of anal intraepithelial neoplasia (AIN).[14] MDT=multidisciplinary team. MSM=men who have sex with men. % circ=percentage of the circumference of the perianal skin/anal canal occupied by lesion

How is anal cancer classified and staged?

The current WHO classification of anal tumours (box) categorises by histological tissue types. Squamous cell carcinoma is the most common type of anal cancer, seen in 80-85% of patients.[w12] Adenocarcinoma of the anus is less common, constituting 5-18% of cases.[20] Other malignancies are very rare.

Squamous cell carcinoma of the anal canal can be graded histologically, but neither the histological type nor the degree of differentiation seem to influence prognosis strongly.[22] Other authors have used anal cancer databases to perform multivariate analysis and establish factors that influence prognosis, which include the patient's sex, tumour stage, node involvement, and response to radiotherapy or combined treatment.[23 24 25]After confirmation of the diagnosis of anal cancer, tumour staging is needed. Anal cancers are staged in accordance with the American Joint Committee on Cancer/tumour node metastasis (TNM) classification. Staging provides prognostic significance based on five year survival (table).

Five year survival for anal cancer on the basis of stage at diagnosis[26]

Tumour stage	5 year survival (%)
I	69.5
II	61.8
IIIA	45.6
IIIB	39.6
IV	15.3

How is anal cancer managed?

Anal cancer is a rare malignancy that requires care at specialist referral centres where diagnostic and treatment decisions can be referred to a single multidisciplinary team. This team ensures that treatment decisions are made involving experienced specialists from surgical, radiological, oncological, and gynaecological divisions. Given that 10% or less of patients with anal cancer have metastases at presentation, the mainstay of treatment is usually local control.

Non-surgical treatment

An important change in the recommended approach for treating anal cancer over the past two decades has been that chemoradiotherapy is now the first choice treatment for invasive anal cancer, with surgery reserved for salvage of local recurrence. The reasons for loss of enthusiasm for surgery as first line therapy included the high associated morbidity and frequent recurrence rates, presumably because although surgical resection removed the malignant tissue it could not eradicate the underlying HPV infection.

Six randomised trials of non-surgical treatment have been reviewed in the Association of Coloproctology position statement on anal cancer,[27] which supports the use of combination chemoradiotherapy including 5-fluorouracil and mitomycin C, but also acknowledges that conclusions are based on a cohort of 1628 patients spread across trials with heterogeneous methodology.

Patients who receive chemoradiotherapy may lose fertility and may need a colostomy either before or after treatment. Pelvic radiotherapy can lead to faecal incontinence and the development of rectovaginal fistula. These complications may reduce a patient's quality of life and patients should be counselled about them when treatment is discussed.

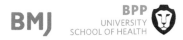

Surgical treatment

Well differentiated anal margin tumours less than 2 cm in diameter (T1 N0) or occupying less than half the anal circumference can initially be treated by local excision, which provides definitive treatment if all resection margins are clear.[28 w13]

Currently the main role for surgery in anal cancer is for "salvage treatment" after failure of chemoradiotherapy. A retrospective review showed that disease relapse is most likely within the first three years and rare after five years.[29]

Renehan and O'Dwyer recently reviewed the management of local disease relapse after treatment for anal cancer.[30] Following examination of 13 studies that had reported oncological outcomes after salvage surgery for relapsed anal cancer they concluded that salvage surgery with abdominoperineal excision offers the only opportunity for cure in these patients. The excision margins for anal cancer surgery are wider than for rectal cancer and therefore perineal reconstruction and the assistance of urological, plastic, and gynaecological surgeons may be required. There are a number of reasons for the wider margins: firstly, to take account of local spread, the perineal skin resection is wider; secondly, the lateral oncological margin for salvage surgery is the level of the ischial tuberosity; thirdly, owing to the preoperative fibrosing effects of radiotherapy, a wide excision margin may be needed to ensure a well vascularised skin edge; and finally, involvement of adjacent pelvic organs is common.

The most frequent operation performed for anal cancer that has failed to respond to chemoradiotherapy is an abdominoperineal resection with perineal reconstruction. This operation involves the removal of the anal canal and rectum and the formation of a permanent stoma, usually sited on the left lower quadrant of the abdomen. Outcomes for this type of surgery have only been described in small, retrospective, single centre studies with heterogeneous methodology, but the results suggest a five year survival between 30% and 69%.[29 w14-w18]

Factors that have been associated with decreased survival include positive lymph nodes at presentation, increased tumour size, advanced age of the patient, comorbidities, and positive resection margins (that is, when pathology shows the tumour extending to the margin of resection, suggesting incomplete excision). Debate continues over whether the presence of persistent or recurrent disease as the reason for surgery has a true effect on survival.[w14-w18]

Perineal reconstruction refers to the use of local and distant tissue flaps or commercial material to fill the defect left after excision. This type of wound repair involves a risk of postoperative complications, with infection and breakdown reported in 35% to 72% of cases.[w15 w16 w18]

Rare anal tumours

Although true anal adenocarcinomas do occur, adenocarcinoma of the anal canal is more commonly a very low rectal cancer that has spread distally. True adenocarcinomas probably originate from the anal glands and then spread outwards to involve the anal

---

WHO HISTOLOGICAL CLASSIFICATION OF TUMOURS OF THE ANAL CANAL

Epithelial tumours
- Intraepithelial neoplasia (dysplasia)
- Squamous or transitional epithelium
- Glandular
- Paget disease

Carcinoma
- Squamous cell carcinoma
- Adenocarcinoma
- Mucinous adenocarcinoma
- Small cell carcinoma
- Undifferentiated carcinoma
- Others
- Carcinoid tumour

Malignant melanomaNon-epithelial tumours

Adapted from Salmo et al[31]

TIPS FOR NON-SPECIALISTS

- Maintain a high index of suspicion for anal intraepithelial neoplasia in patients presenting with anal pruritus or discharge and a suspicious scaly lesion or condylomata
- Ask the patient about sexual history, previous diagnosis of HPV, cervical or vaginal intraepithelial pathology, HIV status, and previous excision of anal warts
- Refer patients with bleeding from the anus that has lasted longer than six weeks, a palpable mass on rectal examination, or anaemia for urgent specialist consultation, using the two week cancer referral rule in the UK
- Explain to patients that chemoradiotherapy is the first line treatment and may allow surgery to be avoided. However, a colostomy may still be needed before or after treatment and radiotherapy can lead to faecal incontinence and recto-vaginal fistula

---

ADDITIONAL EDUCATIONAL RESOURCES

For health professionals
- Association of Coloproctology of Great Britain and Ireland guidelines (www.acpgbi.org.uk/resources/guidelines)—contains an up to date evidence based and detailed guideline on all aspects of care for patients with anal cancer
- European Society for Medical Oncology (http://annonc.oxfordjournals.org/content/21/suppl_5/v87.full)—a more concise set of guidelines for the diagnosis, treatment, and follow-up of anal cancer
- *A Companion to Specialist Surgical Practice—Colorectal Surgery*, 4th ed (ed Robin K S Phillips, Saunders for Elsevier, 2009)—the chapter on anal cancer contains everything a gastrointestinal surgeon would need to know about anal cancer in order to diagnose and arrange treatment for patients

For patients
- Macmillan cancer support website (www.macmillan.org.uk/Cancerinformation/Cancertypes/Anal/Analcancer.aspx)—provides a clear explanation of what anal cancer is and what the treatment options are, along with a telephone number for patients to ask questions and receive support
- Cancer Research UK (www.cancerhelp.org.uk/type/anal-cancer/about)—offers quick guidance about the symptoms, risks, and treatments of anal cancer and pragmatic advice about seeing a doctor.

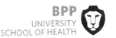

sphincter. This is a very rare tumour that is sensitive to chemoradiotherapy.[w19 w20]

Malignant melanoma accounts for 1% of malignant anal canal tumours. In presentation, they may mimic a thrombosed haemorrhoid. Anal melanoma is an aggressive disease with early infiltration and distant spread resulting in poor overall prognosis. It is not sensitive to chemotherapy or radiotherapy. Review of 85 patients treated at a single centre showed a median survival of 19 months.[w21] A recent systematic review compared abdominoperineal resection of the rectum with wide local excision and found no distinct survival advantage for either procedure.[w22] As chances of cure are minimal, radical surgery should not be considered as a primary treatment, but local excision may provide useful palliation.

Contributors: JADS was responsible article concept, design, drafting and revision. JHS was responsible for revising the article critically and final approval of the published version.

Competing interests: All authors have completed the ICMJE uniform disclosure form at www.icmje.org/coi_disclosure.pdf (available on request from the corresponding author) and declare: no support from any organisation for the submitted work; no financial relationships with any organisations that might have an interest in the submitted work in the previous three years; no other relationships or activities that could appear to have influenced the submitted work.

Provenance and peer review: Not commissioned, externally peer reviewed.

1   Parkin DM. The global health burden of infection-associated cancers in the year 2002. *Int J Cancer*2006;118:3030-44.
2   WHO/ICO Information Centre on HPV and Cervical Cancer (HPV Information Centre). Human Papillomavirus and Related Cancers in United Kingdom. Summary Report. 2010. http://apps.who.int/hpvcentre/statistics/dynamic/ico/country_pdf/GBR.pdf?CFID=27804&CFTOKEN=18959369.
3   Daling JR, Madeleine MM, Johnson LG, Schwartz SM, Shera KA, Wurscher MA, et al. Human papillomavirus, smoking, and sexual practices in the etiology of anal cancer. *Cancer*2004;101:270-80.
4   Critchlow CW, Hawes SE, Kuypers JM, Goldbaum GM, Holmes KK, Surawicz CM, et al. Effect of HIV infection on the natural history of anal human papillomavirus infection. *Aids*1998;12:1177-84.
5   Edgren G, Sparen P. Risk of anogenital cancer after diagnosis of cervical intraepithelial neoplasia: a prospective population-based study. *Lancet Oncol*2007;8:311-6.
6   Brewster DH, Bhatti LA. Increasing incidence of squamous cell carcinoma of the anus in Scotland, 1975-2002. *Br J Cancer*2006;95:87-90.
7   Robinson D, Coupland V, Moller H. An analysis of temporal and generational trends in the incidence of anal and other HPV-related cancers in Southeast England. *Br J Cancer*2009;100:527-31.
8   Daling JR, Weiss NS, Hislop TG, Maden C, Coates RJ, Sherman KJ, et al. Sexual practices, sexually transmitted diseases, and the incidence of anal cancer. *N Engl J Med*1987;317:973-7.
9   Patel P, Hanson DL, Sullivan PS, Novak RM, Moorman AC, Tong TC, et al. Incidence of types of cancer among HIV-infected persons compared with the general population in the United States, 1992-2003. *Ann Intern Med*2008;148:728-36.
10   Bartelink H, Roelofsen F, Eschwege F, Rougier P, Bosset JF, Gonzalez DG, et al. Concomitant radiotherapy and chemotherapy is superior to radiotherapy alone in the treatment of locally advanced anal cancer: results of a phase III randomized trial of the European Organization for Research and Treatment of Cancer Radiotherapy and Gastrointestinal Cooperative Groups. *J Clin Oncol*1997;15:2040-9.
11   UKCCCR Anal Cancer Trial Working Party, UK Co-ordinating Committee on Cancer Research. Epidermoid anal cancer: results from the UKCCCR randomised trial of radiotherapy alone versus radiotherapy, 5-fluorouracil, and mitomycin. *Lancet*1996;348:1049-54.
12   Renehan AG, O'Dwyer ST. Initial management through the anal cancer multidisciplinary team meeting. *Colorectal Dis* 2011;13(suppl 1):21-8.
13   Carter JJ, Madeleine MM, Shera K, Schwartz SM, Cushing-Haugen KL, Wipf GC, et al. Human papillomavirus 16 and 18 L1 serology compared across anogenital cancer sites. *Cancer Res*2001;61:1934-40.
14   Scholefield JH, Harris D, Radcliffe A. Guidelines for management of anal intraepithelial neoplasia. *Colorectal Dis*2011;13(suppl 1):3-10.
15   Zbar AP, Fenger C, Efron J, Beer-Gabel M, Wexner SD. The pathology and molecular biology of anal intraepithelial neoplasia: comparisons with cervical and vulvar intraepithelial carcinoma. *Int J Colorectal Dis*2002;17:203-15.
16   Carter PS, de Ruiter A, Whatrup C, Katz DR, Ewings P, Mindel A, et al. Human immunodeficiency virus infection and genital warts as risk factors for anal intraepithelial neoplasia in homosexual men. *Br J Surg*1995;82:473-4.
17   Chauveinc L, Buthaud X, Falcou MC, Mosseri V, De la Rochefordiere A, Pierga JY, et al. Anal canal cancer treatment: practical limitations of routine prescription of concurrent chemotherapy and radiotherapy. *Br J Cancer*2003;89:2057-61.
18   Renehan AG, Saunders MP, Schofield PF, O'Dwyer ST. Patterns of local disease failure and outcome after salvage surgery in patients with anal cancer. *Br J Surg*2005;92:605-14.
19   Scholefield JH, Castle MT, Watson NF. Malignant transformation of high-grade anal intraepithelial neoplasia. *Br J Surg*2005;92:1133-6.
20   Licitra L, Spinazze S, Doci R, Evans TR, Tanum G, Ducreux M. Cancer of the anal region. *Crit Rev Oncol Hematol*2002;43:77-92.
21   Salmo E, Haboubi N. Anal cancer: pathology, staging and evidence-based minimum data set. *Colorectal Dis* 2011;13(suppl 1):11-20.
22   Hill J, Meadows H, Haboubi N, Talbot IC, Northover JM. Pathological staging of epidermoid anal carcinoma for the new era. *Colorectal Dis*2003;5:206-13.
23   Scott NA, Beart RW, Jr., Weiland LH, Cha SS, Lieber MM. Carcinoma of the anal canal and flow cytometric DNA analysis. *Br J Cancer*1989;60:56-8.
24   Peiffert D, Bey P, Pernot M, Hoffstetter S, Marchal C, Beckendorf V, et al. Conservative treatment by irradiation of epidermoid carcinomas of the anal margin. *Int J Radiat Oncol Biol Phys*1997;39:57-66.
25   Ajani JA, Winter KA, Gunderson LL, Pedersen J, Benson AB, 3rd, Thomas CR Jr, et al. Prognostic factors derived from a prospective database dictate clinical biology of anal cancer: the intergroup trial (RTOG 98-11). *Cancer*2010;116:4007-13.
26   Edge SB, American Joint Committee on Cancer. AJCC cancer staging manual. 7th ed. Springer, 2009.
27   Kronfli M, Glynne-Jones R. Chemoradiotherapy in anal cancer. *Colorectal Dis* 2011;13(suppl 1):33-8.
28   Glynne-Jones R, Northover JM, Cervantes A. Anal cancer: ESMO Clinical Practice Guidelines for diagnosis, treatment and follow-up. *Ann Oncol*2010;21(suppl 5):v87-92.
29   Pocard M, Tiret E, Nugent K, Dehni N, Parc R. Results of salvage abdominoperineal resection for anal cancer after radiotherapy. *Dis Colon Rectum* 1998;41:1488-93.
30   Renehan AG, O'Dwyer ST. Management of local disease relapse. *Colorectal Dis*2011;13(suppl 1):44-52.

Related links

bmj.com/archive
Previous articles in this series
- Management of deep vein thrombosis and prevention of post-thrombotic syndrome (2011;343:d5916)
- Diagnosis and management of autism in childhood (2011;343:d6238)
- Diagnosis and management of maturity onset diabetes of the young (MODY) (2011;343:d6044)
- Actinomycosis (2011;343:d6099)
- Managing perioperative risk in patients undergoing elective non-cardiac surgery (2011;343:d5759)

bmj.com
- Get CME points at BMJ Learning

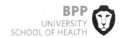

Endometrial cancer

Srdjan Saso clinical research fellow[1], Jayanta Chatterjee clinical research fellow[1], Ektoras Georgiou clinical research fellow[2], Anthony M Ditri general practitioner[3], J Richard Smith gynaecological surgeon[4], Sadaf Ghaem-Maghami senior lecturer and honorary consultant in gynaecological oncology[5]

[1]Division of Surgery, Oncology, Reproductive Biology and Anaesthetics, Institute of Reproductive and Developmental Biology, Imperial College London, Hammersmith Hospital Campus, London W12 0NN, UK

[2]Department of Biosurgery and Surgical Technology, Imperial College London

[3]Carshalton, Surrey, UK

[4]West London Gynaecological Cancer Centre, Queen Charlotte's and Chelsea Hospital, Imperial College London, London

[5]Imperial College London

Correspondence to: S Saso srdjan.saso@imperial.ac.uk

Cite this as: BMJ 2011;342:d3954

<DOI> 10.1136/bmj.d3954
http://www.bmj.com/content/343/bmj.d3954

The International Agency for Research on Cancer recently estimated that endometrial carcinoma is the commonest gynaecological cancer in the developed world,[1] with a rising incidence in postmenopausal women. In 2007, 7536 new endometrial cancers were diagnosed in the UK, making it the fourth most common cancer in women after breast, lung, and colorectal cancers.[2] Cancer of the endometrium is the commonest cancer of the uterine corpus (about 92%, the remainder being uterine carcinosarcomas and sarcomas), according to the Surveillance, Epidemiology and End Results programme of the US National Cancer Institute, which has collected data on cancer from various locations and sources since 1973.[3]

Cure is possible and the overall five year survival rate for all stages is currently around 80%. Most women present early in the course of the disease when cure is more likely, so primary care practitioners need to be vigilant for potential indicators. We discuss the epidemiology, diagnosis, and treatment of endometrial cancer on the basis of a review of observational research, randomised trials, reviews, and meta-analyses.

Who gets endometrial cancer and what causes it?

Cancer Research UK, which pools data from several UK registries (cancer statistics registrations for England, Wales, and Northern Ireland; cancer incidence, mortality and survival data for NHS Scotland) estimates that around 90% of all women diagnosed as having endometrial carcinoma are postmenopausal, with the mean age at diagnosis of about 60 years.[4] A retrospective observational study of observed and modelled trends in 13 European countries showed that in recent years the incidence of endometrial cancer has been increasing in postmenopausal women, whereas it seems to be stable or decreasing in premenopausal and perimenopausal women.[5]

The precise cause of endometrial cancer is unknown, although various associated factors have been identified. Box 1 summarises recognised endogenous and exogenous risk factors for endometrial cancer. A prospective case-control study of 173 patients linked the action of chronic unopposed oestrogen on the endometrium to abnormal endometrial cell proliferation and carcinogenesis.[6] Indeed, the best established risk factors ,such as obesity and nulliparity, relate to chronic exposure to oestrogen.

Excess unopposed oestrogen is also a risk factor for endometrial hyperplasia, a premalignant condition that can predispose to endometrial carcinoma. It can be typical (simple or complex) or atypical. Simple and complex hyperplasias have a 1% and 3% risk of progression to cancer, respectively. However, 30-40% of patients found to have atypical hyperplasia will have a concurrent adenocarcinoma, and the rest are at very high risk of developing the cancer.[8]

What types are there?

Endometrial cancer can been divided into two major types. Type 1 cancers, which account for 80-90%, are usually oestrogen dependent endometrioid adenocarcinomas, which generally have a good prognosis. Type 2 tumours usually

SOURCES AND SELECTION CRITERIA

We searched PubMed to identify peer reviewed original research articles, meta-analyses, and reviews. Search terms were endometrial cancer, cancer of the endometrium, endometrial adenocarcinoma, neoplasm and endometrium, and endometrial neoplasm. Only papers written in English were considered.

SUMMARY POINTS

- Endometrial cancer is the most common gynaecological cancer in more developed countries and its incidence is increasing in postmenopausal women
- Postmenopausal bleeding is the hallmark symptom
- The main risk factors for the development of endometrioid endometrial carcinoma are obesity and chronic unopposed oestrogen stimulation of the endometrium
- All women with suspected endometrial cancer require transvaginal ultrasonography and most will undergo endometrial biopsy; more sophisticated radiological examinations are required for accurate preoperative staging.
- Treatment is usually surgical, comprising total hysterectomy and bilateral salpingo-oophorectomy.
- Adjuvant therapy with radiotherapy, chemotherapy, or hormonal therapy is considered in more advanced or high risk disease

BOX 1 RISK FACTORS AND PROTECTIVE FACTORS FOR ENDOMETRIAL CANCER[6][7]

Endogenous risk factors

- Increasing age
- Obesity and physical inactivity
- Early menarche and late menopause
- Low parity or infertility
- Polycystic ovarian syndrome
- Family history
- Lynch syndrome (hereditary nonpolyposis colorectal cancer)
- Oestrogen secreting tumours (granulosa or thecal cell tumours of ovary)
- Diabetes mellitus
- Hypertension
- History of breast cancer
- Immunodeficiency

Exogenous risk factors

- Unopposed oestrogen only hormone replacement therapy
- Tamoxifen therapy
- Dietary factors
- Previous radiotherapy

Protective factors

- Cigarette smoking
- Combined oral contraception for at least one year
- Grand multiparity

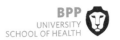

BOX 2 HISTOPATHOLOGICAL SUBTYPES

Type 1
- Endometrioid adenocarcinoma
- With squamous differentiation
- Villoglandular
- Secretory
- With ciliated cells

Type 2
- Papillary serous adenocarcinoma
- Clear cell adenocarcinoma
- Mucinous adenocarcinoma
- Undifferentiated carcinoma
- Mixed carcinoma

WHO/International Society of Gynecological Pathology classification.

---

present late, behave more aggressively, and carry a poor prognosis.[9] They are not oestrogen driven and the risk of relapse and metastasis is high.[7] Within this category, the commonest histological types are uterine papillary serous carcinoma and clear cell carcinoma (box 2).[9]

How does a patient with endometrial cancer present?

Patients with endometrial cancer classically present with postmenopausal bleeding, which is defined as bleeding that occurs at least a year after the last menstrual period. The reported absolute risk of endometrial cancer in non-users of hormone replacement therapy (HRT) who present with postmenopausal bleeding ranges from 5.7% to 11.5%.[2] [3][4][5] About 20% of patients with postmenopausal bleeding are found to have a malignancy, which is most commonly endometrial but can be cervical.[10][11][12] Premenopausal and perimenopausal women may present with intermenstrual bleeding, often with a background of irregular, dysfunctional menstruation that suggests anovulation. Pain, vaginal discharge, and pyometra are rarer symptoms and tend to be secondary to advanced cancer.

How is the diagnosis made?

In the UK, recommendations for diagnosis and referral are based on three sets of guidelines (evidence level IV): National Institute for Health and Clinical Excellence (NICE),[10] European Society for Medical Oncology (ESMO),[11] and Uterus Commission of the German Gynecological Oncology Working Group (AGO-S2k).[12] They recommend that the clinician obtains a detailed account of the presenting symptoms, a full drug history (HRT, oral contraceptive pill, tamoxifen), and a gynaecological history (early menarche/late menopause, known endometrial hyperplasia, parity). Medical and surgical history may be relevant (obesity, treatment for breast cancer, diabetes mellitus, hypothyroidism, hypertension, and Lynch-type syndrome). If the patient reports postmenopausal bleeding, general practitioners in the UK should refer them to a rapid access gynaecology clinic to be seen within two weeks.[10][13] A premenopausal patient older than 40 years who presents with a recent onset abnormal bleeding pattern, or a premenopausal patient of any age with an abnormal bleeding pattern and any of the above risk factors for endometrial cancer, should be referred to a gynaecologist.[10][11][12] The gynaecologist will normally carry out a pelvic examination to rule out other possible sources of vaginal bleeding such as lesions of the vulva, vagina, or cervix.

Two investigations are mandatory in women with suspected endometrial cancer: a transvaginal ultrasound scan and an endometrial biopsy. Transvaginal ultrasound scan is an accurate and precise screening method for endometrial cancer. A retrospective study of 339 patients found that calculating endometrial thickness was easier with transvaginal ultrasound than with transabdominal ultrasound.[14] A meta-analysis of 35 studies using a 5 mm threshold to define abnormal endometrial thickening showed that 96% of women with cancer had endometrial thickness greater than 5 mm; the study reported a negative likelihood ratio of 0.08. Transvaginal ultrasound was also highly reliable in identifying postmenopausal women with vaginal bleeding who were unlikely to have carcinomatous disease (endometrial thickness of <5 mm), which would mean that unnecessary endometrial sampling could be avoided.[15] A meta-analysis of data from 9031 patients concluded that endometrial thickness of less than 4-5 mm in the presence of endometrial pathology poses a very low but not negligible risk of malignancy, although this does not apply to patients who are on regular HRT or tamoxifen for breast carcinoma.[16] A recent meta-analysis showed that the specificity of an abnormal transvaginal ultrasound result dropped from 92% to 77% when used in patients on HRT.[15] The upper endometrial thickness limit for these patients is 8 mm if asymptomatic, but if vaginal bleeding is present a biopsy should be taken if the thickness is greater than 5 mm.

A definitive diagnosis of endometrial cancer is histological. A sample of endometrial tissue can be obtained either in the gynaecology outpatient setting using a Pipelle curette[17] or by hysteroscopy and dilatation and curettage under general anaesthesia. A systematic review of 13 diagnostic evaluations showed that a Pipelle biopsy leads to a high overall diagnostic accuracy when an adequate specimen is obtained (post-test probability of endometrial cancer of 81.7% for a positive test and 0.9% for a negative test).[17] These findings encourage further evaluation in cases of abnormal uterine bleeding where symptoms persist despite negative biopsy. Hysteroscopy tends to be reserved for patients who cannot tolerate outpatient examination and biopsy, patients with cervical stenosis, and patients in whom outpatient biopsy was inadequate. The accuracy of hysteroscopy in diagnosing endometrial cancer and hyperplasia in women with abnormal uterine bleeding was determined by a systematic review of data on 26 346 women.[18] A positive hysteroscopy result (likelihood ratio 60.9) increased the probability of cancer to 71.8% from a pre-test probability of 3.9%, whereas a negative hysteroscopy result (likelihood ratio 0.15) reduced the probability of cancer to 0.6%. Interestingly, diagnostic accuracy tended to be higher for endometrial cancer among postmenopausal women and in the outpatient setting.[18]

Referral to a gynaecologic oncology specialist centre

As outlined by guidelines,[10][11][12] patients with confirmed endometrial cancer require immediate referral to a specialised gynaecology oncological centre (fig 1). Here, further imaging such as computed tomography and magnetic resonance imaging (MRI) is performed to assess the extent of disease and plan for optimal management according to staging. A specialist team will choose the type of treatment (surgical or non-surgical approach) and make a decision about the appropriateness of adjuvant therapy on the basis of results of imaging. MRI is able to assess the depth of myometrial invasion, pelvic lymph node enlargement, and presence of cervical invasion. A meta-analysis of 47 studies that compared the usefulness of computed tomography,

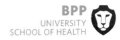

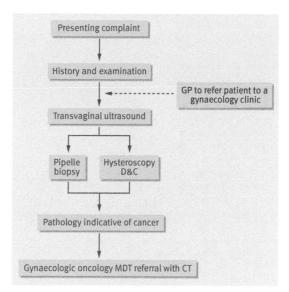

Fig 1 Diagnostic flowchart, NICE guidelines. D&C=dilatation and curettage, MDT=multidisciplinary team, CT=computed tomography

ultrasound, and MRI in staging of endometrial cancer found that contrast enhanced dynamic MRI was the most reliable method of identifying patients at high risk of tumour metastasis and presence of local lymphadenopathy.[19] Computed tomography is mainly used to detect disease outside the pelvis.

FIGO stage I
About 80% of patients present with stage I disease and can be treated surgically with a total abdominal hysterectomy and bilateral salpingo-oophorectomy. Palpation and imaging of para-aortic and pelvic lymph nodes can assess for tumour spread.[26] A study by a gynaecological oncology group looked at the histopathology of 621 patients and found lymph node metastases in about 10% of women who clinically had cancer confined to the uterus.[27]

The subject of pelvic lymphadenectomy is disputed across the Atlantic. In the UK, pelvic lymphadenectomy is not routinely performed along with total abdominal hysterectomy and bilateral salpingo-oophorectomy in women with stage I disease. This stance is supported by a Cochrane Collaboration review,[28] which pooled data from two randomised controlled trials[29] [30] (one of them being the often quoted ASTEC trial[30]) and examined in greater depth the value of lymphadenectomy in women with stage I disease. It found no evidence supporting a survival benefit or a reduction in the risk of disease recurrence compared with not performing it.

In the United States, however, the opposite applies and pelvic lymphadenectomy is routinely performed alongside total abdominal hysterectomy and bilateral salpingo-oophorectomy. A large retrospective observational study of 39 396 patients drawn from the Surveillance, Epidemiology, and End Results programme (1988 to 2001) compared patients who had a lymphadenectomy with those who did not. The results indicate that lymphadenectomy is advisable for stage I grade 3 disease and more advanced endometrioid uterine cancers.[31]

Both arguments have their strengths and weaknesses. The UK bases its approach on data from two randomised controlled trials but a total of only 1945 patients, whereas the United States' argument is based on findings from a study that had a weaker design but included outcomes of a much larger number of patients. As concluded by the Cochrane Collaboration review, lymphadenectomy is associated with substantial short and long term morbidity. It prolongs intraoperative time, thereby increasing the risk of deep venous thrombosis and pulmonary embolism, and increases the risk of lymphoedema and pelvic lymphocyst formation.[28] Nevertheless, it provides useful prognostic information and further randomised trials are needed to evaluate the benefits, if any, of lymph node sampling.

FIGO stages II-IV
Stage II disease is managed with an extended or modified radical hysterectomy, bilateral salpingo-oopherectomy, and lymph node dissection. Maximal surgical cytoreduction is offered to patients who are suitable candidates for surgery as this provides a survival benefit.[32] [33] According to ESMO, patients with stage III disease solely on the basis of positive peritoneal cytology are treated as patients with stage I or II disease, based on other clinicopathological data,[10] because positive cytology has not been found to be an independent prognostic indicator.

How is endometrial cancer staged?
Staging of endometrial cancer is determined by the International Federation of Gynecology and Obstetrics (FIGO). Staging may be based on surgical, clinical, radiological, or histopathological criteria. However, according to the 6th annual FIGO report, which pooled data on 9386 patients (from 34 countries) treated between 1999 and 2001, surgical staging has shown better prognostic value than clinical staging.[20] To incorporate this finding, FIGO staging of endometrial cancer was updated in 2009 to reflect more accurately prognosis at each stage (table).[21] Despite this, a recent prospective analysis examined the extent to which the stage specific overall survival altered in the 2009 system and concluded that the revised system for stage I disease did not improve its predictive ability over the 1988 system.[22]

How is treatment decided?
The guidelines we present here focus specifically on the most common type of endometrial cancer—endometrioid endometrial adenocarcinoma. The management of a patient diagnosed with endometrial cancer is usually decided within a multidisciplinary team setting (fig 2).

What is the preferred surgical approach?
Surgical treatment of endometrial cancer comprises total abdominal hysterectomy, bilateral salpingo-oophorectomy, and peritoneal washings.[10] [11] [12] In some cases, pelvic and para-aortic lymphadenectomy and omentectomy may be performed. Surgery can be open, via laparotomy (entry via a transverse or midline incision), or laparoscopic (normal

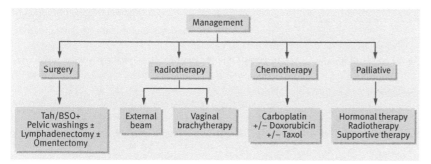

Fig 2 Summary of current management of endometrial cancer

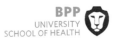

Stage	Description	Five year survival
Stage I*	Tumour confined to corpus uteri	85%
Stage IA*	No myometrial invasion or less than half	
Stage IB*	Invasion equal to or more than half the myometrium	
Stage II*	Tumour invades cervical stroma but does not extend beyond uterus†	75%
Stage III*	Local and/or regional spread of the tumour	45%
Stage IIIA*	Tumour invades serosa of corpus uteri and/or adnexae‡	
Stage IIIB*	Vaginal and/or parametrial involvement‡	
Stage IIIC*	Metastases to pelvic and/or para-aortic lymph nodes‡	
Stage IIIC1	Positive pelvic nodes	
Stage IIIC2	Positive para-aortic lymph nodes with or without positive pelvic lymph nodes	
Stage IV*	Tumour invades bladder and/or bowel mucosa and/or distant metastases	25%
Stage IVA*	Tumour invasion of bladder and/or bowel mucosa	
Stage IVB*	Distant metastases, including intra-abdominal metastases and/or inguinal lymph nodes	

FIGO staging system for carcinoma of the uterine corpus[21]

*Grade 1, 2, or 3.
†Endocervical glandular involvement should be considered only as stage I and no longer as stage II.
‡Positive cytology has to be reported separately without changing the stage.

or robotically assisted). Two extensive meta-analyses and a quantitative review showed no significant difference in terms of recurrence and survival between these two surgical options.[23] [24] [25]

What is the role of radiotherapy and chemotherapy?

The broad consensus is that radiotherapy has no role for early stage low risk disease.[34] Traditionally, external pelvic radiotherapy, commonly with vaginal brachytherapy, has been the adjuvant treatment of choice for patients with early stage high risk disease. A meta-analysis by the ASTEC/EN.5 study group,[35] which analysed data from two randomised controlled trials—the GOG [w1] (392 patients) and PORTEC [w2] (714 patients) studies—reported no benefit in terms of overall, disease specific, and disease specific recurrence-free survival for patients with early endometrial cancer (FIGO stage IA-C, of any grade and histological subtype) receiving adjuvant external beam radiotherapy. Furthermore, any decrease in the incidence of local recurrence was small.[35] These findings definitively refute previous trends based on conclusions from meta-analyses and quantitative analyses favouring the use of radiotherapy for patients with multiple high risk features, such as stage IC and grade 3 disease. [w3,w4]

The value of chemotherapy in stage I disease is not yet clear. Recent data from different studies (prospective, retrospective, and a randomised controlled trial) of patients with stage I or II disease suggest that chemotherapy may improve overall survival in those with high risk features, such as high grade disease, lymphovascular space involvement, or greater than 50% myometrial invasion. [w5-w7] A randomised controlled trial of 345 patients reported no difference between radiotherapy and chemotherapy for early stage high risk disease, but this is a controversial finding since only a third of the study patients actually had early stage disease. [w8]

How should patients be followed up?

Survival outcomes vary with each FIGO stage (table). In general, prognosis depends mainly on the age and health of the patient and the histological grade and stage of the tumour. Screening of the general population is currently not practised because no benefit with regards to patient outcomes has been identified. As neatly explained by AGO-S2k, no screening methods are able to detect uterine hyperplasia or cancer with acceptable sensitivity and specificity.[7] [12]

Any pelvic pain or vaginal or rectal bleeding could indicate disease recurrence and should be investigated promptly. Both patients and healthcare professionals should be alert for general symptoms of malignancy and metastasis such as anorexia, unexplained weight loss, and bowel, urinary, or respiratory symptoms. ESMO recommends follow-up consultations every four months with careful history and pelvic examination at each visit in the first two years after diagnosis. Appointments every six months are recommended for the next three years.[11]

Finally, the importance of facilitating a supportive environment for the patient and their family cannot be stressed enough. The general practitioner can act as the lynchpin, ensuring that the patient is aware of all support networks from the cancer nurse specialist to the local cancer centre.

Contributors: SS wrote the first draft of the article. SS, JC, and EG reviewed the evidence on which the paper is based. AMD gave advice from a GP perspective. JRS and SGM acted as senior authors and are the guarantors for this paper.

Funding: None.

ADDITIONAL EDUCATIONAL RESOURCES

For healthcare professionals

- British Gynaecological Cancer Society (www.bgcs.org.uk)—Research information from Britain's largest gynaeoncological organisation
- National Institute for Health and Clinical Excellence (www.nice.org.uk)—National body providing evidence based guidance on specific diseases and conditions
- Kitchener HC. Chapter 57: cancer of the uterine corpus. In: Edmonds DK, ed. *Dewhurst's Textbook of Obstetrics and Gynaecology.* 7th ed. Blackwell Publishing, 2007
- Smith JR, del Priore G, Coleman RL, eds. *An Atlas of Gynaecological Oncology: Investigation and Surgery.* 3rd ed. InformaHealth care, 2011
- ASTEC study group, Kitchener H, Swart AM, Qian Q, Amos C, Parmar MK. Efficacy of systematic pelvic lymphadenectomy in endometrial cancer (MRC ASTEC trial): a randomised study. *Lancet* 2009;373:125-36
- ASTEC/EN.5 study group, Blake P, Swart AM, Orton J, Kitchener H, Whelan T, et al. Adjuvant external beam radiotherapy in the treatment of endometrial cancer (MRC ASTEC and NCIC CTG EN.5 randomised trials): pooled trial results, systematic review, and meta-analysis. *Lancet* 2009;373:137-46

For patients

- Cancer Advice (www.canceradvice.co.uk/uterine-cancer)—Website designed to inform patients concerning the present state of knowledge of particular cancers and to highlight modern aspects of treatment
- Cancer Research UK (www.cancerresearchuk.org)—World's leading charity dedicated to research activities designed to combat cancer, with information about cancer, treatments, novel therapies, support groups, and fundraising events
- Macmillan Cancer Support (www.macmillan.org.uk)—Organisation offering nursing support for patients with any type of cancer
- Maggie's Centres (www.maggiescentres.org)—Charity organisation that provides help with information, benefits advice, psychological support both individually and in groups, courses, and stress reducing strategies
- Patient UK (www.patient.co.uk)—Comprehensive source of health and disease information for patients

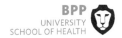

TIPS FOR NON-SPECIALISTS

- Early presentation renders endometrial cancer highly curable with an overall five year survival of about 80%
- Postmenopausal women who start to bleed per vaginum and 40-50 year old women with intermenstrual bleeding should be referred within two weeks to a gynaecologist for an urgent Pipelle biopsy and transvaginal ultrasound
- Also consider speedy referral in younger women who report unusual bleeding if they have received chronic unopposed oestrogen or are obese
- In women who have been treated for endometrial cancer, pelvic pain or vaginal or rectal bleeding could indicate recurrence. Be vigilant for general symptoms of malignancy and metastasis such as anorexia, unexplained weight loss, and bowel, urinary, or respiratory symptoms.

ONGOING RESEARCH

- The transatlantic debate about the diagnostic and therapeutic value of pelvic lymphadenectomy in endometrial cancer could be resolved by further randomised trials.
- The Gynaecologic Oncology Group has created a large prospective biospecimen bank with the aim of helping to identify biological cancer targets. This will in turn facilitate the development of novel antagonistic-type agents that could be used against such targets.
- Laparoscopic and robot assisted laparoscopic surgery may be increasingly used in gynaecological oncology surgery because of early encouraging results that show several advantages over open surgery. Results of a randomised controlled trial of laparoscopic surgery versus open surgery in endometrial cancer are awaited.

Competing interests: All authors have completed the Unified Competing Interest form at www.icmje.org/coi_disclosure.pdf (available on request from the corresponding author) and declare: no support from any organisation for the submitted work; no financial relationships with any organisations that might have an interest in the submitted work in the previous three years; no other relationships or activities that could appear to have influenced the submitted work.

Provenance and peer review: Not commissioned, externally peer reviewed.

1 Sankaranarayanan R, Ferlay J. Worldwide burden of gynaecological cancer: the size of the problem. *Best Pract Res Clin Obstet Gynaecol*2006;20:207-25.
2 Office for National Statistics. Cancer registration statistics England 2007. 2009. www.statistics.gov.uk/StatBase/Product.asp?vlnk=7720.
3 Kosary CL. Cancer of the corpus uteri. In: Ries LAG, Young JL, Keel GE, Eisner MP, Lin YD, Horner M-J, eds. SEER survival monograph: cancer survival among adults: U.S. SEER program, 1988-2001, patient and tumor characteristics. NIH Pub No 07-6215 ed. National Cancer Institute, SEER Program, 2007.
4 Cancer Research UK. Uterine (womb) cancer statistics—UK. http://info.cancerresearchuk.org/cancerstats/types/uterus.
5 Bray F, Dos Santos Silva I, Moller H, Weiderpass E. Endometrial cancer incidence trends in Europe: underlying determinants and prospects for prevention. *Cancer Epidemiol Biomarkers Prev*2005;14:1132-42.
6 Jick SS, Walker AM, Jick H. Estrogens, progesterone, and endometrial cancer. *Epidemiology*1993;4:20-4.
7 Amant F, Moerman P, Neven P, Timmerman D, Van Limbergen E, Vergote I. Endometrial cancer. *Lancet*2005;366:491-505.
8 Mills AM, Longacre TA. Endometrial hyperplasia. *Semin Diagn Pathol*2010;27:199-214.
9 Kitchener HC. Chapter 57: cancer of the uterine corpus. In: Edmonds DK, ed. Dewhurst's textbook of obstetrics and gynaecology. 7th ed. Blackwell Publishing, 2007.
10 National Institute for Health and Clinical Excellence. Referral guidelines for suspected cancer. 2005. www.nice.org.uk/nicemedia/pdf/cg027niceguideline.pdf.
11 Baekelandt MM, Castiglione M, ESMO Guidelines Working Group. Endometrial carcinoma: ESMO clinical recommendations for diagnosis, treatment and follow-up. *Ann Oncol*2009;4:29-31.
12 Emons G, Kimmig R. Uterus commission of the gynecological oncology working group (AGO). Interdisciplinary S2k guidelines on the diagnosis and treatment of endometrial carcinoma. *J Cancer Res Clin Oncol*2009;135:1387-91.
13 Butler J, Kehoe S, Shepherd J, Barton D, Bridges J, Ind T, et al. Referrals to secondary care: Referral rates for postmenopausal bleeding are not respectable. *BMJ*2010;341:c7407.
14 Gull B, Karlsson B, Milsom I, Granberg S. Can ultrasound replace dilatation and curettage? A longitudinal evaluation of postmenopausal bleeding and transvaginal sonographic measurement of the endometrium as predictors of endometrial cancer. *Am J Obstet Gynecol* 2003;188:401-8.
15 Smith-Bindman R, Kerlikowske K, Feldstein VA, Subak L, Scheidler J, Segal M, et al. Endovaginal ultrasound to exclude endometrial cancer and other endometrial abnormalities. *JAMA*1998;280:1510-7.
16 Gupta JK, Chien PF, Voit D, Clark TJ, Khan TS. Ultrasonographic endometrial thickness for diagnosing endometrial pathology in women with postmenopausal bleeding: a meta-analysis. *Acta Obstet Gynecol Scand*2002;81:799-816.
17 Clark TJ, Mann CH, Shah N, Khan KS, Song F, Gupta JK. Accuracy of outpatient endometrial biopsy in the diagnosis of endometrial cancer: a systematic quantitative review. *BJOG*2002;109:313-21.
18 Clark TJ, Voit D, Gupta JK, Hyde C, Song F, Khan KS. Accuracy of hysteroscopy in the diagnosis of endometrial cancer and hyperplasia: a systematic quantitative review. *JAMA*2002;288:1610-21.
19 Kinkel K, Kaji Y, Yu KK, Segal MR, Lu Y, Powell CB, et al. Radiologic staging in patients with endometrial cancer: a meta-analysis. *Radiology*1999;212:711-8.
20 Creasman WT, Odicino F, Maisonneuve P, Quinn MA, Beller U, Benedet JL, et al. Carcinoma of the corpus uteri. FIGO 6th annual report on the results of treatment in gynecological cancer. *Int J Gynecol Obstet*2006;95:S105-43.
21 Creasman W. Revised FIGO staging for carcinoma of the endometrium. *Int J Gynecol Obstet*2009;105:109.
22 Abu-Rustum NR, Zhou Q, Iasonos A, Alektiar KM, Leitao MM Jr, Chi DS, et al. The revised 2009 FIGO staging system for endometrial cancer: should the 1988 FIGO stages IA and IB be altered? *Int J Gynecol Cancer*2011;21:511-6.
23 Lin F, Zhang QJ, Zheng FY, Zhao HQ, Zeng QQ, Zheng MH, et al. Laparoscopically assisted versus open surgery for endometrial cancer - a meta-analysis of randomized controlled trials. *Int J Gynecol Cancer*2008;18:1315-25.
24 de la Orden SG, Reza MM, Blasco JA, Andradas E, Callejo D, Perez T. Laparoscopic hysterectomy in the treatment of endometrial cancer: a systematic review. *J Minim Invasive Gynecol*2008;15:395-401.
25 Ju W, Myung SK, Kim Y, Choi HJ, Kim SC, Korean Meta-Analysis Study Group. Comparison of laparoscopy and laparotomy for management of endometrial carcinoma: a meta-analysis. *Int J Gynecol Cancer*2009;19:400-6.
26 Nout RA, Smit VT, Putter H, Jurgenliemk-Schulz IM, Jobsen JJ, Lutgens LC, et al. Vaginal brachytherapy versus pelvic external beam radiotherapy for patients with endometrial cancer of high-intermediate risk (PORTEC-2): an open-label, non-inferiority, randomised trial. *Lancet*2010;375:816-23.
27 Creasman WT, Morrow CP, Bundy BN, Homesley HD, Graham JE, Heller PB. Surgical pathologic spread patterns of endometrial cancer. A Gynecologic Oncology Group Study. *Cancer*1987;60:2035-41.
28 May K, Bryant A, Dickinson HO, Kehoe S, Morrison J. Lymphadenectomy for the management of endometrial cancer. *Cochrane Database Syst Rev*2010;20:CD007585.
29 Benedetti Panici P, Basile S, Maneschi F, Alberto Lissoni A, Signorelli M, Scambia G, et al. Systematic pelvic lymphadenectomy vs. no lymphadenectomy in early-stage endometrial carcinoma: randomized clinical trial. *J Natl Cancer Inst*2008;100:1707-16.
30 ASTEC study group. Kitchener H, Swart AM, Qian Q, Amos C, Parmar MK. Efficacy of systematic pelvic lymphadenectomy in endometrial cancer (MRC ASTEC trial): a randomised study. *Lancet*2009;373:125-36.
31 Chan JK, Wu H, Cheung MK, Shin JY, Osann K, Kapp DS. The outcomes of 27,063 women with unstaged endometrioid uterine cancer. *Gynecol Oncol*2007;106:282-8.
32 Lambrou NC, Gomez-Marin O, Mirhashemi R, Beach H, Salom E, Almeida-Parra Z, et al. Optimal surgical cytoreduction in patients with stage III and stage IV endometrial carcinoma: a study of morbidity and survival. *Gynecol Oncol*2004;93:653-8.
33 Ayhan A, Taskiran C, Celik C, Yuce K, Kucukali T. The influence of cytoreductive surgery on survival and morbidity in stage IVB endometrial cancer. *Int J Gynecol Cancer*2002;12:448-53.
34 Brown AK, Madom L, Moore R, Granai CO, DiSilvestro P. The prognostic significance of lower uterine segment involvement in surgically staged endometrial cancer patients with negative nodes. *Gynecol Oncol*2007;105:55-8.
35 ASTEC/EN.5 Study Group, Blake P, Swart AM, Orton J, Kitchener H, Whelan T, et al. Adjuvant external beam radiotherapy in the treatment of endometrial cancer (MRC ASTEC and NCIC CTG EN.5 randomised trials): pooled trial results, systematic review, and meta-analysis. *Lancet*2009;373:137-46.

Related links

bmj.com/archive

Previous articles in this series
- Clinical management of stuttering in children and adults (2011; 342:d3742)
- Diagnosis and management of ectopic pregnancy (2011;342:d3397)
- Diagnosis and management of premenstrual disorders (2011;342:d2994)
- The assessment and management of insomnia in primary care (2011;342:d2899)

bmj.com/cme
- Get CME points

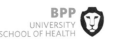
Prostate cancer screening and the management of clinically localized disease

Timothy J Wilt professor of medicine, section of general internal medicine[1], Hashim U Ahmed Medical Research Council clinician scientist and clinical lecturer in urology[23]

[1]Minneapolis VA Center for Chronic Disease Outcomes Research, Minneapolis Veterans Affairs (VA) Health Care System, and the University of Minnesota School of Medicine, Minneapolis, USA

[2]Division of Surgery and Interventional Science, University College London, London, UK

[3]Department of Urology, University College London Hospitals NHS Foundation Trust, London, UK

Correspondence to: T Wilt tim.wilt@va.gov

Cite this as: BMJ 2013;346:f325

‹DOI› 10.1136/bmj.f325
http://www.bmj.com/content/346/bmj.f325

Prostate cancer is an important health problem. More than 40 000 incident cases of prostate cancer and more than 10 000 prostate cancer related deaths occur each year in the United Kingdom.[1] Prevention, detection, and treatment of localized prostate cancer remain controversial. Although screening for prostate cancer with serum prostate specific antigen (PSA) testing is not approved in the UK, informal screening is common and has led to a threefold increase in the incidence of prostate cancer. In the United States, since the introduction of PSA screening more than 1.3 million men have been diagnosed with prostate cancer and one million of these have undergone treatment.[2] We update a previous review, highlighting new findings that deal with clinical questions and future research needs for the prevention, detection, and treatment of clinically localized prostate cancer.[3]

Who is at risk of prostate cancer?

Established risk factors for prostate cancer include increasing age, black ethnic origin, and a family history of prostate cancer in a close male relative. The last two factors convey modest risk compared with age. Prostate cancer is rare before 50 years of age, and about 80% of cases and 90% of deaths occur in men over 65.[3] Lower urinary tract symptoms (poor flow, urgency, frequency, hesitancy, nocturia) are common in older men but not related to prostate cancer development. Testosterone supplementation for hypogonadism does not clearly increase prostate cancer development. Although prostate cancer rates show regional variations and differences between socioeconomic groups, these are mainly due to differences in rates of PSA testing.[1]

The greatest risk factor associated with a prostate cancer diagnosis is undergoing a PSA blood test.[2][3] Using lower thresholds to indicate abnormality and obtaining larger numbers of tissue core samples sets off a cascade of events that more than doubles the incidence of prostate cancer through tumors that would otherwise never come to clinical attention (overdiagnosis).

Can prostate cancer be prevented?

Epidemiologic evidence indicates that the most effective way to reduce prostate cancer incidence is to decrease PSA testing, raise thresholds used to define an abnormal PSA result (fig 1),[4] and lower the number of tissue core samples obtained in men undergoing a prostate biopsy. In men who receive a PSA test, use of risk calculators that take other clinical parameters (age, prostate volume, free to total PSA ratio) into account or a triage test may help identify men who could avoid a prostate biopsy and detection of clinically insignificant disease, while still detecting potentially lethal disease that requires intervention.[5][6]

The only other strategy shown to reduce prostate cancer incidence involves 5-α reductase inhibitors (5ARI), which are approved for treating symptoms of benign prostate enlargement. Large randomized controlled trials (RCTs) and a systematic review have shown that 5ARI reduces prostate cancer incidence but may increase the detection of high risk cancers.[7] These drugs are not approved for prostate cancer prevention. RCTs indicate that antioxidants, particularly vitamin E and selenium, do not reduce prostate cancer incidence and should not be used.[8] Other widely used options including aspirin, statins, low fat or soy based diets, and aerobic or weight based exercise are not clearly effective.

Should men be screened for prostate cancer with the PSA blood test?

Although such screening is common, the UK National Screening Committee and the US Preventive Services Task Force (USPSTF) recommend against it because the benefit is at best small (fig 2) and not greater than the harms.[9][10] Both groups recognize that some men will continue to request screening and some physicians continue to offer it. All major organizations advise that PSA testing should not be conducted without an informed discussion of benefits and harms.

The goal of screening programs is to reduce disease specific and overall morbidity and mortality, not just to detect and treat more disease. This goal is difficult to achieve because screening tests are applied to people without symptoms in the hope of preventing future health

---

SUMMARY POINTS

- Increasing age is the most important risk factor for developing prostate cancer
- The most effective way to reduce prostate cancer incidence is to reduce prostate specific antigen (PSA) testing or raise thresholds that define abnormality
- Prostate cancer screening with the PSA blood test results in at most a small reduction in prostate cancer mortality and leads to considerable diagnostic and treatment related harms
- Physicians should recommend against PSA screening for prostate cancer
- Most men with prostate cancer detected by PSA testing have tumours that will not cause health problems (overdiagnosed), but almost all undergo early treatment (overtreated)

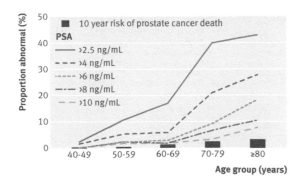

Fig 1 Impact of age on the proportion of men found to have an abnormal serum prostate specific antigen concentration depending on threshold used. The bars represent the 10 year risk of a prostate cancer related death in each age group[4]

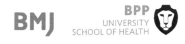

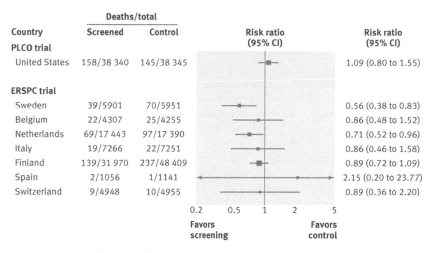

| | Deaths/total | | Risk ratio | Risk ratio |
Country	Screened	Control	(95% CI)	(95% CI)
PLCO trial				
United States	158/38 340	145/38 345		1.09 (0.80 to 1.55)
ERSPC trial				
Sweden	39/5901	70/5951		0.56 (0.38 to 0.83)
Belgium	22/4307	25/4255		0.86 (0.48 to 1.52)
Netherlands	69/17 443	97/17 390		0.71 (0.52 to 0.96)
Italy	19/7266	22/7251		0.86 (0.46 to 1.58)
Finland	139/31 970	237/48 409		0.89 (0.72 to 1.09)
Spain	2/1056	1/1141		2.15 (0.20 to 23.77)
Switzerland	9/4948	10/4955		0.89 (0.36 to 2.20)

Fig 2 Forest plot showing the risk ratio with 95% confidence intervals from the two (of five) randomized prostate cancer screening trials judged to be at least "fair methodological quality" and of "low risk of bias" (PLCO and ERSPC). The vertical line represents no benefit[10]

problems. Although any potential benefit occurs in just a few people, all are subjected to the harms of screening.

The effect of PSA screening on prostate cancer and overall mortality has been investigated in five large long term randomized trials.[10 11] None has reported a reduction in overall mortality. Only the European Randomized Study of Screening for Prostate Cancer (ERSPC), which included results from seven countries using different screening protocols, identified a significant reduction in death from prostate cancer. Positive results mainly came from data from two countries that found large effects using PSA screening every two to four years. Although the precise lifetime effect of PSA screening on prostate cancer mortality remains uncertain, the reduction in prostate cancer mortality after 10-14 years is 0-1 per 1000 men screened, even for men in the optimal age range of 55-69 years.[11]

A raised PSA blood test initiates a cascade of diagnostic and treatment events that have harms and should be considered before testing (fig 3). Over 10 years, 15-20% of men will have a PSA test result that triggers a biopsy. About 80% of PSA tests will be false positive results at widely used cut-off points (2.5-4.0 ng/mL). Harms and errors related to the diagnostic transrectal prostate biopsy are common and often serious. The sampling needles are inserted through the (contaminated) rectum, with inconsistent use of local anesthetic. The UK Prostate Testing for Cancer and Treatment (ProtecT) study and other studies have shown that around a third of men having a prostate biopsy will have moderate or major bothersome symptoms, including pain, fever, bleeding, temporary urinary difficulties, and infection (with sepsis rates of 2-4% from multiresistant bacteria); 1% will be admitted to hospital and nearly 0.1% will die.[12]

Transrectal prostate biopsies are limited by random and systematic errors. Random errors occur because eight to 12 samples are taken randomly (the location of the cancer is unknown) and systematic ones occur because certain parts of the gland are sampled in preference to others. As a result, indolent disease is detected by chance and clinically important cancers missed. These errors lead to poor risk attribution; a man with low risk cancer on transrectal ultrasound guided biopsy has a one in three chance of harboring higher grade disease, with the prospect of undertreatment.[12] This error in risk stratification can be used to advise against observation or active surveillance and recommend surgery or radiotherapy.[13]

There has been little progress in finding new blood or urinary biomarkers that could complement or replace PSA because biomarker development and validation depend on the inaccurate PSA-transrectal biopsy pathway. Imaging, such as multi-parametric magnetic resonance imaging (MRI), has shown promise, especially as it does not detect small low grade cancers.[14] The exact role for MRI is being evaluated in the PROstate Mr Imaging Study (PROMIS) using a reference standard biopsy test—template prostate mapping—that systematically samples the whole prostate.[15]

The major harms of PSA screening relate to treatment of detected cancers—about half of those detected would never cause clinical problems in a man's lifetime even in the absence of treatment (overdiagnosis).[10 11] Men with such cancers cannot benefit from detection and treatment and can only be harmed. Around one in three men over the age of 50 years has prostate cancer that is unlikely to cause harm during their lifetime; this greatly exceeds the 3% lifetime risk of dying of prostate cancer even if left untreated. The use of surgery or radiotherapy to treat most of these men leads to overtreatment. Treatment related harms are common and include serious perioperative complications (rarely death) and long term erectile, urinary, and bowel dysfunction.

Comparing harms and benefits of any screening test involves trade-offs that can be difficult to quantify and often involve differing preferences and values. A recent decision modelling analysis attempted to derive a common metric to assess the benefits and harms of screening and subsequent treatment by assessing quality of life and quality adjusted life years gained or lost. It used selected findings from the European screening trial and other published data.[16] The analysis found that PSA screening may reduce or increase quality adjusted survival, depending on patient values for different health states. The findings were sensitive to assumptions used. The small reported gains in quality adjusted survival would probably have disappeared if mortality and morbidity results from all screening and treatment trials had been incorporated.

What treatments should I recommend for clinically localized prostate cancer?

Treatment options for clinically localized prostate cancer include watchful waiting or observation, active surveillance, radical prostatectomy (RP), external beam radiation therapy, interstitial radiation implants (brachytherapy), cryoablation,

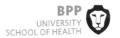

androgen deprivation therapy (ADT), high intensity focused ultrasound, and focal therapy.[3] Treatment recommendations and selection involve patients' values and their weighting of the trade-offs in benefits and harms, as well as physician preferences. A multidisciplinary approach that includes the patient's primary care provider and incorporates the latest findings from randomized trials or higher quality observational studies can help a patient make a well informed decision. Comparative effectiveness remains controversial, partly because few randomized treatment trials with mortality outcomes (only one in the PSA era) have been completed. Trials have been difficult to complete owing to the large size and long term follow-up needed, as well as patients' and clinicians' reluctance to participate. Despite evidence indicating excellent long term disease specific survival with observation, nearly 90% of men with PSA detected prostate cancer in the US receive early treatment. In the UK, 3000-4000 RPs are carried out each year, and two to three times this number of men undergo radiotherapy.[17] In the UK, 60% of men diagnosed with low risk disease undergo immediate treatment; this figure is 70-90% in the US.[18]

Two randomized trials compared RP to observation but were conducted before widespread PSA testing.[19] [20] One failed to find a difference in overall mortality after more than 20 years.[21] The Scandinavian Prostate Cancer Group-4 trial (SPCG-4 trial) demonstrated absolute differences in all cause and prostate cancer related mortality at 15 years of 6.6% and 6.1%, respectively, in favor of RP. Benefits were confined to men under 65 years.[20] Another randomized trial comparing external beam radiotherapy with watchful waiting, also in men diagnosed before PSA testing, reported no significant difference in overall or prostate cancer related mortality over at least 16 years.[22] Prostate cancer mortality

in these two trials was much higher than in men with PSA detected prostate cancer.

The Prostate cancer Intervention Versus Observation Trial (PIVOT) found that RP did not significantly reduce all cause or prostate cancer mortality compared with observation over 15 years (fig 4).[23] Absolute differences were less than 3%. Treatment effects did not differ according to age, race, comorbidity, health status, or cancer grade. In men with PSA values of 10 ng/mL or less or those with low risk disease, prostate cancer mortality was rare (<3%) in men managed by observation. Radical prostatectomy was possibly associated with reduced all cause and prostate cancer mortality in men with PSA greater than 10 ng/mL and high risk disease (fig 5). Complications within 30 days of surgery occurred in 21.4% of men and included one death. Patient reported urinary incontinence and erectile dysfunction, but not bowel dysfunction, were more common at two years in men randomized to surgery.

The current practice of repeated PSA testing, lower PSA thresholds triggering biopsies, obtaining more tissue biopsy samples, and repeating biopsies after initial negative findings increases detection of smaller volume indolent cancers.[24] Therefore, in men diagnosed currently, RP will probably result in smaller absolute reductions in metastases and mortality and a longer time needed to identify a reduction than were reported in PIVOT or SPCG-4.

In contrast to observation, active surveillance involves repeat prostate biopsies every one to two years, in addition to PSA testing and digital rectal examination every three to four months. If these indicate reclassification to a higher risk status, treatment with curative intent is often started. Clinical experience with active surveillance suggests there is an estimated risk of metastasis of less than 1% at two to eight years.[25] 5ARI has shown promising results in reducing

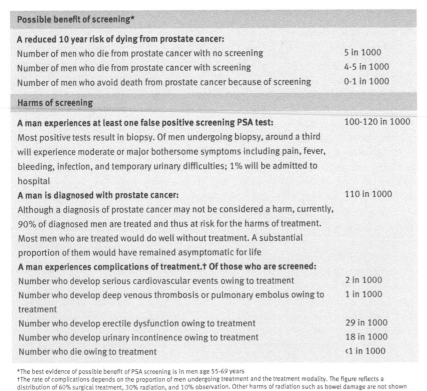

Possible benefit of screening*	
A reduced 10 year risk of dying from prostate cancer:	
Number of men who die from prostate cancer with no screening	5 in 1000
Number of men who die from prostate cancer with screening	4-5 in 1000
Number of men who avoid death from prostate cancer because of screening	0-1 in 1000
Harms of screening	
A man experiences at least one false positive screening PSA test:	100-120 in 1000
Most positive tests result in biopsy. Of men undergoing biopsy, around a third will experience moderate or major bothersome symptoms including pain, fever, bleeding, infection, and temporary urinary difficulties; 1% will be admitted to hospital	
A man is diagnosed with prostate cancer:	110 in 1000
Although a diagnosis of prostate cancer may not be considered a harm, currently, 90% of diagnosed men are treated and thus at risk for the harms of treatment. Most men who are treated would do well without treatment. A substantial proportion of them would have remained asymptomatic for life	
A man experiences complications of treatment.† Of those who are screened:	
Number who develop serious cardiovascular events owing to treatment	2 in 1000
Number who develop deep venous thrombosis or pulmonary embolus owing to treatment	1 in 1000
Number who develop erectile dysfunction owing to treatment	29 in 1000
Number who develop urinary incontinence owing to treatment	18 in 1000
Number who die owing to treatment	<1 in 1000

*The best evidence of possible benefit of PSA screening is in men age 55-69 years
†The rate of complications depends on the proportion of men undergoing treatment and the treatment modality. The figure reflects a distribution of 60% surgical treatment, 30% radiation, and 10% observation. Other harms of radiation such as bowel damage are not shown

Fig 3 Benefits and harms of screening men aged 55-69 years* with a prostate specific antigen (PSA) test every 1-4 years for 10 years. Calculations rely on assumptions and are imprecise. Estimates should be considered in the full context of clinical decision making and used to stimulate shared decision making[10]

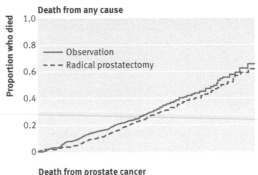

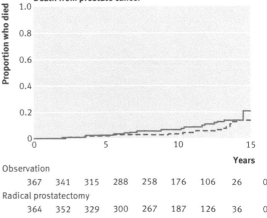

Fig 4 Kaplan-Meier curves showing death from any cause and death from prostate cancer in the Prostate Cancer Intervention versus Observation Trial (PIVOT) comparing radical prostatectomy with observation[24]

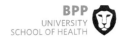

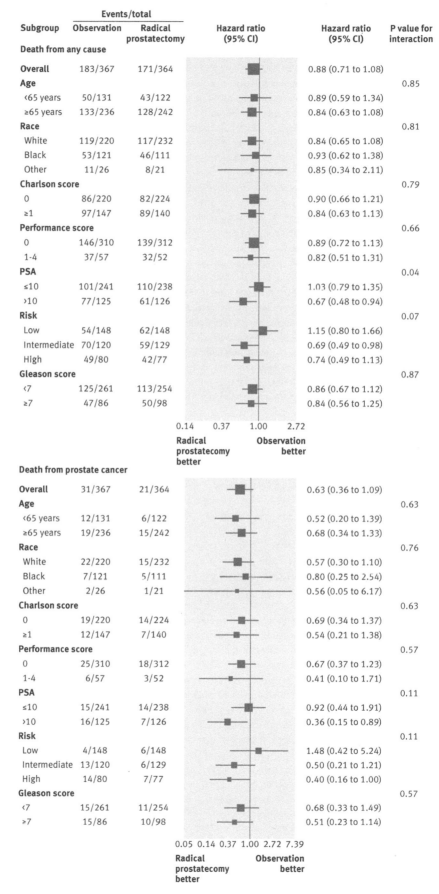

Subgroup	Events/total		Hazard ratio (95% CI)	Hazard ratio (95% CI)	P value for interaction
	Observation	Radical prostatectomy			
Death from any cause					
Overall	183/367	171/364		0.88 (0.71 to 1.08)	
Age					0.85
<65 years	50/131	43/122		0.89 (0.59 to 1.34)	
≥65 years	133/236	128/242		0.84 (0.63 to 1.08)	
Race					0.81
White	119/220	117/232		0.84 (0.65 to 1.08)	
Black	53/121	46/111		0.93 (0.62 to 1.38)	
Other	11/26	8/21		0.85 (0.34 to 2.11)	
Charlson score					0.79
0	86/220	82/224		0.90 (0.66 to 1.21)	
≥1	97/147	89/140		0.84 (0.63 to 1.13)	
Performance score					0.66
0	146/310	139/312		0.89 (0.72 to 1.13)	
1-4	37/57	32/52		0.82 (0.51 to 1.31)	
PSA					0.04
≤10	101/241	110/238		1.03 (0.79 to 1.35)	
>10	77/125	61/126		0.67 (0.48 to 0.94)	
Risk					0.07
Low	54/148	62/148		1.15 (0.80 to 1.66)	
Intermediate	70/120	59/129		0.69 (0.49 to 0.98)	
High	49/80	42/77		0.74 (0.49 to 1.13)	
Gleason score					0.87
<7	125/261	113/254		0.86 (0.67 to 1.12)	
≥7	47/86	50/98		0.84 (0.56 to 1.25)	

0.14   0.37   1.00   2.72

Radical prostatecomy better   **Observation better**

Death from prostate cancer					
Overall	31/367	21/364		0.63 (0.36 to 1.09)	
Age					0.63
<65 years	12/131	6/122		0.52 (0.20 to 1.39)	
≥65 years	19/236	15/242		0.68 (0.34 to 1.33)	
Race					0.76
White	22/220	15/232		0.57 (0.30 to 1.10)	
Black	7/121	5/111		0.80 (0.25 to 2.54)	
Other	2/26	1/21		0.56 (0.05 to 6.17)	
Charlson score					0.63
0	19/220	14/224		0.69 (0.34 to 1.37)	
≥1	12/147	7/140		0.54 (0.21 to 1.38)	
Performance score					0.57
0	25/310	18/312		0.67 (0.37 to 1.23)	
1-4	6/57	3/52		0.41 (0.10 to 1.71)	
PSA					0.11
≤10	15/241	14/238		0.92 (0.44 to 1.91)	
>10	16/125	7/126		0.36 (0.15 to 0.89)	
Risk					0.11
Low	4/148	6/148		1.48 (0.42 to 5.24)	
Intermediate	13/120	6/129		0.50 (0.21 to 1.21)	
High	14/80	7/77		0.40 (0.16 to 1.00)	
Gleason score					0.57
<7	15/261	11/254		0.68 (0.33 to 1.49)	
>7	15/86	10/98		0.51 (0.23 to 1.14)	

0.05 0.14 0.37 1.00 2.72 7.39

Radical prostatecomy better   **Observation better**

Fig 5 Forest plots demonstrating subgroup effects (hazard ratio with 95% confidence intervals and P value for interaction) in the Prostate Cancer Intervention versus Observation Trial (PIVOT) comparing radical prostatectomy with observation. The vertical line indicates no effect. The size of the boxes indicates the weight of the effects[24]

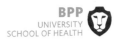

risk reclassification on active surveillance, but follow-up is too short to make definitive recommendations.[21] Active surveillance is being compared with surgery or radiotherapy in the UK's ProtecT randomized trial.[26]

No randomized trials have assessed mortality outcomes of external beam radiotherapy or brachytherapy versus other management strategies in men with PSA detected prostate cancer. Treatment of localized prostate cancer is not an approved indication for ADT.

Radical surgery, external beam radiotherapy, or interstitial radiotherapy can cause serious harm because they treat the whole prostate regardless of risk, volume, or location of the cancer. This leads to collateral damage to the external urinary sphincter, neurovascular bundles, and rectal mucosa. Although rates of side effects vary between treatment modalities, urinary incontinence occurs in 10-20%, erectile dysfunction in 50%, and rectal toxicity (diarrhea, bleeding, pain) in 10-20%.[27] Despite refinements in radiotherapy (conformal, intensity modulation, robotic radiosurgery) and radical prostatectomy (laparoscopic or robot assisted) these harms have not changed. No large long term RCTs have evaluated the clinical and cost effectiveness outcomes of these newer techniques. ADT is associated with an increased risk for impotence, hot flashes, metabolic syndrome, gynecomastia, and other serious harms. A recent meta-analysis of eight randomized trials in men with non-metastatic high risk prostate cancer found that ADT was not associated with increased mortality from cardiac disease.[28]

What are the future research needs?
The past few years have provided important new information on prostate cancer prevention, detection, and treatment. Several key research endeavors are needed to close important knowledge gaps.

Firstly, we need to develop and evaluate novel research methods that can be used to obtain comparative effectiveness data in a timely and cost efficient manner but are adaptive to the incremental technological changes that occur over the lifetime of a study. Such studies may include designs that feature point of care enrolment and use of cohort multiple RCT methods.[29] Recent findings show that RCTs are vital for accurately assessing the benefits and harms of prevention, detection, and treatment strategies.

Secondly, we need better methods for population screening and diagnostic strategies that avoid diagnosing men with clinically insignificant prostate cancer but still identify those with clinically important disease. Few, if any, biomarkers have been identified that could replace or complement PSA. One strategy that could be readily evaluated is the impact of using higher PSA thresholds (such as 6-10 ng/mL) to define abnormality, trigger prostate biopsy, and recommend early treatment. The current strategy of using transrectal biopsy or histologic outcomes from surgery as a means to validate new biomarkers is probably flawed because of the inherent spectrum and selection biases that result. Biomarkers require validation against a reference standard that can be applied to all men at risk. The target condition for detection should focus on clinically significant cancers.[30 31] Imaging research that allows the targeting (for biopsy or treatment) of clinically significant lesions has shown promise and requires additional study.[32]

Thirdly, active surveillance protocols and communication about the benefits of observation and active surveillance need to be improved to be acceptable to physicians and patients. The use of a clinical examination that is inaccurate (digital rectal examination), a blood test that lacks specificity (PSA), and a histologic verification test (transrectal biopsy) that is temporally unstable and can cause considerable harm may contribute to this lack of acceptability. Results of the ongoing ProtecT study are urgently needed to assess the trade-offs between active surveillance versus surgery or radiotherapy, especially in men with higher PSA concentrations or higher risk disease. Research that uses imaging and tissue biomarkers as surveillance tools and prognostic markers is needed.

Fourthly, comparativeness effectiveness research, especially assessing minimally invasive treatments, using novel RCT designs to enhance recruitment is needed before implementation. Despite considerable overdetection and overtreatment, evidence indicates that interventions can alter the natural course of prostate cancer and may have clinically important benefits in some men. Men most likely to benefit include those with a long life expectancy (age <65 years, excellent health status, and few comorbidities) and those with tumors likely to cause serious health problems (palpable prostate cancer or PSA values greater than 10 ng/mL). Even in these men, however, the harms of current treatments are considerable and the absolute benefit modest. The role of minimally invasive treatments, such as cryosurgery and high intensity focused ultrasound, has recently been identified by the National Institute for Health and Clinical Excellence as a priority for NHS evaluation in clinical trials or as part of cohort registry studies.[33 34 35] Early proof-of-concept studies have shown that tissue preserving focal therapy—in which the treatment is directed at the tumor rather than the whole organ—has a low rate of side effects and may be sufficiently effective.[36]

Fifthly, physicians need sufficient information, educational resources, and communication skills to confidently and accurately provide prevention, detection, and treatment recommendations. Although some information exists, health service research is needed to develop efficient and effective tools to communicate scientific findings showing that observation and not PSA screening is the preferred treatment approach for most men diagnosed as having prostate cancer. These tools will help primary care providers in their role as a patient's healthcare resource regarding prostate cancer.

What is the prognosis for men with clinically localized prostate cancer?
The long term prognosis for most men with clinically localized prostate cancer is excellent, even with no early treatment. This is particularly true for men with prostate cancer that is detected by PSA screening and not palpable (most men diagnosed currently); in men with PSA values of 10 ng/mL or less; or those with "low risk disease" defined by PSA levels (≤10 ng/mL), tumor stage (T1 or T2a), and histologic grade (Gleason score <6). Prostate cancer mortality over at least 15 years in these men treated with observation is 5% or less. Nonetheless, prostate cancer remains a leading cause of cancer related morbidity and mortality. Men with PSA values greater than 10 ng/mL or with high risk disease (PSA >20 ng/mL; tumor stage >T2b; Gleason score 8-10) have a worse prognosis. Their 15 year risk of prostate cancer mortality when managed expectantly is 20% or more. In this group surgery seems to reduce overall and disease mortality and bone metastases. Patients, their families, physicians, and the public seek answers to reduce the physical, social, and financial costs of this disease. We need better markers

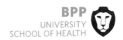

PROSTATE CANCER SCREENING MESSAGES FOR MEN

- Major evidence based guidelines recommend against the prostate specific antigen (PSA) blood test for prostate cancer screening because:
- The test is unlikely to prevent you from dying of prostate cancer over 10-15 years or help you live longer
- Elevated PSA values are common and lead to additional tests that have harms
- PSA testing finds many cancers that will not cause health problems
- Once we find cancer it is hard not to treat it
- Treatments have harms that occur early, can be serious, and may persist, but have very little, if any, benefit
- By choosing not to have the PSA test you can live a similar length of life, have little to no difference in your risk of dying from prostate cancer, and avoid the harms associated with tests, procedures, and treatments

ADDITIONAL EDUCATIONAL RESOURCES FOR HEALTHCARE PROFESSIONALS AND PATIENTS

- These websites provide evidence based guidelines and recommendations from the United States and United Kingdom on screening and treatment for clinically localized prostate cancer. These resources are mainly developed by and for primary care providers and patients seen in primary care settings. Additional society guidelines and recommendations from other countries also exist. Each listed resource contains links to informational tools for both clinicians and patients to help in making well informed decisions about screening and treatment for prostate cancer
- Cancer Research UK. www.cancerresearch.org
- UK National Screening Committee. www.screening.nhs.uk
- US Preventive Services Task Force. www.uspreventiveservicestaskforce.org/prostatecancerscreening.htmAmerican
- Cancer Society. www.cancer.org/healthy/informationforhealthcareprofessionals/prostatemdcliniciansinformationsource/index
- Foundation for Informed Medical Decision Making.
- http://informedmedicaldecisions.org/imdf_decision_aid/deciding-if-the-psa-test-is-right-for-you/

UNANSWERED QUESTIONS

- The role of new methods in conducting randomized controlled trials where recruitment has proved difficult
- The role of new screening strategies such as the impact of different thresholds of prostate specific antigen (PSA) abnormality and risk calculators on the trade-off between benefits and harms
- Discovery, development, and validation of tissue and imaging (novel ultrasound, functional magnetic resonance imaging) biomarkers to detect clinically important prostate cancer using accurate reference standards that minimize spectrum and selection bias
- The role of novel tissue and imaging biomarkers in men with localized prostate cancer undergoing active surveillance
- The clinical and cost effectiveness of minimally invasive whole gland and focal treatments for men with intermediate to high risk disease.
- Health services research to integrate findings from PSA screening and treatment trials into primary care

of prognosis, determinants of treatment effectiveness, and methods to effectively communicate and implement prognostic information. We need safer and more effective strategies and more rational use of existing options.

What should we tell patients who request screening?

Physicians can improve the health of their male patients by recommending against PSA screening for prostate cancer. However, PSA screening is common, and some men will continue to request and some physicians will continue to offer such screening. A decision to start or continue PSA screening should reflect an explicit understanding of the possible benefits and harms and respect for patient preferences. The box gives examples of screening messages that can be delivered in primary care to patients who ask about PSA screening. Figure 3 provides information about the potential benefits and harms of testing and treatment. Community, employer based, and clinician ordered PSA

A PATIENT'S PERSPECTIVE

I was diagnosed with prostate cancer on my 60th birthday, with a Gleason score of 3+4, not the most welcome of birthday presents. I had been urinating more frequently, so my general practitioner suggested doing a prostate specific antigen (PSA) test. The result was 10 ng/mL, so my local urologist arranged a biopsy. When it came back positive, he fully explained the meaning of the results, the potential prognosis, and treatment options. My wife accompanied me, but we could not remember much. Mention of the word "cancer" blanked out everything else. Fortunately, the consultant jotted down the main points on several sheets of paper. We were told that there were three treatment options—surgery, radiotherapy, and hormone treatment—watchful waiting not being considered appropriate. The main reason I chose surgery was that if it failed it could be followed by radiotherapy, which in turn could be followed by hormone treatment. Our choice was also colored by an emotional response. I had this "thing" growing inside me, and I wanted it got rid of and cut out quickly.

Although the postoperative PSA concentration fell to near zero, some adverse features were seen on histologic analysis. We decided not to wait for the PSA to rise (indicating failure), but to have pre-emptive radiotherapy to the pelvic and prostate bed area three months after surgery.

Three years later my PSA is below 0.1 ng/mL; in the short term the treatments seemed successful. The intervening period has given me time to reflect on what has happened. I found the surgery less stressful than the radiotherapy. Although the radical prostatectomy was a major operation, recovery seemed to follow an uphill path, with symptoms such as incontinence getting better over time. Radiotherapy seemed much more insidious, at first seemingly benign, only later revealing the true extent of the side effects. Bowel movements took some time to return to near normal, and incontinence was somewhat worse than it had been two months after surgery.

Although we were fully informed at every consultation about the potential side effects, we did not fully take this on board. When I was diagnosed, we focused on the effectiveness of the treatment against the cancer. The potential side effects seemed a minor matter. Three years later I am not so sure. Incontinence is still a problem as I use pads. I find myself acutely aware of the nearest toilet, becoming anxious in new places. With modern technology, erectile dysfunction is manageable, but sex is not what it once was.

One unanticipated consequence is the effect of the six monthly PSA tests on me. When first told about this regimen, I was happy, thinking that if anything developed it could be caught at an early stage. While accepting this logic, I dread the approach of each test, wondering if it will herald the re-emergence of the cancer. However, although I get depressed, I do realize that this is something that has to be done.

Has this affected the quality of my life? To some extent it has, but I am still here, and I am grateful for that. Given the situation when diagnosed, I am not sure that we would have done anything differently.

testing in the absence of well informed decision making should be discontinued. Physicians should use higher thresholds to define abnormalities that trigger a diagnostic prostate biopsy in men who have undergone a PSA test, thereby reducing overdiagnosis and overtreatment.

Compared with early intervention with surgery or radiotherapy, observation can help most men with early stage prostate cancer detected by PSA testing live a similar length of life and avoid death from prostate cancer, as well as prevent treatment related harms. Physicians should encourage patient participation in RCTs examining new prevention, screening, and treatment approaches.

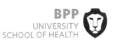

Contributors: TJW conceived the idea for the article and wrote the first draft. HUA and TJW both contributed to further drafts. TJW is guarantor.

Funding: No special funding received.

Competing interests: All authors have completed the ICMJE uniform disclosure form at www.icmje.org/coi_disclosure.pdf (available on request from the corresponding author) and declare: HUA is co-principal investigator in several investigator led diagnostic and focal therapy trials in prostate cancer supported by the MRC (UK), National Institute for Health Research Health Technology Assessment programme, Pelican Cancer Foundation charity, and Prostate Cancer UK charity; HUA receives funding from USHIFU and Advanced Medical Diagnostics for clinical trials; HUA has received consultancy payments in the past from Steba Biotech and Oncura/GE Healthcare and payment for conference travel from USHIFU; TJW is a volunteer member of the US Preventive Services Task Force and chairman of the Prostate cancer Intervention Versus Observation Trial (PIVOT).

Provenance and peer review: Commissioned; externally peer reviewed.

The PROMIS trial is funded by the NIHR Health Technology Assessment programme (project number 09/22/67) and will be published in full in *Health Technology Assessment*. The views and opinions expressed therein and in any media associated with this study are those of the authors and do not necessarily reflect those of the HTA programme, NIHR, NHS, or the Department of Health.

Patient consent obtained.

1 Cancer Research UK. Prostate cancer statistics. 2012. www.cancerresearchuk.org/cancer-info/cancerstats/types/prostate/.

2 Welch HG, Albertsen PC. Prostate cancer diagnosis and treatment after the introduction of prostate-specific antigen screening: 1986-2005. *J Natl Cancer Inst*2009;101:1325-9.

3 Wilt TJ, Thompson IM. Clinically localised prostate cancer. *BMJ*2006;333:1102-6.

4 Welch HG, Schwartz LM, Woloshin S. Prostate-specific antigen levels in the United States: implications of various definitions for abnormal. *J Natl Cancer Inst*2005;97:1132-7.

5 Zhu X, Albertsen PC, Andriole GL, Roobol MJ, Schroder FH, Vickers AJ. Risk-based prostate cancer screening. *Eur Urol*2012;61:652-61.

6 Bossuyt PM, Irwig L, Craig J, Glasziou P. Comparative accuracy: assessing new tests against existing diagnostic pathways. *BMJ*2006;332:1089-92.

7 Wilt TJ, Macdonald R, Hagerty K, Schellhammer P, Tacklind J, Somerfield MR, et al. 5-alpha-Reductase inhibitors for prostate cancer chemoprevention: an updated Cochrane systematic review. *BJU Int*2010;106:1444-51.

8 Dennert G, Zwahlen M, Brinkman M, Vinceti M, Zeegers MPA, Horneber M. Selenium for preventing cancer. Cochrane Database Syst Rev 2011;5: CD005195.

9 Burford DC, Kirby M, Austoker J. Prostate cancer risk management programme information for primary care; PSA testing in asymptomatic men. Evidence document. 2010. www.cancerscreening.nhs.uk/prostate/pcrmp02.pdf

10 Moyer VA. Screening for prostate cancer: US Preventive Services Task Force recommendation statement. *Ann Intern Med*2012;157:120-34.

11 Chou R, Croswell JM, Dana T, Bougatsos C, Blazina I, Fu R, et al. Screening for prostate cancer: a review of the evidence for the US Preventive Services Task Force. *Ann Intern Med*2011;155:762-71.

12 Onik G, Miessau M, Bostwick DG. Three-dimensional prostate mapping biopsy has a potentially significant impact on prostate cancer management. *J Clin Oncol*2009;27:4321-6.

13 Ganz PA, Barry JM, Burke W, Col NF, Corso PS, Dodson E, et al. National Institutes of Health state-of-the-science conference: role of active surveillance in the management of men with localized prostate cancer. *Ann Intern Med*2012;156:591-5.

14 Ahmed HU, Kirkham A, Arya M, Illing R, Freeman A, Allen C, et al. Is it time to consider a role for MRI before prostate biopsy? *Nat Rev Clin Oncol*2009;6:197-206.

15 Medical Research Council Clinical Trials Unit. PROMIS—prostate MRI imaging study: evaluation of multi-parametric magnetic imaging in the diagnosis and characterisation of prostate cancer. www.ctu.mrc.ac.uk/promis.aspx.

16 Heijnsdijk EA, Wever EM, Auvinen A, Hugosson J, Ciatto S, Nelen V, et al. Quality-of-life effects of prostate-specific antigen screening. *N Engl J Med*2012;367:595-605.

17 McVey GP, McPhail S, Fowler S, McIntosh G, Gillatt D, Parker CC. Initial management of low-risk localized prostate cancer in the UK: analysis of the British Association of Urological Surgeons Cancer Registry. *BJU Int*2010;106:1161-4.

18 Cooperberg MR, Lubeck DP, Meng MV, Mehta SS, Carroll PR. The changing face of low-risk prostate cancer: trends in clinical presentation and primary management. *J Clin Oncol*2004;22:2141-9.

19 Iversen P, Madsen PO, Corle DK. Radical prostatectomy versus expectant treatment for early carcinoma of the prostate. Twenty-three year follow-up of a prospective randomized study. *Scand J Urol Nephrol Suppl*1995;172:65-72.

20 Bill-Axelson A, Holmberg L, Ruutu M, Garmo H, Stark JR, Busch C, et al. Radical prostatectomy versus watchful waiting in early prostate cancer. *N Engl J Med*2011;364:1708-17.

21 Fleshner NE, Lucia MS, Egerdie B, Aaron L, Eure G, Nandy I, et al. Dutasteride in localised prostate cancer management: the REDEEM randomised, double-blind, placebo-controlled trial. *Lancet*2012;379:1103-11.

22 Widmark A, Tomic R, Modig H, Thellenberg Karlsson C, Lundbeck F, Hoyer M, et al. Prospective randomized trial comparing external beam radiotherapy versus watchful waiting in early prostate cancer (T1b-T2, pN0, grade 1-2 Mo). 53rd Annual ASTRO Meeting, 2-6 October 2011, Florida.

23 Wilt TJ, Brawer MK, Jones KM, Barry MJ, Aronson WJ, Fox S, et al. Radical prostatectomy versus observation for localized prostate cancer. *N Engl J Med*2012;367:203-13.

24 Van der Kwast TH. The trade-off between sensitivity and specificity of clinical protocols for identification of insignificant prostate cancer. *Eur Urol*2012;62:469-71.

25 Dahabreh IJ, Chung M, Balk EM, Yu WW, Mathew P, Lau J, et al. Active surveillance in men with localized prostate cancer: a systematic review. *Ann Intern Med*2012;156:582-90.

26 Donovan J, Hamdy F, Neal D, Peters T, Oliver S, Brindle L, et al. Prostate Testing for Cancer and Treatment (ProtecT) feasibility study. *Health Technol Assess*2003;7:1-88.

27 Sanda MG, Dunn RL, Michalski J, Sandler HM, Northouse L, Hembroff L, et al. Quality of life and satisfaction with outcome among prostate-cancer survivors. *N Engl J Med*2008;358:1250-61.

28 Nguyen PL, Je Y, Schutz FA, Hoffman KE, Hu JC, Parekh A, et al. Association of androgen deprivation therapy with cardiovascular death in patients with prostate cancer: a meta-analysis of randomized trials. *JAMA*2011;306:2359-66.

29 Relton C, Torgerson D, O'Cathain A, Nicholl J. Rethinking pragmatic randomised controlled trials: introducing the "cohort multiple randomised controlled trial" design. *BMJ*2010;340:c1066.

30 Ahmed HU, Hu Y, Carter T, Arumainayagam N, Lecornet E, Freeman A, et al. Characterizing clinically significant prostate cancer using template prostate mapping biopsy. *J Urol*2011;186:458-64.

31 Lord SJ, Staub LP, Bossuyt PM, Irwig LM. Target practice: choosing target conditions for test accuracy studies that are relevant to clinical practice. *BMJ*2011;343:d4684.

32 Dickinson L, Ahmed HU, Allen C, Barentsz JO, Carey B, Futterer JJ, et al. Magnetic resonance imaging for the detection, localisation, and characterisation of prostate cancer: recommendations from a European consensus meeting. *Eur Urol*2011;59:477-94.

33 National Institute for Health and Clinical Excellence. Prostate cancer. CG58. 2008. http://guidance.nice.org.uk/CG58.

34 National Institute for Health and Clinical Excellence. Focal therapy using cryoablation for localised stage prostate cancer. IPG423. 2012. www.nice.org.uk/nicemedia/live/13512/58915/58915.pdf.

35 National Institute for Health and Clinical Excellence. Focal therapy using high-intensity focused ultrasound (HIFU) for localised prostate cancer. IPG424. 2012. http://publications.nice.org.uk/focal-therapy-using-high-intensity-focused-ultrasound-for-localised-prostate-cancer-ipg424.

36 Ahmed HU, Hindley RG, Dickinson L, Freeman A, Kirkham AP, Sahu M, et al. Focal therapy for localised unifocal and multifocal prostate cancer: a prospective development study. *Lancet Oncol*2012;13:622-32.

Related links

bmj.com
- Listen to a linked podcast at bmj.com/multimedia

bmj.com/archive
Previous articles in this series
- Bed bug infestation (2013;346:f138)
- Developmental assessment of children (2013;346:e8687)
- Thunderclap headache (2013;346:e8557)
- Bipolar disorder (2012;345:e8508)
- Diagnosis and management of supraventricular tachycardia (2012;345:e7769)

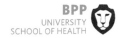

Malignant and premalignant lesions of the penis

Manit Arya senior lecturer and honorary consultant in urological oncology[1], Jas Kalsi consultant urologist [2], John Kelly professor and consultant in urological oncology [3], Asif Muneer consultant urological surgeon and andrologist [3]

[1]University College Hospital, London, and Barts Cancer Institute, London, UK

[2]Wexham Park Hospital, Slough, UK

[3]University College Hospital, London, UK

Correspondence to: M Arya manit_arya@hotmail.com

Cite this as: BMJ 2013;346:f1149

‹DOI› 10.1136/bmj.f1149
http://www.bmj.com/content/346/bmj.f1149

Penile cancer can have devastating mutilating and psychological consequences for those affected. It is important for clinicians to be aware of the condition. Differentiation of benign genital dermatoses from premalignant penile lesions and early stage penile cancer, with prompt specialist referral, usually prevents progression, improves prognosis, and results in improved functional and cosmetic outcomes for affected men. A retrospective single centre study of all penile cancer cases in a specialist unit over five years found that general practitioners initiated most referrals, but that about 20% of patients were initially referred to specialties other than urology, such as genitourinary medicine, dermatology, or plastic surgery.[1] This error delayed diagnosis by up to six months and potentially adversely affected quality of life, prognosis, and survival. Our article, written for the non-specialist, aims to provide an evidence based review of the causes and current trends in the diagnosis and management of premalignant and malignant penile lesions.

How common are penile cancer and premalignant lesions of the penis?

Current understanding of penile cancer is based mainly on small non-randomised retrospective case series. However, there is now a push for research into penile cancer by the International Rare Cancers Initiative (IRCI), a strategic collaboration between Cancer Research UK, the UK National Cancer Research Network (NCRN), the US National Cancer Institute (NCI), and the European Organisation for Research and Treatment of Cancer (EORTC).

The mean age at diagnosis of penile cancer is about 60 years. However, a prospective study of 100 consecutive patients from one institution in the United Kingdom suggested that 25% of men were under 50 years of age at diagnosis.[2] The age standardised incidence is 0.3-1 per 100 000 men in European countries and the United States, according to European Association of Urology guidelines.[3] Incidence is much higher in developing countries—3 per 100 000 in parts of India, 8.3 per 100 000 in Brazil, and even higher in Uganda.[3] In Uganda it is the most commonly diagnosed cancer in men, accounting for 10-20% of all tumours. The incidence and prevalence of premalignant penile lesions and their geographical variation is not well established. However, as a European example, a retrospective analysis using two nationwide registries estimated the age specific incidence rate of premalignant penile conditions in Denmark to be 0.9 per 100 000 men in 2006-08.[4] No similar robust data have been published from developing countries where the cancer is more common.

What are the risk factors for penile cancer?

An extensive systematic review of publications (case-control studies, cohort studies, ecological studies, cross sectional studies, case series, and case reports) from 1966 to 2000 and their citations found an association between the presence of a foreskin and tumour development.[5] Researchers in North America observed this association in a population based case-control study.[6] They found a 3.2 times greater risk in men who were never circumcised and a 3.0 times greater risk in men who were circumcised after the neonatal period compared with those circumcised as neonates. Adult circumcision seems to have no protective effect. In addition, penile cancer is rarer in countries with subpopulations who practise childhood circumcision, such as India and Nigeria. Early circumcision protects against phimosis, poor penile hygiene, and retention of smegma (desquamated epidermal cells and urinary products). These conditions are proposed to result in chronic inflammation of the glans and prepuce, which is thought to promote the development of penile cancer.[5] However, well conducted longitudinal studies are needed to fully elucidate the protective role of early circumcision.

Human papillomavirus (HPV) infection also plays a role in the development of this tumour. A systematic review of the major penile cancer studies published from 1986 to 2008 established that about 50% of cancers were associated with HPV, with the main subtype being HPV-16 (involved in 60% of cases) followed by HPV-18 (13% of cases).[7]

Table 1 summarises other risk factors for penile cancer.

How does penile cancer present and what are the indications for specialist referral?

Presentation is often delayed because of embarrassment about the lesion. A retrospective UK study suggested a delay of 5.8 months from the onset of symptoms to presentation

SUMMARY POINTS

- Penile cancer has potentially devastating functional and psychological consequences for the patient
- Penile cancer is thought to be associated with foreskin and genital infection with human papillomavirus types 16 and 18
- Most patients present with a penile lump (47%), ulcer (35%), or erythematous lesion (17%)
- Carcinoma in situ of the penis is treated initially with topical chemotherapy or lasers; surgery is reserved for unresponsive cases and men with extensive premalignant changes
- In invasive penile cancer, penile preserving surgery minimises voiding and sexual dysfunction and psychological sequelae; more radical penile surgery is reserved for advanced cases
- Metastatic inguinal lymph node involvement is the most important prognostic factor

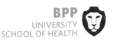

Table 1 Risk factors for penile cancer

Risk factor	Relative increased risk of penile cancer
Not circumcised (associated with phimosis, poor penile hygiene, smegma retention)	×3.2 relative to neonatal circumcision[5]
HPV infection (most commonly types 16 and 18)[6]	—
Genital warts	5.9 times[5]
Multiple sexual partners and early age of first intercourse	3-5 times[4]
HIV infection	8 times[8]*
Smoking (dose dependent effect)	×2.8 relative to non-smokers[5]
Psoralen plus ultraviolet light A (PUVA) treatment for psoriasis	×58.8 times[9]†
Penile injury (small tears or abrasions)	3.9 times[5]

*A retrospective review of a cancer database over 18 years in patients with HIV/AIDs.
†A 12.3 year prospective cohort study in a single centre of men with psoriasis treated with PUVA.
HPV=human papillomavirus.

Table 2 Histological variants of primary penile cancer

Histological subtype	Relative frequency (%)
Squamous cell variants	95
Usual type	60-70
Papillary	7
Condylomatous	7
Basaloid	4-10
Verrucous	7
Sarcomatoid	1-4
Others	5
Malignant melanoma	2
Basal cell carcinoma	2
Extramammary Paget's disease	<1
Sarcoma	<1

to a medical professional.[1] Most men present with a lump (47%), ulcer (35%), or erythematous lesion (17%). Men may also present with bleeding or discharge from a lesion concealed by a phimotic foreskin.

The diagnosis of penile cancer is therefore often obvious because lesions are directly visible or palpable under a phimotic foreskin. If penile cancer is suspected, urgently refer the man to a urology department, ideally a supraregional referral centre for penile cancer. Arrange an emergency admission if there are coexistent complications—such as voiding dysfunction, urinary retention, or extensive metastatic disease—so that adequate urinary drainage and investigations can be instigated without delay.

How can premalignant lesions be differentiated from benign genital dermatoses?

Differentiating erythematous premalignant lesions from benign genital dermatoses is a challenge. Maintain a high index of suspicion and remember that follow-up is extremely important. Benign lesions such as eczema, psoriasis, lichen planus, and Zoon's balanitis are common and normally respond to treatment with a combination of topical steroids and emollients. However, patients treated for these benign conditions must be closely followed up to ensure that the lesions resolve completely. If an erythematous area or ulcer does not heal after two to three weeks of conservative treatment with steroids or antifungals, urgent referral to

a urologist or dermatologist with an interest in genital dermatology is essential because a diagnostic biopsy is mandatory to exclude premalignant disease. However, if the initial lesion is exophytic or raised and irregular, prompt urological referral from the outset is preferable because this may be an invasive carcinoma.

What are the histological subtypes of penile cancer and staging system?

Table 2 summarises the histological subtypes of penile cancer. Squamous cell carcinoma accounts for most cases and is the main focus of this article. Sarcomatoid and basaloid subtypes are rarer, more aggressive, and have a poorer prognosis. The box shows the TNM staging of this cancer.[10]

What premalignant conditions are associated with penile cancer?

Several premalignant lesions of the penis have been described (tables 3 and 4), although the risk of progression to invasive penile cancer depends on the site and type of lesion. Penile intraepithelial neoplasia (PIN), classified as PIN I-III, is commonly associated with high risk HPV types 16 and 18.[7] The pathological features of PIN II are similar to Bowenoid papulosis and those of PIN III are synonymous with erythroplasia of Queyrat (fig 1) and Bowen's disease, both of which are also referred to as carcinoma in situ (CIS). Bowenoid papulosis is mainly located on the penile shaft and presents as multiple red velvety maculopapular areas. Erythroplasia of Queyrat presents as velvety bright red patches located on the mucosal surfaces of the penis, whereas lesions in Bowen's disease are solitary well defined red plaques located on the penile shaft, often with areas of crusting or ulceration.

The most common non-HPV related premalignant condition is lichen sclerosus et atrophicus, otherwise known as balanitis xerotica obliterans (fig 2). Lichen sclerosus is seen in uncircumcised men and is secondary to a chronic inflammatory process affecting the glans and prepuce. A pathological phimosis normally develops, and in severe cases both the meatus and urethra can be affected. The largest published series (retrospective study of 522 patients in a single centre) reported that 2.3% of patients diagnosed with lichen sclerosus had squamous cell carcinoma of the penis,[11] whereas synchronous lichen sclerosus is found in 28-50% of patients treated for penile cancer. Lichen sclerosus can therefore be considered a risk factor for the development of penile cancer, albeit with a latency time of 12-17 years. Other non-HPV related premalignant lesions include leucoplakia and cutaneous penile horn (table 4).

TNM PATHOLOGICAL CLASSIFICATION OF PENILE CANCER (N CATEGORIES ARE BASED ON BIOPSY OR SURGICAL EXCISION)[10]

Primary tumour (T)
- TX: Primary tumour cannot be assessed
- T0: No evidence of primary tumour
- Tis: Carcinoma in situ
- Ta: Non-invasive verrucous carcinoma, not associated with destructive invasion
- T1: Tumour invades subepithelial connective tissue
- T2: Tumour invades corpus spongiosum or corpora cavernosa
- T3: Tumour invades urethra
- T4: Tumour invades other adjacent structures

Regional lymph nodes (N)
- NX: Regional lymph nodes cannot be assessed
- N0: No regional lymph node metastasis
- N1: Intranodal metastasis in a single inguinal lymph node
- N2: Metastasis in multiple or bilateral inguinal lymph nodes
- N3: Metastasis in pelvic lymph node(s); unilateral, bilateral, or extranodal extension of regional lymph node metastasis

Distant metastasis (M)
- M0: No distant metastasis
- M1: Distant metastasis

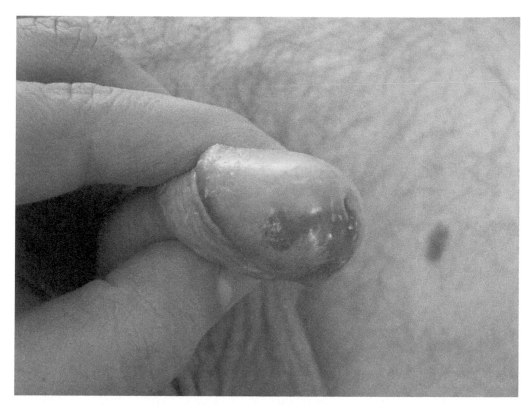

Fig 1 Erythroplasia of Queyrat, which is also known as carcinoma in situ of the glans penis

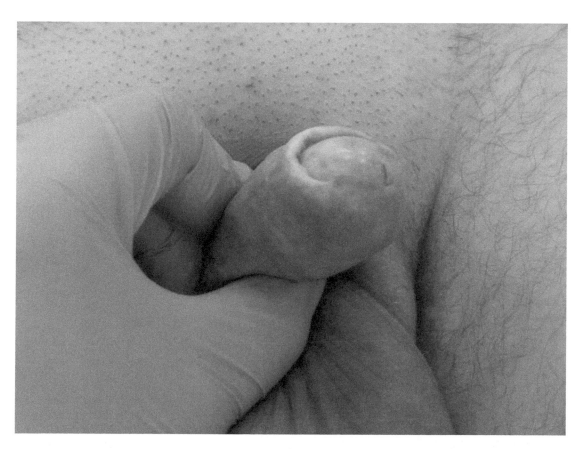

Fig 2 Balanitis xerotica obliterans, also known as lichen sclerosus et atrophicus

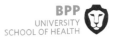

Table 3 HPV related premalignant penile lesions

Lesion	Location and appearance	Progression rate to invasive cancer (%)*
Erythroplasia of Queyrat (PIN III; non-keratinising CIS)	Velvety red plaques on the glans penis and inner prepuce	30
Bowen's disease (PIN III; keratinising CIS)	Pigmented lesions affecting follicle bearing areas of the penile shaft and scrotum	5
Bowenoid papulosis	Multiple brown-red maculopapular areas	1
Buschke-Löwenstein "tumour" (giant condyloma acuminatum)	Confluence of warty exophytic cauliflower-like growths	30

*Progression rates are not well documented and are based on small retrospective case series.
CIS=carcinoma in situ; HPV=human papillomavirus; PIN=penile intraepithelial neoplasia.

Table 4 Non-HPV related premalignant lesions

Lesion	Location and appearance	Progression rate to invasive cancer (%)*
Lichen sclerosus et atrophicus (also known as balanitis xerotica obliterans)	White sclerotic patches affecting the prepuce, glans, or meatus; often result in phimosis	Not known
Leucoplakia	White verrucous plaques on mucosal surfaces	Not known
Cutaneous penile horn	Conical and exophytic lesion associated with areas of chronic inflammation	30 (mostly low grade)

*Progression rates are not well documented and are based on small retrospective case series.
HPV=human papillomavirus.

How is penile cancer investigated?

Penile cancer should be managed in high volume supraregional referral centres. Premalignant conditions need only an incisional or excisional biopsy to confirm the diagnosis and exclude invasive elements. However, invasive tumours require staging of the primary penile lesion and inguinal and pelvic lymph nodes. Tumours are most commonly seen on the glans (48%) or prepuce (21%) (fig 3). Such tumours require no further imaging unless it is unclear whether the tumour is limited to the corpus spongiosum or extends into the corpus cavernosum. Local staging can be performed by using intracavernosal prostaglandin (PGE1) to induce an artificial erection after magnetic resonance imaging (MRI) using T2 and T1 precontrast and postcontrast sequences. The largest study on the use of MRI retrospectively analysed the correlation between MRI and the final histological findings in 55 patients in a single tertiary referral centre.[12] Although corpus cavernosum involvement was correctly predicted in two cases, the technique over-staged six cases of T1 tumour as T2.[12] Ultrasound of the glans penis can also be used to identify involvement of the corpus cavernosum.

Clinical examination of the inguinal region will detect enlarged inguinal lymph nodes as a result of metastatic disease (cN+) and staging computed tomography (CT) is performed to detect further abnormal lymphadenopathy in the inguinal and pelvic region, together with any distant metastatic disease. However, the sensitivity of both conventional CT and MRI for clinically impalpable disease (cN0) is poor because these techniques classify abnormal lymphadenopathy on the basis of size and morphology criteria. Alternative imaging modalities for cN0 and cN+ disease include ultrasonography combined with fine needle aspiration cytology and positron emission tomography-CT with fluorine-18 labelled FDG. A recent meta-analysis reported that this last technique had a pooled sensitivity of 96.4% for cN+ disease and 56.5% for cN0 disease.[13] MRI with lymphotrophic nanoparticles using intravenous ferumoxtran-10 showed promising results in detecting occult metastases in a case series of seven patients with penile carcinoma.[14] However, use of these nanoparticles is currently not authorised in Europe. Bilateral dynamic sentinel lymph node biopsy (fig 4; see below) is used in some specialist centres in Europe and North America for detecting lymph node metastasis in cN0 disease, but the technique is not yet standard in many countries.

What treatments are available for premalignant and malignant disease of the penis?

Treatment of premalignant disease

All men with suspected premalignant disease of the penis will have undergone a diagnostic biopsy. If this was an excisional biopsy and histological analysis indicates that the lesion was excised completely, the patient is placed under close surveillance after circumcision (which is strongly recommended internationally). If incisional biopsy was performed rather than excision, after circumcision further treatment will be needed to completely eradicate the lesion. Not only does circumcision remove a preputial lesion, it also aids surveillance (including self examination) and allows topical treatment to be applied.

The most common first line topical treatment for CIS or PIN of the penis is 5% 5-fluorouracil, an antimetabolite chemotherapeutic agent. Treatment protocols vary, but it is generally applied to the lesion on alternate days for four to six weeks. In the largest study to date—a single centre retrospective review of 42 cases of penile CIS treated with 5-fluorouracil identified from a prospective database over 10 years—50% achieved a complete response and 31% a partial response.[15] Persistent lesions can be treated with second line immunotherapy using topical 5% imiquimod, although its use is supported only by uncontrolled cohort studies and case reports, so its effectiveness is unclear. Topical chemotherapy is most effective for solitary lesions in immunocompetent patients, but clinicians must be alert to recurrence in partial responders.

Premalignant lesions have also been treated using lasers (carbon dioxide; Nd:YAG (neodymium-doped yttrium aluminium garnet; Nd:Y3Al5O12); and KTP (potassium titanyl phosphate)) with good functional and cosmetic results. Published studies have included only modest numbers, but in one study 19 patients with premalignant penile disease who were treated with lasers were free from cancer after two years.[16]

Surgical excision is reserved for refractory cases or for patients who have developed extensive CIS of the glans penis. Both intractable in situ disease and non-invasive verrucous disease can be effectively treated by excising the diseased area. This involves excision of the epithelial and subepithelial tissues of the glans penis with preservation of the underlying corpus spongiosum, followed by coverage of the denuded glans penis with a split thickness skin graft. This surgical technique is called glans resurfacing.

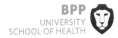

Treatment of invasive cancer

The treatment of invasive penile lesions involves surgical excision of the primary penile lesion combined with a risk adapted approach to performing inguinal lymphadenectomy. Depending on the extent of the tumour, surgery is divided into penile preserving surgery or radical surgery.

Penile preserving surgery

Single centre case series that retrospectively analysed resection margins after partial and total penectomy showed that the conventional 2 cm resection margin from the primary tumour is not needed to achieve long term oncological control and disease specific survival.[17] [18] This finding has formed the basis of penile preserving surgery, which allows surgical excision of the tumour while maintaining penile length and minimising anatomical, functional, and psychological disruption.

T1-T2 lesions confined to the glans penis

Wide local excision of the cancer followed by primary closure may be possible if the lesion is small. For larger tumours, a partial or total excision of the penile glans combined with reconstruction using a split skin graft can be performed. A retrospective analysis of a case series of 72 consecutive patients undergoing glansectomy and reconstruction reported a local recurrence rate of 6% after a mean follow-up of 27 months.[19] Provided that local recurrences are excised, the long term prognosis remains unchanged for this group of patients.

Surgery for advanced tumours (T2, T3, T4)

The management of stage T4, high grade stage T3, or advanced stage T2 disease requires radical surgery in the form of a partial penectomy or total penectomy, with formation of a perineal urethrostomy (a form of urine diversion).

Radiotherapy and chemotherapy

The use of radiotherapy (external beam radiotherapy or brachytherapy) is now uncommon for penile carcinoma and is most appropriate for small T1 or T2 lesions in patients unfit or unwilling to undergo surgery.

Unlike other squamous cell carcinomas, penile cancer is an aggressive cancer with a limited response to chemotherapy regimens. Data on the use of chemotherapy in penile cancer are lacking, so evidence based recommendations are limited and the optimal chemotherapy regimen has yet to be defined.

How important is lymph node disease?

Anatomical and lymphoscintigraphic studies have shown that lymph from the penis drains bilaterally to the inguinal lymph nodes in most patients. Once metastatic disease involves the inguinal lymph nodes, further spread of metastatic cells occurs in a step wise manner to the pelvic lymph nodes, then distant sites such as the lungs, bone, and para-aortic lymph nodes. In a retrospective analysis of 118 patients with penile cancer treated at the Netherlands Cancer Institute from 1956 to 1989, inguinal lymph node involvement was the most important prognostic indicator.[20] In the same study, patients with metastatic disease in one

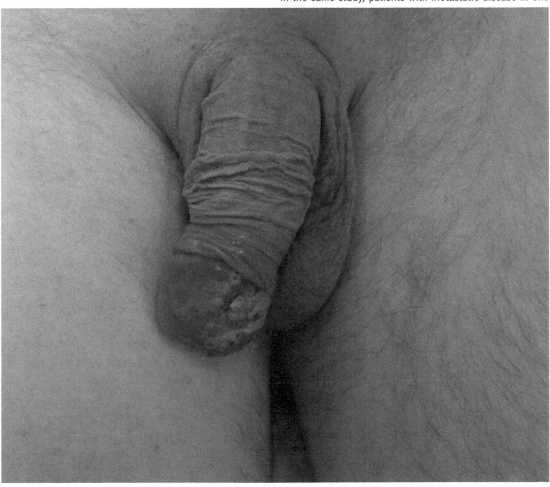

Fig 3 Penile tumour on glans penis

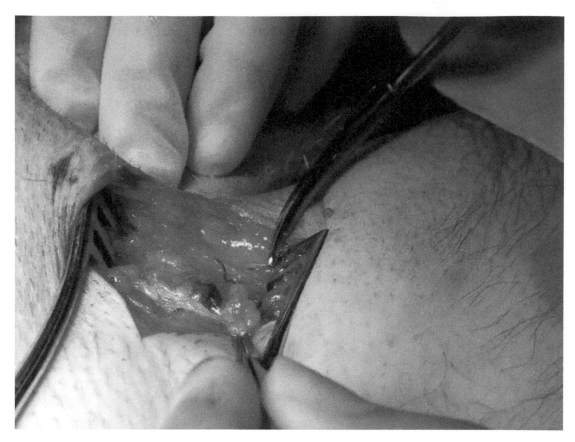

Fig 4 Dynamic inguinal sentinel lymph node biopsy. This involves injection of patent blue dye and a 99m-technetium labelled nanocolloid around the primary penile tumour. During surgery a γ ray detection probe helps localise the sentinel lymph node together with the patent blue, which deeply stains the node (shown)

or two inguinal lymph nodes had a five year survival rate of about 80%.[20] A separate retrospective analysis of 201 patients over a 24 years period reported that extension of metastatic disease into the pelvic nodes was associated with a five year survival of 0-21%.[21]

Management of cN+ disease (clinically node positive)
About 20% of patients in Western countries present with palpable inguinal lymph nodes, which almost always signify metastatic disease and will require a radical inguinal lymphadenectomy (a procedure associated with high morbidity).

Management of cN0 disease (clinically node negative)
About 80% of patients present with clinically impalpable inguinal lymph nodes. However, 20-25% of these patients will have occult metastasis, and it is this group of men who need accurate nodal staging. To avoid overtreatment of these patients, alternative options such as close surveillance, modified superficial inguinal lymphadenectomy, or bilateral dynamic sentinel lymph node biopsy (fig 4) can be offered.

What are the psychological effects of penile cancer?
The penis is functionally important for micturition and sexual purposes. The effects of any disfiguring surgery to this organ can have a psychological impact on self image and self esteem, but research in this area is lacking. Embarrassment, anxiety, and fear may result in delayed presentation. In a retrospective study of 30 patients followed up for a median of 80 months after treatment for penile cancer, 50% had mental health symptoms, most commonly anxiety related conditions.[22] These patients were also less satisfied with regard to subjective wellbeing and showed decreased social

activity. Another systematic focused review of the literature on quality of life after penile cancer surgery identified 128 men from six studies.[23] It found that treatment for penile cancer had negative effects on wellbeing in 37.5-40%, with psychiatric symptoms in about 50% and 36-67% of patients reporting a decrease in sexual function. In dedicated units in the UK, penile cancer nurse specialists are available to provide patient support and guidance and to arrange psychosocial services as needed.

A PATIENT'S PERSPECTIVE
The first thing that I noticed was a rash on the tip of my penis. I ignored it for a while, but it seemed to get larger and wouldn't go away. I decided to see my general practitioner who prescribed a cream that I applied on a regular basis. The rash didn't get any better so my doctor referred me to a dermatologist. The dermatologist took one look at the rash and said that she suspected it may be a cancerous growth. When I realised that this was potentially a cancer on my penis I was devastated. I didn't realise that cancer could affect that part of a man's body, especially at my age—I was in my 30s. Nobody else I knew had heard of this problem or experienced it. I was urgently referred to a urology department that specialised in treating penile cancer. I was told that I needed surgery to remove the cancer and I was initially worried about the impact that surgery might have on my relationship with my wife and whether the cancer could spread elsewhere. The surgery that I underwent removed the tip of my penis and sampled the lymph nodes in my groin. Thankfully, the cancer had not spread to these lymph nodes and five years after surgery I am still clear of cancer. I can urinate normally and have normal erections for sexual intercourse. I have long been back at work, although I continue to see the specialists for regular check-ups.

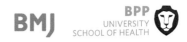

Preventive strategies

Public health education on the risks of smoking, poor genital hygiene, and sexually transmitted diseases in relation to penile cancer is essential. Since 2005, three well designed randomised control trials of more than 10 000 men conducted in South Africa, Kenya, and Uganda have evaluated male circumcision for prevention of sexually transmitted infections.[24][25][26] The trials found that circumcision decreases HIV infection by 53-60% and the prevalence of oncogenic high risk HPV by 32-35%. Although these trials were not designed to investigate the potential for circumcision programmes to reduce the incidence of penile cancer, it may be possible in future to assess whether circumcision has affected penile cancer rates in these regions.

Another potential preventive strategy is HPV vaccination, which has been introduced for girls to prevent cervical cancer. HPV vaccination has also been proposed for boys to reduce the total HPV burden in the population (herd effect) and to prevent HPV related cancers. Currently, decisions on routine vaccination in boys are awaiting the results of the female HPV vaccination programme.

The 2009 International Consultation on Urologic Disease Consensus Publishing Group suggested that circumcision and early treatment of phimosis, together with important changes in global health policy, were the most useful measures to prevent penile cancer.[27]

MA would like to thank Orchid (male cancer charity based in the UK) and the Barts and the London Charity. JK would like to thank the UCLH Biomedical Research Centre.

Funding: No special funding received.

Competing interests: All authors have completed the ICMJE uniform disclosure form at www.icmje.org/coi_disclosure.pdf (available on request from the corresponding author) and declare: no support from any organisation for the submitted work; no financial relationships with any organisations that might have an interest in the submitted work in the previous three years; no other relationships or activities that could appear to have influenced the submitted work.

Patient consent obtained.

Provenance and peer review: Not commissioned; externally peer reviewed.

TIPS FOR NON-SPECIALISTS

- Refer patients with suspected penile cancer to a specialist supraregional penile cancer centre via the two week wait pathway
- Have a high index of suspicion in men with a persistent erythematous lesion or ulcer on the penis that does not heal with conservative treatment within two to three weeks or in patients who have a phimotic foreskin with underlying bleeding and discharge
- All patients with a suspected premalignant or malignant lesion on the penis need an initial diagnostic biopsy
- Early referral to a urologist at a specialist centre is more likely to allow penile preserving surgery
- Offer psychological and emotional support to all patients diagnosed and treated for penile cancer
- All patients with penile cancer should be managed in a high volume specialist centre

ONGOING RESEARCH

PEPC (Patients' Experiences of Penile Cancer): A UK multicentre observational study funded by the National Institute for Health Research Central Commissioning Facility, which aims to improve the understanding of patients' experiences after treatment for penile cancer (recruitment now closed)

Penile TPF (docetaxel, cisplatin, and 5-fluorouracil): A UK multicentre phase II trial funded by Cancer Research UK looking at the role of docetaxel, cisplatin, and 5-fluorouracil chemotherapy in locally advanced and metastatic carcinoma of the penis (recruitment now closed)

Videoscopic Versus Open Inguinal Lymphadenectomy for Cancer: Randomised, prospective interventional study based in the US that includes patients with penile cancer. The trial will randomise participants to videoscopic or traditional open inguinal lymphadenectomy to determine any differences in wound complication rate and, as a secondary endpoint, time to recurrence

ADDITIONAL EDUCATIONAL RESOURCES

Resources for healthcare professionals

- Pompeo ACL, Heyns CF, Abrams P, eds. International consultation on penile cancer. Société Internationale d'Urologie, 2009. www.icud.info/penilecancer.html. Consensus recommendations of the major international urological associations on the management of penile cancer
- Muneer A, Arya M, Horenblas S, eds. *Textbook of penile cancer*. Springer, 2011. Comprehensive, stand alone, and up to date volume on penile cancer
- Kayes O, Ahmed HU, Arya M, Minhas S. Molecular and genetic pathways in penile cancer. *Lancet Oncol* 2007;8:420-9. Detailed review of the molecular biology of penile cancer

*Resources for patients*These websites are free resources that provide reliable and balanced material for patients

- Orchid (male cancer charity) (www.orchid-cancer.org.uk)
- Cancer Research UK (www.cancerhelp.org.uk)
- National Cancer Institute (www.cancer.gov)
- Cancer.net (www.cancer.net)
- Macmillan Cancer Support (www.macmillan.org.uk)
- Patient.co.uk (www.patient.co.uk)

1. Lucky MA, Rogers B, Parr NJ. Referrals into a dedicated British penile cancer centre and sources of possible delay. *Sex Transm Infect* 2009;85:527-3.
2. Hegarty PK, Kayes O, Freeman A, Christopher N, Ralph DJ, Minhas S. A prospective study of 100 cases of penile cancer managed according to European Association of Urology guidelines. *BJU Int* 2006;98:526-31.
3. European Association of Urology. Online guidelines. 2012. www.uroweb.org/guidelines/online-guidelines/.
4. Baldur-Felskov B, Hannibal CG, Munk C, Kjaer SK. Increased incidence of penile cancer and high-grade penile intraepithelial neoplasia in Denmark 1978-2008: a nationwide population-based study. *Cancer Causes Control* 2012;23:273-80.
5. Dillner J, von Krogh G, Horenblas S, Meijer CJ. Etiology of squamous cell carcinoma of the penis. *Scand J Urol Nephrol Suppl* 2000;205:189-93.
6. Maden C, Sherman KJ, Beckmann AM, Hislop TG, Teh CZ, Ashley RL, et al. History of circumcision, medical conditions, and sexual activity and risk of penile cancer. *J Natl Cancer Inst* 1993;85:19-24.
7. Miralles-Guri C, Bruni L, Cubilla AL, Castellsagué X, Bosch FX, de Sanjosé S. Human papillomavirus prevalence and type distribution in penile carcinoma. *J Clin Pathol* 2009;62:870-8.
8. Engels EA, Pfeiffer RM, Goedert JJ, Virgo P, McNeel TS, Scoppa SM, et al; for the HIV/AIDS Cancer Match Study. Trends in cancer risk among people with AIDS in the United States 1980-2002. *AIDS* 2006;20:1645-54.
9. Stern RS. Genital tumors among men with psoriasis exposed to psoralens and ultraviolet A radiation (PUVA) and ultraviolet B radiation. The Photochemotherapy Follow-up Study. *N Engl J Med* 1990;322:1093-7.
10. Sobin LH, Gospodariwics MK, Wittekind C, eds. TNM classification of malignant tumours (UICC International Union Against Cancer). 7th ed. Wiley-Blackwell, 2009.
11. Depasquale I, Park AJ, Bracka A. The treatment of balanitis xerotica obliterans. *BJU Int* 2000;86:459-65.
12. Kayes O, Minhas S, Allen C, Hare C, Freeman A, Ralph D. The role of magnetic resonance imaging in the local staging of penile cancer. *Eur Urol* 2007;51:1313-8.
13. Sadeghi R, Gholami H, Zakavi SR, Kakhki VR, Horenblas S. Accuracy of 18F-FDG PET/CT for diagnosing inguinal lymph node involvement in penile squamous cell carcinoma: systematic review and meta-analysis of the literature. *Clin Nucl Med* 2012;37:436-41.
14. Tabatabaei S, Harisinghani M, McDougal WS. Regional lymph node staging using lymphotropic nanoparticle enhanced magnetic resonance imaging with ferumoxtran-10 in patients with penile cancer. *J Urol* 2005;174:923-7.
15. Alnajjar HM, Lam W, Bolgeri M, Rees RW, Perry MJ, Watkin NA. Treatment of carcinoma in situ of the glans penis with topical chemotherapy agents. *Eur Urol* 2012;62:923-8.
16. Malek RS. Laser treatment of premalignant and malignant squamous cell lesions of the penis. *Lasers Surg Med* 1992;12:246-53.
17. Agrawal A, Pai D, Ananthakrishnan N, Smile SR, Ratnakar C. The histological extent of the local spread of carcinoma of the penis and its therapeutic implications. *BJU Int* 2000;85:299-301.
18. Minhas S, Kayes O, Hegarty P, Kumar P, Freeman A, Ralph D. What surgical resection margins are required to achieve oncological control in men with primary penile cancer? *BJU Int* 2005;96:1040-3.
19. Smith Y, Hadway P, Biedrrzcki O, Perry MJA, Corbishley C, Watkin NA. Reconstructive surgery for invasive squamous carcinoma of the glans penis. *Eur Urol* 2007;52:1179-1185.
20. Horenblas S, van Tinteren H. Squamous cell carcinoma of the penis. IV. Prognostic factors of survival: analysis of tumor, nodes and metastasis classification system. *J Urol* 1994;151:1239-43.

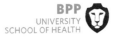

21 Ravi R. Correlation between the extent of nodal involvement and survival following groin dissection for carcinoma of the penis. *Br J Urol*1993;72:817-9.

22 Opjordsmoen S, Fosså SD. Quality of life in patients treated for penile cancer. A follow-up study. *Br J Urol*1994;74:652-7.

23 Maddineni SB, Lau MM, Sangar VK. Identifying the needs of penile cancer sufferers: a systematic review of the quality of life, psychosexual and psychosocial literature in penile cancer. *BMC Urol*2009;9:8.

24 Auvert B, Taljaard D, Lagarde E, Sobngwi-Tambekou J, Sitta R, Puren A. Randomized, controlled intervention trial of male circumcision for reduction of HIV infection risk: the ANRS 1265 Trial. *PLoS Med*2005;2:e298.

25 Bailey RC, Moses S, Parker CB, Agot K, Maclean I, Krieger JN, et al. Male circumcision for HIV prevention in young men in Kisumu, Kenya: a randomised controlled trial. *Lancet*2007;369:643-56.

26 Gray RH, Kigozi G, Serwadda D, Makumbi F, Watya S, Nalugoda F, et al. Male circumcision for HIV prevention in men in Rakai, Uganda: a randomised trial. *Lancet*2007;369:657-66.

27 Minhas S, Manseck A, Watya S, Hegarty PK. Penile cancer—prevention and premalignant conditions. *Urology*2010;76:S24-35.

Related links

bmj.com/archive

- Postpartum management of hypertension (2013;346:f894)
- Diagnosis and management of pulmonary embolism (2013;346:f757)
- Anaphylaxis: the acute episode and beyond (2013;346:f602)
- Ulcerative colitis (2013;346:f432)
- Prostate cancer screening and the management of clinically localized disease (2013;346:f325)
- Bed bug infestation (2013;346:f138)

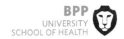

Melanoma—Part 2: management

Christina Thirlwell specialist registrar, medical oncology[1], Paul Nathan consultant medical oncologist[2]

[1]Royal Free Hospital, London NW3 2QG

[2]Mount Vernon Cancer Centre, Northwood HA6 2RN

Correspondence to: P Nathan
nathan.pd@gmail.com

Cite this as: BMJ 2008;337:a2488

‹DOI› 10.1136/bmj.a2488
http://www.bmj.com/content/337/bmj.a2488

Most melanomas that are detected and treated early are cured. However, advanced disease carries a dismal diagnosis, and timely intervention from members of the multidisciplinary skin cancer team at all stages of the disease is essential to maximise cure rates. The management of patients with incurable disease is highly specialised and requires the input of surgeons, medical and clinical oncologists, palliative care teams, and clinical nurse specialists. In the second of this two part series on melanoma we review its management from primary lesion through to metastatic disease.

How is melanoma managed in primary care?

In the past, suspicious lesions were often removed in primary care. However, recent national guidance recommends that patients with suspicious pigmented lesions are referred to a specialist member of the hospital based skin cancer team using the two week cancer wait procedure.[1][2] This has been the subject of much debate and if fully implemented will result in a change in practice for many general practitioners.

Primary melanoma is often difficult to diagnose, even for those with a specialist training. A prospective study showed that dermatologists were better than general practitioners at recognising melanoma.[3] However, a systematic review failed to identify a statistically significant advantage in favour of specialists,[4] but the amount of available evidence for review was limited. Several studies have shown that the incomplete excision rate is higher in patients treated by general practitioners than by specialists and that general practitioners send fewer lesions for histopathological review[5][6][7]. Training programmes using internet based tutorials have improved diagnostic accuracy in the United States.[8][9] Dermatoscopy improves diagnostic accuracy for experienced users but not for inexperienced users.[10]

Primary care doctors who wish to treat skin cancer and be part of the multidisciplinary team can train as general practitioners with a special interest in dermatology. The Department of Health has recently defined the training needed.[11]

The seven point check list (box)[12] may help identify melanoma. Worrying signs are a new mole growing quickly in patients over the age of puberty; change in shape, colour, or size of a long standing mole; a mole with three or more colours or which has lost its symmetry; a mole that has changed and is also itching or bleeding; any new skin lesion or nodule persisting for more than eight weeks, especially if it is growing and pigmented or vascular in appearance; a new pigmented line in a nail, especially where there is nail damage; a lesion growing under a nail. Any of these signs warrants a prompt referral for a specialist opinion.

How should a suspicious lesion be managed?

Primary excision

Guidance from the United Kingdom states that lesions suspected to be melanoma should be excised completely, with a clinical margin of 2 mm of normal skin and a cuff of fat.[1][2] This allows confirmation of the diagnosis by examination of the entire lesion, so that definitive treatment can be based upon histological features.

Shave biopsies are discouraged because they may lead to incorrect diagnosis as a result of sampling error and make accurate pathological staging of the lesion impossible. Incisional or punch biopsies are sometimes acceptable—for example, in the differential diagnosis of lentigo maligna on the face or of acral melanoma—but incisional biopsy of a suspicious pigmented lesion has no place outside the skin cancer multidisciplinary team.

Staging

Staging of primary melanoma is based on the histological features of the lesion. Accurate staging is vital to determine appropriate treatment, follow-up, and calculation of risk of recurrence. The current American Joint Committee on Cancer (AJCC) staging is based on measurement of the invasive component of the tumour (the Breslow thickness) and the presence or absence of microscopic ulceration.[14] The staging system is in the process of being revised and

SOURCES AND SELECTION CRITERIA

We used Medline (1966-2008), Cochrane Library, and Embase (1980-2008) to identify studies and meta-analyses for this review. The search string included the terms melanoma, adjuvant and metastatic therapy, wide local excision, and sentinel lymph node biopsy. We accessed the websites of the National Institute for Health and Clinical Excellence, National Cancer Research Network, and National Cancer Research Institute for guidelines and current trials in the United Kingdom.

SUMMARY POINTS

- The seven point checklist is useful for identifying suspicious lesions
- Suspicious pigmented lesions should be excised by specialists
- Rapid referral for surgery and further management are imperative to improve outcomes
- Multidisciplinary specialist teams should manage patients with high risk or advanced disease
- Systemic treatment options have modest effectiveness, so patients should be offered entry into clinical trials of new agents

MELANOMA SEVEN POINT CHECKLIST

Major features
- Change in size
- Irregular shape
- Irregular colour

Minor features
- Largest diameter 7 mm or more
- Inflammation
- Oozing
- Change in sensation
- Lesions with any of the major features or three of the minor ones are suspicious of melanoma[13]

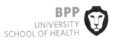

Table 1 Staging and survival for primary melanoma

Pathological stage	Breslow thickness (mm)	Microscopic ulceration	5 year survival (%)	10 year survival (%)
Ia	≤1.0	No	95.3	87.9
Ib	1.01-2.0	No	89.0	79.2
	≤1.0	Yes	90.9	83.1
IIa	2.01-4.0	No	78.7	63.8
	1.01-2.0	Yes	77.4	64.4
IIb	>4.0	No	67.4	53.9
	2.01-4.0	Yes	63.0	50.8
IIc	>4.0	Yes	45.1	32.3

Table 2 Recommended wide local excision margins[1]

Breslow thickness	Excision margins
In situ	5 mm margins to achieve complete histological excision
<1 mm	1 cm
1-2 mm	1-2 cm
2.1-4 mm	2-3 cm
>4 mm	2-3 cm

an update is expected in 2009. Additional histological features such as number of mitoses per mm², which have independent prognostic value, are likely to be included.[2] Melanocytic lesions can be notoriously difficult to diagnose, and expert dermatopathological assessment is needed. The National Institute for Health and Clinical Excellence has recommended double reporting of all melanomas if the report can be produced within 14 days. The Royal College of Pathologists has produced a minimum dataset, which defines the histological features of a melanoma that should be included in the histopathology report.[15]

The risk of death from a primary melanoma increases dramatically with increasing stage (table 1), reinforcing the importance of early diagnosis and treatment.

What are the benefits of wide local excision and sentinel lymph node biopsy?

Wide local excision of a cuff of normal tissue after excision biopsy reduces local recurrence rates. Up until the 1980s, disfiguring radical wide local excision margins of 4-5 cm were used on the basis of anecdotal evidence from 1907.[16] Prospective studies carried out in the US and Europe under the World Health Organization melanoma programme determined that a 1 cm excision margin could be safely used for melanomas less than 2 mm thick.[17] Further prospective studies in the US and the UK showed that 2 cm and 3 cm excision margins were safe for lesions greater than 2 mm and 4 mm thick, respectively.[18] [19] Table 2 outlines the current guidelines for wide local excision margins. Wide local excision reduces local recurrence rates but has no statistically significant effect on survival.[19] [20] Decisions on the size of the margin are therefore usually taken by members of the multidisciplinary team, who balance the morbidity of the procedure with the potential benefit to the patient.

Sentinel lymph node biopsy, a procedure that identifies and removes the lymph node(s) immediately draining the area of the primary tumour for histological analysis, has been the subject of much debate. The procedure provides powerful prognostic information. Microscopic lymph node involvement is an integral part of the AJCC staging system,[14] and sentinel node status is therefore used to stratify patients who enrol into current clinical trials of adjuvant treatment. However, completion lymphadenectomy, in which the locoregional lymph nodes are removed when a sentinel node biopsy is positive, has not been shown to improve overall survival.[21] [22] Whether sentinel lymph node biopsy can identify a group of patients who are particularly likely to benefit from adjuvant treatment needs to be examined prospectively.

What adjuvant treatments are available?

Adjuvant treatments increase the chance of cure in patients at risk of recurrence after potentially curative surgery. Despite much effort, no treatment has yet been shown to be efficacious enough to become routine.

Interferon alfa

The value of adjuvant interferon alfa, which is given intravenously or subcutaneously depending on the dose and regimen used, has been widely discussed. After initial reports of a highly significant overall survival benefit,[23] later reports and further studies have found this drug to be less active.

A recent meta-analysis of individual patient data from randomised controlled trials of adjuvant interferon alfa found no dose-response relation but did show a proportional benefit in overall survival of 3% at five years (95% confidence interval 1% to 5%).[24] Results indicated that patients whose primary lesion was ulcerated were more likely to benefit from adjuvant interferon, but this observation requires prospective assessment.

Preliminary results from the EORTC (European Organisation for Research and Treatment of Cancer) 18991 study randomising weekly pegylated interferon alfa versus observation were recently reported.[25] They showed a significant improvement in relapse-free survival (hazard ratio 0.82, 0.71 to 0.96) but not in distant metastasis-free survival or overall survival. Subgroup analysis of patients with N1 disease (microscopic nodal disease—those with a positive sentinel lymph node biopsy) suggested that these patients may benefit most, and a planned EORTC study will look at this question.

There is currently no accepted adjuvant standard of care in the UK, so patients should be referred for entry into clinical trials. The current UK National Cancer Research Network adjuvant phase III study is examining whether bevacizumab (Avastin), a humanised anti-vascular endothelial growth factor antibody, reduces the risk of relapse in high risk primary and resected locoregional disease.

How do I treat metastatic disease?

Metastases can occur virtually anywhere and at any time after a diagnosis of melanoma. Common sites are nodal basins, liver, lung, bone, and brain.

NICE guidance is that all patients diagnosed with distant metastases should be referred to a specialist oncologist and have access to a clinical nurse specialist and palliative care team. All new diagnoses of metastatic disease should be discussed by the specialist multidisciplinary team.[2]

In advanced disease, no intervention has been shown to have a significant effect on overall survival. Management of various clinical scenarios is outlined below.

Metastasectomy in oligometastatic relapse may be considered in highly selected patients who have been disease free for a long time.[26] [27]

Cutaneous metastases, in-transit metastases (deposits from a focus of cells moving along regional lymphatic

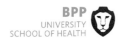

channels), or nodal metastases are generally treated surgically with palliative intent. A carbon dioxide laser[28] and radiotherapy can also help provide an element of local control.

Multiple cutaneous deposits in a single limb (with no distant metastases) can be treated by isolated limb perfusion or infusion using melphalan as a single agent or combined with other cytotoxic and biological agents.[29][30] This can have excellent results in appropriately selected patients but can cause considerable morbidity.

Metastases to the central nervous system carry a poor prognosis. Surgery may be indicated for isolated lesions if amenable.[31][32] Stereotactic radiotherapy including newer techniques such as γ knife treatment can also be used.[33] No survival benefit has been proved for whole brain radiotherapy or chemotherapy, although both are commonly used as standard of care.

Systemic treatment in melanoma is unsatisfactory—few drugs are available and response rates are limited. Patients with metastatic disease have a median survival of six to nine months.[14]

Despite many studies over the past 20 years investigating various chemotherapy regimens, dacarbazine remains the standard of care. It has a response rate of 5-15% and improves progression-free survival by a few months at best. There is no randomised evidence for an improvement in overall survival. Patients with raised lactate dehydrogenase are less likely to benefit from systemic treatment.[34]

Adding interferon alfa and interleukin-2 to chemotherapy increases response rates and toxicity, but does not significantly improve overall survival[35]; it is therefore not recommended. High dose interleukin-2 did not extend overall survival in a randomised clinical trial, although a small number of patients experience durable complete responses.[36]

What therapeutic agents are being investigated?

Significant advances have been made in understanding the pathways that drive the growth and survival of melanoma cells.[37] Activating mutations in two cell signalling pathways have been identified, and targeted treatments are in early phase clinical development. Current opinion is that inhibition of signalling through both pathways may be required. Single agent sorafenib, a multitarget kinase inhibitor with modest activity against b-raf, was not significantly active.[38] Combination studies with chemotherapy are currently under way after phase II studies showed some promise.[39] Agents that induce apoptosis[40] and potentiate the activity of chemotherapy[41] are also being investigated in large clinical trials. New activators of the immune system have shown promise in a subset of patients with advanced disease, and studies are planned in the adjuvant setting.[42][43] Because current therapeutic options are so limited, patients should be offered entry into clinical trials.

Conclusions and future directions

Treatments for melanoma are limited. The main emphasis must be in primary prevention, prompt identification, and referral of suspicious lesions. Surgery has a central role in the management of melanoma. Advances in understanding the molecular pathology of melanoma and in immunotherapeutics provide some hope for future improvements in the treatment of advanced disease and in the adjuvant setting for patients at high risk of relapse.

> **ADDITIONAL EDUCATIONAL RESOURCES**
>
> **Resources for healthcare professionals**
>
> - World Health Organization (www.who.int/uv/publications/sunbedpubl/en/index.html)—Guidance on the use of artificial tanning sun beds
> - National Institute for Health and Clinical Excellence (www.nice.org.uk/Guidance/CSGSTIM/Guidance/pdf/English)—UK National guidance on the management and organisation of services for all stages of melanoma
> - Cancer Research UK (www.cancerhelp.org.uk/help/default.asp?page=2788)—Information for doctors and patients that includes information on clinical trials currently funded by Cancer Research UK
> - Cochrane review: Crosby T, Fish R, Coles B, Mason MD. Systemic treatments for metastatic cutaneous melanoma. 2008. www.cochrane.org/reviews/en/ab001215.html
>
> **Resources for patients**
>
> - Macmillan Cancer Support (www.cancerbackup.org.uk)—Up to date cancer information, practical advice, and support for cancer patients, their families, and carers
> - National Cancer Research Network (www.ncrn.org.uk) and National Cancer Research Institute (www.ncri.org.uk)—Both websites have open access portfolios of clinical trials in melanoma currently open for enrolment
> - British Association of Dermatologists (www.bad.org.uk/public/cancer/)—Advice on the use of sunscreens and on suspicious lesions

Thanks to Veronique Bataille for helpful comments in the preparation of the manuscript.

Contributors: PN and CT contributed equally to the planning, research, and writing of this paper. PN is guarantor.

Competing interests: None declared.

Provenance and peer review: Commissioned; externally peer reviewed.

1   Roberts DL, Anstey AV, Barlow RJ, Cox NH, Newton Bishop JA, Corrie PG, et al. UK guidelines for the management of cutaneous melanoma. Br J Dermatol2002;146:7-17.
2   National Institute for Health and Clinical Excellence. Improving outcomes for people with skin tumours including melanoma: the manual.2006. www.nice.org.uk/Guidance/CSGSTIM/Guidance/pdf/English.
3   Brochez L, Verhaeghe E, Bleyen L, Naeyaert JM. Diagnostic ability of general practitioners and dermatologists in discriminating pigmented skin lesions. J Am Acad Dermatol2001;44:979-86.
4   Chen SC, Bravata DM, Weil E, Olkin I. A comparison of dermatologists' and primary care physicians' accuracy in diagnosing melanoma: a systematic review. Arch Dermatol2001;137:1627-34.
5   Khorshid SM, Pinney E, Bishop JA. Melanoma excision by general practitioners in north-east Thames region, England. Br J Dermatol1998;138:412-7.
6   Herd RM, Hunter JA, McLaren KM, Chetty U, Watson AC, Gollock JM. Excision biopsy of malignant melanoma by general practitioners in south east Scotland 1982-91. BMJ1992;305:1476-8.
7   McWilliam LJ, Knox F, Wilkinson N, Oogarah P. Performance of skin biopsies by general practitioners. BMJ1991;303:1177-9.
8   Gerbert B, Bronstone A, Wolff M, Maurer T, Berger T, Pantilat S, et al. Improving primary care residents' proficiency in the diagnosis of skin cancer. J Gen Intern Med1998;13:91-7.
9   Gerbert B, Bronstone A, Maurer T, Berger T, McPhee SJ, Caspers N. The effectiveness of an internet-based tutorial in improving primary care physicians' skin cancer triage skills. J Cancer Educ2002;17:7-11.
10   Kittler H, Pehamberger H, Wolff K, Binder M. Diagnostic accuracy of dermoscopy. Lancet Oncol2002;3:159-65.
11   Department of Health. Guidance and competencies for the provision of services using GPs with special interests (GPwSIs). Dermatology and skin surgery.2007. www.pcc.nhs.uk/uploads/pwsis/gpwsis_dermatology.pdf.
12   Mackie RM, Doherty VR. Seven-point checklist for melanoma. Clin Exp Dermatol1991;16:151-3.
13   Du Vivier AW, Williams HC, Brett JV, Higgins EM. How do malignant melanomas present and does this correlate with the seven-point check-list? Clin Exp Dermatol1991;16:344-7.
14   Balch CM, Buzaid AC, Soong SJ, Atkins MB, Cascinelli N, Coit DG, et al. Final version of the American Joint Committee on Cancer staging system for cutaneous melanoma. J Clin Oncol2001;19:3635-48.

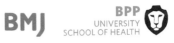

15 Royal College of Pathologists. *Standards and minimum datasets for reporting skin cancers.* 2002. www.rcpath.org/resources/pdf/skincancers2802.pdf.

16 Handley W. The pathology of melanotic growths in relation to their operative treatment. *Lancet*1907;1:927-33.

17 Veronesi U, Cascinelli N. Narrow excision (1-cm margin). A safe procedure for thin cutaneous melanoma. *Arch Surg*1991;126:438-41.

18 Balch CM, Soong SJ, Smith T, Ross MI, Urist MM, Karakousis CP, et al. Long-term results of a prospective surgical trial comparing 2 cm vs 4 cm excision margins for 740 patients with 1-4 mm melanomas. *Ann Surg Oncol*2001;8:101-8.

19 Thomas JM, Newton-Bishop J, A'Hern R, Coombes G, Timmons M, Evans J, et al. Excision margins in high-risk malignant melanoma. *N Engl J Med*2004;350:757-66.

20 Lens MB, Nathan P, Bataille V. Excision margins for primary cutaneous melanoma: updated pooled analysis of randomized controlled trials. *Arch Surg*2007;142:885-91; discussion 891-3.

21 Morton DL, Thompson JF, Cochran AJ, Mozzillo N, Elashoff R, Essner R, et al. Sentinel-node biopsy or nodal observation in melanoma. *N Engl J Med*2006;355:1307-17.

22 Thomas JM. Prognostic false-positivity of the sentinel node in melanoma. *Nat Clin Pract Oncol*2008;5:18-23.

23 Kirkwood JM, Resnick GD, Cole BF. Efficacy, safety, and risk-benefit analysis of adjuvant interferon alfa-2b in melanoma. *Semin Oncol*1997;24(1 suppl 4):S16-23.

24 Wheatley K. Interferon-alpha as adjuvant therapy for melanoma: an individual patient data meta-analysis of randomised trials [abstract]. *J Clin Oncol*2007;25(18S):8526.

25 Eggermont AM. EORTC 18991. Long term adjuvant pegylated IFN-2b (PEG-IFN) compared to observation on resected stage III melanoma, final results of a randomised phase III trial [abstract]. *J Clin Oncol*2007;25(18S):8504.

26 Overett TK, Shiu MH. Surgical treatment of distant metastatic melanoma. Indications and results. *Cancer*1985;56:1222-30.

27 Meyer T, Merkel S, Goehl J, Hohenberger W. Surgical therapy for distant metastases of malignant melanoma. *Cancer*2000;89:1983-91.

28 Waters RA, Clement RM, Thomas JM. Carbon dioxide laser ablation of cutaneous metastases from malignant melanoma. *Br J Surg*1991;78:493-4.

29 Grunhagen DJ, Brunstein F, Graveland WJ, van Geel AN, de Wilt JH, Eggermont AM. One hundred consecutive isolated limb perfusions with TNF-alpha and melphalan in melanoma patients with multiple in-transit metastases. *Ann Surg*2004;240:939-47; discussion 947-8.

30 Thompson JF, Kam PC, Waugh RC, Harman CR. Isolated limb infusion with cytotoxic agents: a simple alternative to isolated limb perfusion. *Semin Surg Oncol*1998;14:238-47.

31 Mori Y, Kondziolka D, Flickinger JC, Kirkwood JM, Agarwala S, Lunsford LD. Stereotactic radiosurgery for cerebral metastatic melanoma: factors affecting local disease control and survival. *Int J Radiat Oncol Biol Phys*1998;42:581-9.

32 Zacest AC, Besser M, Stevens G, Thompson JF, McCarthy WH, Culjak G. Surgical management of cerebral metastases from melanoma: outcome in 147 patients treated at a single institution over two decades. *J Neurosurg*2002;96:552-8.

33 Selek U, Chang EL, Hassenbusch SJ 3rd, Shiu AS, Lang FF, Allen P, et al. Stereotactic radiosurgical treatment in 103 patients for 153 cerebral melanoma metastases. *Int J Radiat Oncol Biol Phys*2004;59:1097-106.

34 Eton O, Legha SS, Moon TE, Buzaid AC, Papadopoulos NE, Plager C, et al. Prognostic factors for survival of patients treated systemically for disseminated melanoma. *J Clin Oncol*1998;16:1103-11.

35 Ives NJ, Stowe RL, Lorigan P, Wheatley K. Chemotherapy compared with biochemotherapy for the treatment of metastatic melanoma: a meta-analysis of 18 trials involving 2621 patients. *J Clin Oncol*2007;25:5426-34.

36 Tarhini AA, Kirkwood JM, Gooding WE, Cai C, Agarwala SS. Durable complete responses with high-dose bolus interleukin-2 in patients with metastatic melanoma who have experienced progression after biochemotherapy. *J Clin Oncol*2007;25:3802-7.

37 Gray-Schopfer V, Wellbrock C, Marais R. Melanoma biology and new targeted therapy. *Nature*2007;445:851-7.

38 Eisen T, Ahmad T, Flaherty KT, Gore M, Kaye S, Marais R, et al. Sorafenib in advanced melanoma: a phase II randomised discontinuation trial analysis. *Br J Cancer*2006;95:581-6.

39 McDermott D. Randomised phase II study of DTIC with or without sorafenib in patients with advanced melanoma [abstract]. *J Clin Oncol*2007;25(18S):8511.

40 Bedikian AY, Millward M, Pehamberger H, Conry R, Gore M, Trefzer U, et al. Bcl-2 antisense (oblimersen sodium) plus dacarbazine in patients with advanced melanoma: the Oblimersen Melanoma Study Group. *J Clin Oncol*2006;24:4738-45.

41 Gonzalez R, Lawson DH, Weber RW, Hutchins LF, Anderson CM, Williams KN, et al. Phase II trial of elesclomol (formerly STA-4783) and paclitaxel in stage IV metastatic melanoma (MM): subgroup analysis by prior chemotherapy [abstract]. *ASCO Meeting Abstracts*2008;26(15 suppl):9036.

42 Weber J. The efficacy and safety of ipilimumab (MDX 010) in patients with stage III/IV melanoma [abstract]. *J Clin Oncol*2007;25(18S):8523.

43 Saenger YM, Wolchok JD. The heterogeneity of the kinetics of response to ipilimumab in metastatic melanoma: patient cases. *Cancer Immun*2008;8:1.

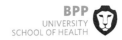

Diagnosis and management of soft tissue sarcoma

Shiba Sinha microsurgery research fellow[1], A Howard S Peach consultant plastic and reconstructive surgeon[2]

[1]O Brien Institute of Microsurgery, St Vincent's Hospital Department of Plastic Surgery, Melbourne, VIC 3065, Australia

[2]General Infirmary at Leeds, Great George Street, Leeds, UK

Correspondence to: S Sinha shibasinha@gmail.com

Cite this as: BMJ 2010;341:c7170

<DOI> 10.1136/bmj.c7170
http://www.bmj.com/content/341/bmj.c7170

Soft tissue sarcomas are a heterogeneous group of tumours of mesodermal origin. Although they are rare, accounting for less than 1% of all malignant tumours, half of patients diagnosed will die from the sarcoma.[1][w1] Lumps are commonly encountered in primary and specialist care, and differentiating benign from possibly malignant lesions can be difficult. The estimated benign:malignant ratio is 100:1. A family doctor will see about one case of soft tissue sarcoma for every 24 years of practice.[w2] However, prognosis is related to size at presentation, so early recognition, referral to a specialist (see National Institute for Health and Clinical Excellence (NICE) guidelines), and appropriate treatment improve outcomes.[2] Evidence from cohort studies suggests that patients experience delays in referral,[w3][w4] and in the United Kingdom referrals to specialist sarcoma centres often fall outside the recommended two week window for suspected cancer.[3][4] We review evidence from national guidelines, randomised trials, and observational studies to provide the non-specialist with a guide to diagnosis, appropriate referral, and management of patients with suspected soft tissue sarcoma, focusing on a multidisciplinary approach. We limit our discussion of management to the treatment of soft tissue sarcoma of the extremities—the most common site.

Who gets soft tissue sarcomas?

International incidence rates vary from 1.8 to 5.0 cases per 100 000 per year.[w5-w7] In the United States, about 10 600 new cases were diagnosed in 2009, with 3820 deaths.[w8] In the UK, 1500-2000 new cases are diagnosed annually.[2] Soft tissue sarcomas can occur at any age, but incidence increases with age. Certain subtypes, such as rhabdomyosarcoma, are more common in children and young adults. These tumours, which account for 7-10% of paediatric cancers, are an important cause of death in those aged 14-29 years.[w9][w10] A US registry based study of 17 364 patients showed an average age for diagnosis of 57.4 years.[5] Large scale epidemiological studies and national cancer registries show that men and women are affected equally.[5][6]

What are the main types of soft tissue sarcoma?

Soft tissue sarcomas are heterogeneous and usually differentiate towards one tissue type. The World Health Organization has defined more than 50 histological subtypes, although these subtypes cannot predict the clinical course.[w11] Table 1 summarises the main sarcomas by line of differentiation.

What causes soft tissue sarcoma?

Published epidemiological studies of soft tissue sarcoma are largely centre based rather than population based and suffer from selection bias. Most sarcomas seem to arise de novo, with no obvious cause. Several inherited genetic diseases have been associated with an increased risk of developing soft tissue sarcoma, including Li-Fraumeni syndrome,[w12] Gardner's syndrome, inherited retinoblastoma,[w13] and neurofibromatosis. Radiation induced soft tissue sarcoma is rare but has been associated with radiotherapy for breast cancer and lymphoma, with an average time between exposure and tumour presentation of about 10 years.[w14] A Finnish population based study of 295 712 subjects and 147 sarcomas found an increased incidence of sarcoma in younger patients (under 55) who had received radiotherapy (odds ratio 2.1, 95% confidence interval 1.6 to 2.6).[w15] Exposure to chemical carcinogens including vinyl chloride, dioxins, and phenoxyacetic herbicides has been associated with an increased incidence of soft tissue sarcoma.[w16][w17] A retrospective cohort study of 21 863 workers exposed to phenoxyherbicides, chlorophenols, and dioxins in 12 countries found a standardised mortality ratio of 2.0 for exposure and development of soft tissue sarcoma compared with national mortality rates.[7] Kaposi's sarcoma is caused by human herpesvirus 8,[w18] and Epstein Barr virus may have a role in the development of soft tissue sarcoma in immunodeficiency.

SOURCES AND SELECTION CRITERIA

We searched Medline, PubMed, Embase, and CINAHL using the terms "soft tissue sarcoma" together with "cancer", "diagnosis", and "treatment". We obtained guidelines from the National Comprehensive Cancer Network and National Institute for Health and Clinical Excellence.

SUMMARY POINTS

- Soft tissue lumps are common, but soft tissue sarcomas account for only 1% of adult cancers
- Distinguishing between malignant and benign lumps is difficult but important because early diagnosis improves outcomes
- Urgently refer patients with a lump that is deep to the fascia, >5 cm, increasing in size, or painful to a specialist surgical team
- Treatment options includes wide surgical excision alone, excision with radiotherapy (before or after surgery), and adjuvant chemotherapy
- Newer techniques of limb salvage surgery and adjuvant radiotherapy have reduced the need for amputation

---

DEPARTMENT OF HEALTH CRITERIA FOR URGENT (TWO WEEK) REFERRAL OF A SOFT TISSUE LESION

- Soft tissue mass >5 cm (golf ball size)
- Painful lump
- A soft tissue lump that is increasing in size
- A lump of any size that is deep to the muscle fascia
- Recurrence of a lump after previous excision

How does soft tissue sarcoma present?

Soft tissue swellings are common and most are benign. Patients typically present with a painless mass that has been growing slowly for months or years. Tumours often do not limit function or affect general health so may be discovered incidentally. This history and presentation, alongside the rarity of these sarcomas, commonly leads

Table 1 Main histological subtypes of soft tissue sarcoma

Sarcoma	Normal counterpart
Myxofibrosarcoma	Fibroblast or myofibroblast
Liposarcoma	Adipocyte
Leiomyosarcoma	Smooth muscle
Rhabdomyosarcoma	Skeletal muscle
Angiosarcoma	Endothelial cell
Malignant peripheral nerve sheath tumour	Schwann cell
Synovial sarcoma	Unknown
Ewing's sarcoma	Unknown

to malignant tumours being considered benign when initially examined. So what points to possible malignancy? A national multicentre cohort study of 4508 adults showed the anatomical distribution of soft tissue sarcomas to be thigh, buttock, and groin (46%); torso (18%); upper extremity (13%); retroperitoneum (13%); and head and neck (9%).[8] The UK Department of Health guidelines highlight the clinical features that should prompt urgent referral to a specialist in soft tissue sarcoma (box). A prospective study of 365 patients with soft tissue sarcoma aimed to see which referral criteria were most useful. It found that depth of tumour seemed to be a sensitive marker of malignancy.[9]

The initial consultation should look for the presence of suspicious features (box). Examine the lump to ascertain its size, anatomical site, and whether it is painful. Note whether on direct palpation the lump is fixed to the skin or situated directly beneath the skin where the margins are relatively easily defined. Restricted movement, accentuated by muscle contraction, implies fixation of the lump to the underlying deep fascia. This information should be contained in any letter of referral.

Guidelines for referral to specialist care

The US National Comprehensive Cancer Network,[10] European Society of Medical Oncology,[11] and recent UK consensus guidelines[12] based on 2006 NICE guidance recommend that general practitioners and non-specialist centres rapidly refer all patients with a suspicious soft tissue mass to a specialist referral centre that provides a protocol driven multidisciplinary approach to diagnosis and treatment.

Cohort studies have shown that these guidelines are often not adhered to.[w3] A prospective study of 216 patients in a UK centre found that 20% of patients experienced a median delay of 14 months before seeing a sarcoma specialist.[w4] An important reported consequence of delayed referral is an increase in tumour size, which affects prognosis.

Two recent studies from different UK sarcoma centres showed that 74-94% of their referrals fell outside the recommended two week window. There is little current evidence that the two week rule is resulting in earlier diagnosis of soft tissue sarcoma. This suggests a lack of awareness of optimal referral pathways by general practitioners and poor public awareness regarding soft tissue lumps.[3 4]

Referral to specialist sarcoma centres also helps to prevent "whoops procedures," where an unsuspected soft tissue lump is excised, usually by a non-specialist, and subsequent histological diagnosis shows soft tissue sarcoma with inadequate excision margins. A retrospective case note review of 104 patients in the US showed that half of patients who had undergone such procedures had done so in a non-specialist centre.[w19] A retrospective study of 203 patients showed that 69% of patients with high grade sarcomas who had "whoops procedures" had microscopic residual disease and increased rates of local recurrence.[w20]

A comparative study of 260 patients treated at specialist sarcoma centres or district general hospitals found that local recurrence occurred in 19% v 39%, respectively. However, five year survival rates did not differ significantly.[13] Although the benefit of treatment in specialist centres is difficult to quantify, it is recommended as best practice.

How is suspected soft tissue sarcoma investigated?

NICE guidelines recommend that patients with suspected soft tissue sarcoma are urgently referred for rapid assessment at a one stop diagnostic clinic where triple assessment with clinical history and examination, ultrasound imaging, tissue biopsy, and specific imaging can be undertaken.[2] Each English cancer network has stated the location of these diagnostic clinics, enabling a more rapid diagnostic pathway from primary care. The recommended first line investigation is not clearly stipulated in the guidelines and depends on local expertise and radiology facilities.[10 11]

Ultrasound

A prospective cohort study of 358 patients with soft tissue masses showed that ultrasound can rapidly triage benign and more suspicious lesions.[14] If clinical suspicion of malignancy exists but referral criteria are not met, an urgent ultrasound can help decide how fast to refer. But for lesions with a high degree of clinical suspicion, do not delay immediate referral to a specialist centre by imaging requests. Ultrasound guided biopsy of the lesion within a specialist centre helps avoid specific anatomical structures and ensures biopsy of viable rather than necrotic tumour tissue.

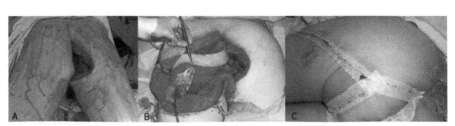

(A) Defect after excision of buttock soft tissue sarcoma. (B) Raising of a pedicled flap. (C) Reconstruction of sarcoma excision with flap

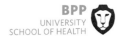

Table 2 American Joint Committee on Cancer grading system

Grade	Characteristic
Tumour (T)	
T0	No evidence of primary tumour
T1	Primary tumour <5 cm (T1a: superficial; T1b: deep)
T2	Primary tumour >5 cm (T2a: superficial; T2b: deep)
Regional lymph nodes (N)	
N0	No regional lymph nodes
N1	Regional lymph nodes involved
Metastases (M)	
M0	No metastases
M1	Distant metastases

Table 3 International Union against Cancer staging system

Stage	Tumour characteristic
1A	Low grade, small, superficial or deep (T1 a-b, No, Mo)
1B	Low grade, large, superficial (T2a, No, Mo)
IIA	Low grade, large, deep (T2b, No, Mo)
IIB	High grade, small, superficial or deep (T1a-b, No, Mo)
IIC	High grade, large, superficial (T2a, No, Mo)
Stage III	High grade, large, deep (T2b, No, Mo)
Stage IV	Any metastasis (any T, N1, or M1)

Table 4 Musculoskeletal Tumour Society staging system

Stage	Grade	Site
IA	Low	Intracompartmental
IB	Low	Extracompartmental
IIA	High	Intracompartmental
IIB	High	Extracompartmental
III	Any	Regional or distant metastases (or both)

Table 5 Classification of surgical margins in soft tissue sarcoma

Type	Surgical dissection	Outcome
Intralesional	Margin runs through the tumour	Microscopic disease remains
Marginal	Surgical margin runs through pseudocapsule or reactive zone	Tumour satellites remain in the reactive tissue—high local recurrence rate
Wide	En bloc resection within the same compartment as the tumour with a cuff of normal tissue	May leave skip lesions—low recurrence rate
Radical	En bloc resection of the entire compartment	No residual—minimal risk of local recurrence

Table 6 Summary of European Society for Medical Oncology guidelines for follow-up in soft tissue sarcoma

Year since diagnosis	Frequency of follow-up
High grade tumours	
1-3	3-4 months
4-5	6 months
More than 5	Annually
Low grade tumours	
3-5	4-6 months
More than 5	Annually

Plain radiography

For lumps that arise in extremities plain radiography can rule out a mass that arises from bone. Certain soft tissue sarcomas, and synovial sarcoma, may show characteristic calcification.

Computed tomography and magnetic resonance imaging

Magnetic resonance imaging is the preferred method of initial imaging for soft tissue sarcoma of the extremities, trunk, and head and neck in most specialist centres. Computed tomography is the gold standard for preoperative staging and is commonly used to assess intra-abdominal masses. Debate about which of the two modalities is superior continues. A multicentre trial, which included 133 evaluable soft tissue sarcomas and correlated radiological findings with histological and intraoperative findings found no statistically significant difference between the two modalities for efficacy of local staging of soft tissue sarcomas of the extremities.[15] Small comparative studies have suggested that magnetic resonance imaging may be slightly better than computed tomography because it provides multiplanar images with better spatial orientation.[w21 w22]. UK consensus guidelines state that high resolution computed tomography has a role in the identification of bony involvement and preoperative assessment to exclude pulmonary metastases.[12] The role of routine positron emission computed tomography scanning for diagnosis and monitoring of soft tissue sarcoma is currently unknown.[w23]

Biopsy

A histological diagnosis is needed to guide treatment planning. Core needle biopsy is the standard approach to diagnosing suspicious lesions, and open incision biopsy, with its high complication rate (12-17%) and association with a more radical resection, is no longer recommended.[16] Several cores are needed to improve diagnostic accuracy. Single centre prospective and retrospective studies have shown that core needle biopsy has a diagnostic sensitivity of 90-95%; it is quicker than open biopsy, cheaper, and morbidity is lower.[w24-w26] A single centre study of 530 patients found a sensitivity of 96.3% in differentiating soft tissue sarcomas from benign tumours, with a complication rate of 0.4%.[w27] Ultrasound and computed tomography guided biopsies are used when the tumour is difficult to palpate or necrotic. In the rare instance that open biopsy is needed it should be undertaken in a specialist centre.

Fine needle aspiration is not recommended in the initial diagnostic evaluation of a suspicious mass. A review of five studies found that this technique had a lower diagnostic accuracy than core biopsy. It may have a role in confirming disease recurrence.[17]

NICE guidelines recommend that biopsy results should be interpreted by a specialist sarcoma pathologist in close conjunction with a surgeon and radiologist.[2] Although histological diagnosis is the gold standard, newer methods such as cytogenetics and immunocytochemistry can aid diagnosis by identifying tumour lineage.[w28]

What affects the prognosis of soft tissue sarcoma?

Stage and grade of tumour

Information on tumour stage can help estimate prognosis and survival and plan management. Several systems are used to stage soft tissue sarcoma. The most widely accepted are those from the American Joint Committee on Cancer (AJCC) (table 2) and International Union against Cancer (IUCC) (table 3), which include information on both tumour grade and stage. The Musculoskeletal Tumour Society staging system (table 4) also takes into account whether the tumour is intracompartmental or extracompartmental and presence of regional and distant metastases.

Tumour grade is related to prognosis. A commonly adopted system in the UK is the Trojani system, which incorporates information on degree of cellular differentiation, tumour necrosis, and mitotic count.[w29] High grade tumours are poorly differentiated or undifferentiated; they carry a high likelihood of metastasis and poor patient survival. A study of 1240 patients from a national database found that tumour grade was the most important prognostic factor in metastatic recurrence.[18]

A recent systematic review found an overall five year survival for patients with soft tissue sarcoma of 60-80%.[19]

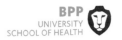

A study of 2136 prospectively followed patients estimated sarcoma specific death to be 36% after 12 years.[20] In the largest population based study assessing survival in patients with soft tissue sarcoma of the extremities, advanced age, large tumour size, and high grade all contributed to adverse prognosis and increased 10 year sarcoma specific mortality.[w30] This agrees with other population based studies[w31] and a large single centre study,[21] both of which found metastatic disease at presentation and tumour depth to be adverse prognostic indicators.

Histological subtype

Several single centre studies have shown that histological subtype may help predict prognosis.[w32-w34] A recent retrospective analysis of 17 364 patients from a population based study showed that within a tumour grade, survival differed according to histological type, but small numbers in some histological groups limited interpretation of the findings.[w34] Advances in genetic diagnosis and in the ability to predict the behaviour of certain histological subtypes of tumour may affect treatment planning and staging in the future.

How are soft tissue sarcomas managed?

Management of soft tissue sarcomas requires a multidisciplinary approach, as stated by national guidelines and protocols.[2 10 11 12] Treatment aims to ensure long term survival, avoid local recurrence, and maximise patient function while minimising morbidity. This is achieved by various combinations of surgery, radiotherapy, and chemotherapy. Treatment decisions are best made by a specialist multidisciplinary team of surgeons, pathologists, radiologists, medical oncologists, and clinical oncologists. The team will take into account the tumour's site and stage plus the patient's comorbidities and treatment preferences.

Surgery

Surgery is the mainstay of treatment in patients with localised disease. It aims to excise the soft tissue sarcoma completely, along with a biological barrier of normal tissue. Table 5 summarises the four categories of surgical margin that have been described histologically.[22] No international consensus exists on what constitutes an acceptable resection margin. Limb salvage surgery, which aims to retain a functional limb (to maintain a good postoperative quality of life) while providing an acceptable resection margin (to ensure a low risk of recurrence), is the standard of care for most patients with soft tissue sarcoma of the extremities. UK consensus guidelines state that 1 cm of normal soft tissue or equivalent (for example, fascia) is an acceptable margin.[12] Single centre retrospective case series have shown that positive margins carry an increased risk of disease recurrence and reduced disease specific survival.[21] In a retrospective study of 248 patients, those with wide surgical margins or margins greater than 2 mm had a five year survival of around 70% compared with 47% in those with positive margins or margins less than 2 mm.[w35] A tumour's proximity to important anatomical structures such as nerves and blood vessels can make it difficult to achieve an acceptable tumour-free margin.

Improved adjuvant radiotherapy and reconstructive surgery have enabled more limited surgery to be performed and function to be preserved. The surgical objective of maintaining a functional limb may require a planned microscopic positive margin and adjuvant radiotherapy. A seminal prospective study showed that less radical surgery had no detrimental effect on overall survival but was associated with a higher rate of local recurrence compared with amputation.[23] When considering more limited surgery make patients aware of the risks of tumour recurrence and the possibility of further surgery, including potential amputation.

Advances in reconstructive techniques have enabled limb preservation in complex cases in the form of pedicled and free tissue transfers (figure). Several single centre studies have shown that surgical flaps can successfully achieve wound closure, minimise surgical dead space, shorten the duration of wound healing, and protect vital structures (blood vessels, nerves, tendons, and joints).[w36-w38] A recent review showed that reconstructive techniques are cost effective.[w39]

Early complications of surgery may include haemorrhage, wound infection, and deep venous thrombosis. Although, microvascular free flap reconstructions have a success rate of greater than 95%, they can fail or experience wound breakdown, which can delay subsequent planned adjuvant treatment. The patient must be told about the risks of these complications before surgery.

European Society of Medical Oncology guidance states that treatment by wide excision surgery is sufficient for low grade tumours that are superficial or deep and less than 5 cm, in addition to high grade superficial tumours.[11] Single centre retrospective case series have shown that surgery alone is suitable for selected patients with soft tissue sarcoma, with one series reporting 10 year outcomes of 93% for local control and 73% for overall survival.[w40 w41] In one prospective trial of patients with T1 tumours and negative surgical margins treated by surgery alone the five and 10 year estimated recurrence rates were 14% (standard deviation 4%) and 16.2% (4.45%), respectively, with an estimated sarcoma specific death rate of 3.2% (2.2%) at 10 years.[24]

In advanced disease, surgery may be an appropriate palliative procedure. A single centre study found amputation rates of 9-14% in patients with recurrent soft tissue sarcoma of the extremities and less than 5% in those with primary disease.[w42 w43] Amputation may be recommended when limb salvage surgery is not possible, after careful discussion with the patient regarding surgical morbidity compared with the pros and cons of other palliative treatment options. Typically such patients have high grade, large, recurrent tumours that often affect anatomically important sites. They are likely to have poor long term survival, and the need to relieve local symptoms such as pain or fungation may outweigh negative factors associated with amputation.

A surgical and reconstructive procedure can take up to 12 hours. A small single centre study assessing the cost effectiveness of limb reconstruction found that the mean length of stay was eight days and 6.6 days for procedures involving upper and lower extremities, respectively.[w39] The duration of postoperative rehabilitation will vary from patient to patient and according to the type of surgery. This will require intensive specialist nursing, physiotherapy, and occupational therapy.

A single centre prospective study found that the preoperative expectations of patients influenced functional outcome—uncertain expectations were associated with worse functional outcomes.[w44] This finding stresses the importance of clear preoperative communication with

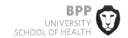
patients regarding the often long and difficult rehabilitative process and functional limitations that they may experience.

Radiotherapy

Prospective and retrospective studies have shown that radiotherapy improves local control in surgically resectable disease.[25][w45][w46] Most intermediate or high grade soft tissue sarcomas, large deep low grade sarcomas, and incompletely resected tumours that are close to important structures (such as nerves and blood vessels) are candidates for radiotherapy.[11][12] The optimum timing of radiotherapy for soft tissue sarcoma of the extremities is unclear. In the UK and other countries, postoperative radiotherapy is the standard approach. Preoperative radiotherapy can reduce the size of some radiosensitive tumours, such as myxoid liposarcoma. A recent systematic review and meta-analysis of five studies that compared preoperative and postoperative radiotherapy in localised resectable soft tissue sarcoma found a lower risk of recurrence in the preoperative radiotherapy group (odds ratio 0.61, 0.42 to 0.89). However, no overall survival benefit was seen.[26] A multicentre, prospective randomised study of 190 patients found an increased incidence of wound complications in those receiving preoperative radiotherapy (35% v 17%), but this risk was negated when reconstruction involved imported vascularised tissue.[25] A randomised phase III trial showed that the timing of radiotherapy had little effect on postoperative function.[27] Further prospective randomised controlled trials are needed to evaluate the role of preoperative radiotherapy. Single centre studies have shown that the complications associated with postoperative radiotherapy include joint stiffness, oedema, and pathological fractures. Five to 10 year local control rates for postoperative radiotherapy range from 82% to 87%.[w45][w47]

The results of the VORTEX randomised controlled trial comparing a single phase of radiotherapy with the standard two phase technique in patients with soft tissue sarcoma of the extremities with the aim of improving postoperative function are awaited.[w48] Other technological advances, including brachytherapy, where radioactive seeds or wires are placed into the tumour bed after tumour resection, and intensity modulated radiotherapy (a method of delivering radiotherapy to protect the soft tissues needed to achieve wound closure) do not yet have a convincing evidence base.[w49]

Chemotherapy

The role of adjuvant chemotherapy in the management of soft tissue sarcoma of the extremities is controversial because the evidence for its use is conflicting. Different histological subtypes vary greatly in chemosensitivity—for example, myxoid liposarcomas are more chemosensitive than some other types. UK consensus guidelines do not advocate chemotherapy as standard management.[12] The use of adjuvant chemotherapy may be considered in specific cases of advanced disease with palliative intent.

Doxorubicin based regimens are the first line drug for most histological subtypes. A large meta-analysis including data from 14 randomised phase III controlled trials showed that adjuvant doxorubicin chemotherapy improved 10 year survival by 7% (P=0.029) compared with no chemotherapy in high risk patients with localised disease.[28] A more recent meta-analysis that included data from the Italian sarcoma group trial supported these findings.[w50] It found a significant increase in overall survival with adjuvant chemotherapy and that the addition of ifosfamide significantly improved

survival.[29] Interestingly, the EORTC trial, which is the largest trial of adjuvant chemotherapy for soft tissue sarcoma, found no improvement in overall survival.[30] Future trials should include homogeneous groups of tumours (of specific histological and molecular subtypes) and patients. There is no recognised second line chemotherapy after failure of doxorubicin and ifosfamide. Most data on newer agents include phase II trials, and as knowledge about the molecular profile of tumours increases, tailored novel agents may emerge.

Several single centre studies and a multicentre phase II trial have suggested that neoadjuvant chemotherapy may be appropriate for patients who have large and high grade tumours (typically synovial sarcoma and liposarcoma) to shrink the tumour before palliative surgery.[31][w51][w52] A randomised phase III trial has shown that regional hyperthermia (heat kills cells by direct thermal toxicity and increases drug efficacy) reduces local progression and death in high risk patients.[w53] Studies in lower risk patients are needed.

Isolated limb perfusion

Isolated limb perfusion is used to treat melanoma. It is widely used in Europe to treat soft tissue sarcoma of the extremities, but it is available in only a few centres in the UK. High concentrations of tumour necrosis factor and melphalan (a chemotherapeutic agent) are delivered under hyperthermic conditions via arterial and venous cannula to a limb isolated by tourniquet compression. This treatment can be used to reduce tumour size to enable limb salvage procedures, or for palliative treatment. Single and multicentre studies of this technique have shown limb salvage rates of 74-87% in selected patients with intermediate or high grade disease.[w54][w55]

How can metastatic disease be treated?

A large population based study found that 40-50% of patients with soft tissue sarcoma develop metastatic disease.[18] Common sites of metastases include lung, local soft tissues, and local and distant lymph nodes. A single centre study of 716 patients found that about 20% of patients with soft tissue sarcoma of the extremities have isolated pulmonary metastases.[w56] The outlook for patients with metastatic disease is poor—estimated five year survival was 8% with pulmonary metastases and 59% with lymph node metastases in a recent small retrospective study.[w57] Metastases in isolated areas or a single organ may be managed with surgery with or without adjuvant treatment. Once metastases are discovered, restaging the tumour will help to determine the risk to benefit ratio of any proposed treatment for the individual patient.

Follow-up for patients with soft tissue sarcoma of the extremities

Follow-up protocols for patients with treated soft tissue sarcoma are based on the rationale that early recognition and treatment of local or distant recurrence can prolong survival. A single centre study of 2123 patients found that two thirds of recurrences developed within two years of initial surgery. This reinforces the need for close surveillance, including regular history and clinical examination to look for local recurrence, with ultrasound or magnetic resonance imaging as needed. Furthermore, 9% of recurrences occurred after a disease-free interval of five years.[32] There is little evidence to favour one follow-up regimen over another, and this area

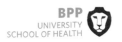

needs further research.[w58] A survey of treatment centres in the UK found varying practices and duration of follow-up.[w59] Chest radiography is the recommended technique for detecting pulmonary metastases and suspicious lesions are further investigated with computed tomography of the chest.[31] Table 6 summarises the follow-up guidelines from the European Society for Medical Oncology.

Contributors: SS planned, researched, co-wrote the article and is guarantor. AHSP co-wrote the article. Damien Grinsell kindly provided images.

AREAS OF ONGOING RESEARCH

- New chemotherapeutic agents: for example, exatecan, a synthetic analogue of topoisomerase I inhibitor (EOTRC study)
- Proton beam therapy: reduces treated volume, enabling a higher radiation dose to be delivered to the tumour and reducing toxicity
- Targeted molecular therapies: drugs that target tumour growth factor pathways and induce apoptosis in tumour cells (for example, Apo2 ligand/TRAIL in osteosarcoma)
- Immunomodulant drugs: looking for tumour antigens to use as vaccines against soft tissue sarcomas

---

ADDITIONAL EDUCATIONAL RESOURCES FOR HEALTHCARE PROFESSIONALS

- National Institute for Health and Clinical Excellence. Improving outcomes for patients with sarcoma. 2006. www.nice.org.uk/csgsarcoma
- National Comprehensive Cancer Network. Clinical practice guidelines in oncology: soft tissue sarcoma. 2008 www.nccn.org/professionals/physician_gls/f_guidelines.asp.
- Badellino F, Toma S. Treatment of soft tissue sarcoma: a European approach. Surg Oncol Clin N Am 2008;17:649-72
- Clark MA, Fisher C, Judson I, Thomas JM. Soft-tissue sarcomas in adults. N Engl J Med 2005;353:701-11

Funding: None.

Competing interests: All authors have completed the Unified Competing Interest form at www.icmje.org/coi_disclosure.pdf (available on request from the corresponding author) and declare: no support from any organisation for the submitted work; no financial relationships with any organisations that might have an interest in the submitted work in the previous three years; no other relationships or activities that could appear to have influenced the submitted work.

Provenance and peer review: Not commissioned; externally peer reviewed.

Patient consent obtained.

1. Rydholm A. Improving the management of soft tissue sarcoma. BMJ 1998;317:93-4.
2. National Institute for Health and Clinical Excellence. Improving outcomes for people with sarcoma. The manual. NICE, 2006.
3. Taylor W St J, Grimer RJ, Carter SR, Tillman RM, Abudu A, Jeys L. "Two-week waits"—are they leading to earlier diagnosis of soft tissue sarcomas? Sarcoma 2010; online 26 September.
4. Pencavel TD, Strauss DC, Thomas GP, Thomas JM, Hayes AJ. Does the two-week rule pathway improve the diagnosis of soft tissue sarcoma? A retrospective review of referral patterns and outcomes over five years in a regional sarcoma centre. Ann R Coll Surg Engl 2010;92:417-21.
5. Canter RJ, Beal S, Borys D, Martinez SR, Bold RJ, Robbins AS. Interaction of histologic subtype and histologic grade in predicting survival for soft-tissue sarcomas 2009. J Am Coll Surg 2010;210:191-8.
6. Wibmer C, Leithner A, Zielonke N, Sperl M, Windhager R. Increasing incidence rates of soft tissue sarcomas? A population-based epidemiologic study and literature review. Ann Oncol 2010;21:1106-11.
7. Kogevinas M, Becher H, Benn T, Bertazzi PA, Boffetta P, Bueno-de-Mesquita HB, et al. Cancer mortality in workers exposed to phenoxy herbicides, chlorophenols, and dioxins. An expanded and updated international cohort study. Am J Epidemiol 1997;145:1061-75.
8. Lawrence W, Donegan WL, Natarajan N, Mettlin C, Beart R, Winchester D. Adult soft tissue sarcomas. A pattern of care survey of the American College of Surgeons. Ann Surg 1987;205:349-59.
9. Hussein R, Smith MA. Soft tissue sarcomas: are current referral guidelines sufficient? Ann R Coll Surg Engl 2005;87:171-3.
10. Demetri GD, Antonia S, Benjamin RS, Bui MM, Conrad EU, DeLaney TF, et al. Soft tissue sarcoma. J Natl Compr Canc Netw 2010;8:630-74.
11. Casali PG, Blay JV; ESMO/CONTICANET/EUROBONET Consensus Panel of Experts. Soft tissue sarcomas: ESMO clinical practice guidelines for diagnosis, treatment and follow-up. Ann Oncol 2010;21:198-203.
12. Grimer R, Judson I, Peake D, Seddon B. Guidelines for the management of soft tissue sarcomas. Sarcoma 2010;506182; online 31 May.
13. Bhangu AA, Beard JAS, Grimer RJ. Should soft tissues sarcomas be treated at a specialist centre? Sarcoma 2004;8:1-6.
14. Lakkaraju A, Sinha R, Garikpati R, Edward S, Robinson P. Ultrasound for initial evaluation and triage of clinically suspicious soft tissue masses. Clin Radiol 2009;64:615-21.
15. Panicek DM, Gatsonis C, Rosenthal DI, Seeger LL, Huvos AG, Moore SG, et al. CT and MR imaging in the local staging of primary malignant musculoskeletal neoplasms: report of the radiology diagnostic group. Radiology 1997;202:237-46.
16. Strauss DC, Qureshi YA, Hayes AJ, Thway K, Fisher C, Thomas JM. The role of core needle biopsy in the diagnosis of suspected soft tissue sarcomas. J Surg Oncol 2010;102:523-9.
17. Rougraff BT, Abouloafia A, Biermann JS, Healey J. Biopsy of soft tissue masses: evidence-based medicine for the musculoskeletal tumor society. Clin Orthop Relat Res 2009;467:2783-91.
18. Coindre JM, Terrier P, Guillou L, Le Doussal V, Collin F, Ranchere D, et al. Predictive value of grade for metastasis development in the main histologic types of adult soft tissue sarcomas: a study of 1240 patients from the French Federation of Cancer Centers Sarcoma Group. Cancer 2001;15:1914-26.
19. Medenhall WN, Indelicato DJ, Scarborough MJ, Zlotecki RA, Gibbs CP, Medenhall NP, et al. The management of adult soft tissue sarcomas. Am J Clin Oncol 2009;32:436-42.
20. Kattan MW, Leing DH, Brennan MF. Post operative nomogram for 12 year sarcoma specific death. J Clin Oncol 2002;20:791-6.
21. Pisters PW, Leung DH, Woodruff J, Shi W, Brennan MF. Analysis of prognostic factors in 1041 patients with localised soft tissue sarcoma of the extremities. J Clin Oncol 1996;14:1679-89.
22. Enneking WF, Spanier SS, Goodman MA. A system for surgical staging of musculoskeletal sarcoma. Clin Orthop Relat Res 2003;415:4-18.
23. Rosenberg SA, Tepper J, Glatstein E, Costa J, Baker A, Brennan M, et al. The treatment of soft-tissue sarcomas of the extremities: prospective randomized evaluations of (1) limb-sparing surgery plus radiation therapy compared with amputation and (2) the role of adjuvant chemotherapy. Ann Surg 1982;196:305-15.
24. Pisters PW, Pollock RE, Lewis VO. Long term results of prospective trial of surgery alone with selective use of radiation for patients with T1 extremity and trunk soft tissue sarcomas. Ann Surg 2007;246:675-81.
25. O'Sullivan B, Davis AM, Turcotte R, Bell R, Catton C, Chabot P, et al. Preoperative versus postoperative radiotherapy in soft tissue sarcoma of the limbs: a randomised trial. Lancet 2002;359:2235-41.
26. Al-Absi E, Farrokhyar F, Sharma R, Whelan K, Corbett TT, Aatel M, et al. A systematic review and meta-analysis of oncologic outcomes of pre versus post operative radiation in localised resectable soft tissue sarcoma. Ann Surg Oncol 2010;17:1367-74.
27. Davis AM, O'Sullivan B, Bell RS, Turcotte R, Catton CN, Wunder JS, et al. Function and health status outcomes in a randomised trial comparing pre-operative and postoperative radiotherapy in extremity soft tissue sarcoma. J Clin Oncol 2002;20: 4472-7.
28. Sarcoma Meta Analysis Collaboration. Adjuvant chemotherapy for localised resectable soft tissue sarcoma of adults: meta-analysis of individual data. Lancet 1997;350:1647-54.
29. Pervaiz N, Colterjohn N, Farrokhyar F, Tozer R, Figueredo A, Ghert M. A systematic meta-analysis of randomised controlled trials of adjuvant chemotherapy for localized resectable soft-tissue sarcoma. Cancer 2008;113:573-81.
30. Woll PJ, van Glabbeke P, Hohenberger A, Le Cesne A, Gronchi A, Hoekstra HJ. Adjuvant chemotherapy with doxorubicin and ifosfamide in resected soft tissue sarcoma: interim analysis of a randomised phase III trial. J Clin Oncol 2007;25:18(s).
31. Gortzak E, Azzarelli A, Buesa J. Bramwell VHC, van Coevorden F, van Geel AN, et al. EORTC. Soft tissue bone sarcoma group and the National Cancer Institute of Canada Clinical Trials Group/Canadian Sarcoma Group. A randomised phase II study on neoadjuvant chemotherapy for "high risk" adult soft tissue sarcoma. Eur J Cancer 2001;37:1096-103.
32. Stojadinovic A, Leung DHV, Allen P, Lewis JJ, Jacques DP, Brennan MF. Primary adult soft tissue sarcoma: time dependent influence of prognostic variables. J Clin Oncol 2002;20:4344-52.

Related links

bmj.com/archive

Previous articles in this series
- Recent advances in the management of rheumatoid arthritis (2010;341:c6942)
- Investigating and managing chronic scrotal pain (2010;341:c6716)
- Commentary: managing oesophageal cancer in a resource poor setting—a Malawian example
- Oesophageal cancer (2010;341:6280)

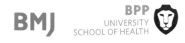
Preservation of fertility in adults and children diagnosed with cancer

Roger Hart associate professor of reproductive medicine[1] medical director[2]

[1]School of Women's and Infants' Health, University of Western Australia, Perth, WA 6008, Australia

[2]Fertility Specialists of Western Australia, Perth, WA 6010

roger.hart@uwa.edu.au

Cite this as: *BMJ* 2008;337:a2045

‹DOI› 10.1136/bmj.a2045
http://www.bmj.com/content/337/bmj.a2045

In the United Kingdom each year 11 000 patients aged 15-40 years are diagnosed with cancer, and more than half of them will live for more than five years.[1] [2] Patients want quality of life, including the ability to have a family, and many request advice on fertility preservation. This review describes the fertility preservation techniques available and recent recommendations from the UK and the United States.[3] [4] [5]

Why should oncology patients consider fertility preservation?

Chemotherapy and radiotherapy reduce the number of germ cells within the ovary and decrease testicular spermatogenesis; this reduction is related to the dose, agent used, and age at treatment. In addition, patients are at risk of permanent gonadal failure.[3] [4] The persistence of menstrual cycles after treatment does not preclude ovarian damage, and the preservation of testosterone production does not confirm the preservation of spermatogenesis.

Who should be referred to discuss fertility preservation options?

UK and American Society of Clinical Oncology (ASCO) guidelines recommend that the implications of oncological treatment for fertility are discussed with patients.[3] [5] The need to refer for fertility advice will depend on the patient's age, disease, prognosis, and time interval before treatment. Many patients seek advice from their general practitioner, oncologist, and allied health professionals, but evidence from several observational studies indicates that many do not receive adequate informed advice.[6]

What options are available for men?

As a result of the systemic effects of cancer, semen quality is often poor, and azoospermia is often present in Hodgkin's lymphoma and testicular cancer before chemotherapy.[4] The sperm count is lowest in the six months after treatment and may need two years to recover.[7] The risk of producing chromosomally abnormal sperm is highest in the few weeks after completion of chemotherapy,[7] so men should wait six months before conception is attempted. Hormonal suppression has not been shown to help reduce testicular damage caused by chemotherapy.[3]

Men and adolescent boys preparing for chemotherapy should be offered semen cryostorage, which has been shown to be effective in many small observational studies[8] [9] [10] and is recommended by the National Institute for Health and Clinical Excellence (NICE) and ASCO.[3] [5] Large prospective studies have found no increase in abnormalities for children born after semen cryopreservation,[11] [12] although sperm that have been frozen may be less effective in assisted reproduction.[13]

It is difficult to discuss the production of semen samples with adolescent boys and we have no reliable method to determine if they are able to produce a sample. Anecdotal evidence suggests that for boys who are unable to ejaculate, taking a urine sample after masturbation may help isolate some sperm.[14]

What options are available for women?

Women in a committed relationship

After chemotherapy the ovary is at risk of permanent gonadal failure,[4] and sensitivity to chemotherapy increases with age. Exposing the ovary to gonadotoxic agents accelerates the age related decline in oocyte number. Women treated with chemotherapy may have premature ovarian failure and may experience the systemic effects of oestrogen deficiency; including osteoporosis, and the psychological impact of a premature menopause, according to the agents used and the duration of treatment.

If sufficient time exists before the woman starts chemotherapy or radiotherapy, she could undergo in vitro fertilisation (IVF) to cryopreserve embryos, providing she has a normal platelet count and can tolerate the anaesthesia needed for oocyte retrieval. As with any IVF cycle, too few oocytes may be collected or the cycle may have to be cancelled because of the risk of hyperstimulation syndrome. This is always distressing, but if this is the woman's only chance of preserving her fertility, it is devastating. Any resulting embryos will be cryopreserved and when required single embryos can be thawed and replaced in the uterus. However, only about 15% of thawed embryos result in a live birth.[15]

Is IVF safe in women with oestrogen receptor positive breast cancer?

In women with oestrogen receptor positive breast cancer, the raised oestrogen concentrations generated by IVF could accelerate the disease process,[4] although this has yet to be confirmed by prospective studies.[16] Performing ovarian stimulation with concurrent administration of an aromatase inhibitor or tamoxifen may temper this effect. This approach

SUMMARY POINTS

- Warn patients of the possible effects that treatment may have on their reproductive capacity
- Provide access to a fertility specialist and supportive counselling
- Sperm banking is an effective and well established technique for adolescent boys and men
- Women should be offered access to oocyte or embryo freezing if sufficient time is available before treatment begins
- Oocyte cryostorage has limited success and freezing of ovarian tissue is still experimental

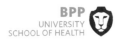

was used in a study of more than 100 patients who were prospectively compared with patients not undergoing fertility preservation. It did not interfere with the IVF cycle and recurrence was not increased.[17] [18] A technique that avoids ovarian stimulation—whereby immature oocytes are collected and matured by in vitro maturation—has been used successfully in some women with polycystic ovary syndrome.[19] This technique might be useful in women with oestrogen receptor positive breast cancer.

After diagnosis women are generally advised not to try to conceive for up to five years[4] because they are taking adjuvant hormonal therapy, although observational evidence derived from large cohorts suggests that conceiving within two years of treatment does not influence survival.[20] [21]

Several retrospective studies and one recent randomised controlled trial of 80 patients showed that suppressing ovarian activity—with a gonadotrophin hormone releasing agonist, for up to six months concurrent with chemotherapy helped preserve ovarian function—although the evidence was not conclusive.[3] [22] [23] [24]

What options are available for single women?

Freezing oocytes

Single women, or women not in a stable relationship, cannot usually cryopreserve embryos because they must be sure that a partner would give permission for their future use. Such women can start an IVF cycle and freeze any oocytes collected, without having them fertilised. However, systematic reviews show that, despite advances in freezing techniques, for each oocyte retrieved the chance of a live birth is only 3-5%.[25] [26] Expert consensus is that this technique is developmental and should not be considered routine; consequently, it is not funded by the NHS.[3] [4]

Alternative strategies for single women, women with insufficient time for embryo cryopreservation, or women who are unable to countenance the further emotional or financial burden of IVF at this difficult time include freezing ovarian tissue or adopting a "wait and see" policy and relying on receiving donated oocytes if unable to conceive in the future.

Oocyte donation

Oocyte donation is a well established form of assisted reproduction—20% of embryos replaced result in a live birth (data derived from national registries).[15] Small observational studies show that both parents bond as well with their child as those couples who conceive spontaneously.[27]

Harvesting and freezing ovarian tissue

The process of harvesting ovarian tissue is less well established and still at the developmental stage.[4] Ovarian cortex is removed during laparoscopy and cryopreserved for potential reimplantation at a later date. Storage of such tissue in the UK is subject to tissue banking regulations (www.hta.gov.uk), and its availability is therefore very restricted, whereas sperm, eggs, and embryos are stored and used in a licensed centre (Human Fertilisation and Embryology Authority; www.hfea.gov.uk). Because ovarian tissue is harvested by a surgical procedure the patient must be fit for theatre and understand the recognised potential risks.[28] [29] The process of tissue removal and subsequent rapid freezing leads to cortical ischaemia, and in a study of eight women, harvested samples had lost a considerable number of follicles.[30] Few women have had the thawed ovarian tissue reimplanted, and to date this has resulted in only two live births.[31] [32] Furthermore, malignant cells could theoretically be seeded; this is a particular concern in women with haematological malignancies.[33]

What are the effects of pelvic irradiation for women?

Uterine effects

Pelvic irradiation may lead to myometrial fibrosis and poor endometrial development. Small observational studies indicate an increased risk of miscarriage, growth restriction, and premature delivery depending upon the site, dose, and duration of treatment.[34] [35] In one study of 33 infants born to women after abdominal irradiation, 10 weighed less than 2500 g and three died during the perinatal period.[35] Furthermore, the prepubertal uterus is thought to be more vulnerable to radiotherapy than the mature one, so radiotherapy might cause irreparable impairment of uterine growth.[34] [36] [37]

Ovarian failure

Patients undergoing pelvic irradiation should be warned of the gonadotoxic effect of radiation, which accelerates the natural process of ovarian ageing.[3] [4] Radiotherapists can predict the likelihood of ovarian failure by using a modified model of natural oocyte decline.[38] Performing laparoscopic ovarian transposition—by moving the ovary on its vascular pedicle laterally from the incident radiation—can minimise exposure to ionising radiation and reduces incident pelvic radiation, according to the site of treatment and the distance the ovary is moved.[39] Subsequent spontaneous conception may occur, but if IVF is needed the ovaries may require repositioning to enable vaginal access, or the patient may need to undergo laparoscopic egg collection.

What are the effects of cranial irradiation?

Cranial irradiation may initiate hypogonadotrophic hypogonadism. If this occurs, ovulation or spermatogenesis will need to be induced with both exogenous follicle stimulating hormone and luteinising hormone or human chorionic gonadotrophin.

What options are available for children and adolescents?

Children pose a difficult ethical problem because although they may have some insight into the potential effect of their cancer treatment on their fertility, it is usually their parents who are more worried about preserving reproductive function.

The prepubertal testicle is more vulnerable to the cytotoxic effects of chemotherapy than the adult testicle.[7] As described, adolescent boys may be able to store a semen sample, but those who cannot produce one by masturbation may find that penile vibratory stimulation is more successful. Ethical board approval may be needed before considering surgery for testicular extraction of sperm in an adolescent boy. The retrieval of precursors of spermatozoa or spermatogonial stem cells for subsequent reimplantation or in vitro maturation for use in IVF has not been used in prepubertal boys, although it has been successful in animal models.[7] The production of testosterone by Leydig cells can be preserved after chemotherapy, and in such cases normal pubertal progression would be expected.[7]

The prepubertal and early adolescent ovary is less vulnerable to the effects of chemotherapy and radiotherapy than the mature ovary. None the less, after counselling, girls may be considered for ovarian tissue harvesting—a hospital ethics committee should help with such decisions.[40]

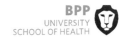
How should a doctor discuss these effects with a patient?

Observational studies indicate that, despite most patients' desire to be informed about the effects of cancer treatment on their fertility,[3] many doctors and family members tend to focus on the immediate treatment of a patient with a life threatening illness,[6] and only a minority of patients receive this advice.[41 42]

The implications of a patient's treatment on their fertility will depend on the patient's age, understanding, the type of cancer, and treatment. Any doctor-patient discussion will be influenced by the wishes of a partner if the patient is in a relationship. The chance of a live birth is substantially better for a woman who freezes embryos than for one who freezes unfertilised eggs. A woman may have to make a difficult decision about the strength of a current relationship as she tries to decide whether to freeze embryos or eggs, set against a background state of distress due to a recent diagnosis of cancer, the threat of chemotherapy and possible menopause. Supportive counselling by a trained fertility counsellor is therefore essential.[3 4]

In the UK, IVF treatment cannot be offered to a couple unless it is in the best interests of the child born from the treatment. Consequently the treating IVF clinician and counselling staff should take a broad view before starting treatment.

Thanks to Martha Hickey for her comments and suggestions in preparing this manuscript.

Competing interests: RH is the medical director and a shareholder of the IVF unit Fertility Specialists of Western Australia.

Provenance and peer review: This review was encouraged but not commissioned; it was externally peer reviewed.

Patient consent obtained.

ONGOING RESEARCH

- Studies are currently investigating the benefit of concurrent treatment with gonadotrophin releasing hormone analogues at the time of chemotherapy
- Techniques of ovarian stimulation that avoid raising oestradiol concentrations in women with breast cancer are being refined
- Surveillance of children born after the technique of in vitro maturation is ongoing
- Refinements to the cryopreservation process aimed at increasing the viability of frozen oocytes are under way
- Women will increasingly be having ovarian tissue reimplanted, and the reporting of outcomes should be encouraged
- Retrieval of tissue from the immature testicle for subsequent reimplantation has been successful in animals and may be developed for future use in boys

---

ADDITIONAL EDUCATIONAL RESOURCES

Resources for healthcare professionals

- Royal College of Physicians, Royal College of Radiologists, Royal College of Obstetricians and Gynaecologists Working Party. *The effects of cancer treatment on reproductive functions. Guidance on management.* www.rcog.org.uk/resources/public/pdf/EffectCancerRepro.pdf
- American Society of Clinical Oncology. *Recommendations on fertility preservation in cancer patients.* http://jco.ascopubs.org/cgi/content/full/24/18/2917
- National Institute for Health and Clinical Excellence. *Fertility: assessment and treatment for people with fertility problems.* 2004. www.nice.org.uk/guidance/index.jsp?action=byID&r=true&o=10936
- Human Fertilisation and Embryology Authority (www.hfea.gov.uk)—The UK's independent regulator overseeing the use of gametes and embryos in fertility treatment and research

Resources for patients

- American Society for Reproductive Medicine. *Patient's fact sheet for fertility preservation.* 2004. www.asrm.org/Patients/FactSheets/cancer.pdf

---

A PATIENT'S PERSPECTIVE

In April 2008, at the age of 32, I was diagnosed with grade 2 invasive ductal carcinoma (oestrogen receptor positive, progesterone receptor positive, and cerbB2 positive). My recommended treatment plan was surgery followed by docetaxel, carboplatin, trastuzumab, adjuvant endocrine therapy, and local radiotherapy. I was warned that the risk of premature ovarian failure was up to 20% and I was referred to Fertility Specialists of Western Australia.

I was due to be married in 2009 and planned to start a family later that year. After counselling, and with my oncologist's consent to postpone the start of chemotherapy, I underwent a cycle of in vitro fertilisation (IVF). Because I had only a few antral follicles on vaginal ultrasound I was not suitable for the technique of in vitro maturation. I was given 112.5 IU of recombinant follicle stimulating hormone together with leuprolide acetate. Oocyte maturity was triggered with recombinant human chorionic gonadotrophin, and the eggs were retrieved on day 12 of the IVF cycle. Thirteen oocytes were retrieved and subsequently inseminated. Seven embryos were frozen for use after completion of the cancer treatment. The next week I started chemotherapy in conjunction with a gonadotrophin releasing hormone analogue.

CK, Perth, Western Australia

1 Office of Cancer Survivorship. *Facts about cancer survivorship.* Bethesda: National Cancer Institute, 2005.
2 Cancer Research UK. *CancerStats key facts all cancers.* 2008. http://info.cancerresearchuk.org/cancerstats/incidence/.
3 Lee SJ, Schover LR, Partridge AH, Patrizio P, Wallace WH, Hagerty K, et al. American Society of Clinical Oncology recommendations on fertility preservation in cancer patients. *J Clin Oncol* 2006;24:2917-31.
4 Royal College of Physicians, Royal College of Radiologists, Royal College of Obstetricians and Gynaecologists. *The effects of cancer treatment on reproductive functions. Guidance on management. Report of a working party.* 2007. www.rcog.org.uk/resources/public/pdf/EffectCancerRepro.pdf.
5 National Institute for Health and Clinical Excellence. *Fertility assessment and treatment for people with fertility problems.* 2004. www.rcog.org.uk/resources/Public/pdf/Fertility_summary.pdf.
6 Quinn GP, Vadaparampil ST, Bell-Ellison BA, Gwede CK, Albrecht TL. Patient-physician communication barriers regarding fertility preservation among newly diagnosed cancer patients. *Soc Sci Med* 2008;66:784-9.
7 Revel A, Revel-Vilk S. Pediatric fertility preservation: is it time to offer testicular tissue cryopreservation? *Mol Cell Endocrinol* 2008;282:143-9.
8 Sanger WG, Olson JH, Sherman JK. Semen cryobanking for men with cancer—criteria change. *Fertil Steril* 1992;58:1024-7.
9 Lass A, Akagbosu F, Brinsden P. Sperm banking and assisted reproduction treatment for couples following cancer treatment of the male partner. *Hum Reprod Update* 2001;7:370-7.
10 Kelleher S, Wishart SM, Liu PY, Turner L, Di Pierro I, Conway AJ, et al. Long-term outcomes of elective human sperm cryostorage. *Hum Reprod* 2001;16:2632-9.
11 Hoy J, Venn A, Halliday J, Kovacs G, Waalwyk K. Perinatal and obstetric outcomes of donor insemination using cryopreserved semen in Victoria, Australia. *Hum Reprod* 1999;14:1760-4.
12 Lansac J, Royere D. Follow-up studies of children born after frozen sperm donation. *Hum Reprod Update* 2001;7:33-7.
13 O'Flaherty C, Vaisheva F, Hales BF, Chan P, Robaire B. Characterization of sperm chromatin quality in testicular cancer and Hodgkin's lymphoma patients prior to chemotherapy. *Hum Reprod* 2008;23:1044-52.
14 Bahadur G, Ling KL, Hart R, Ralph D, Riley V, Wafa R, et al. Semen production in adolescent cancer patients. *Hum Reprod* 2002;17:2654-6.
15 Wang YA Dean JH, Sullivan EA. Assisted reproduction technology in Australia and New Zealand 2005. In: Unit ANPS, ed. *Assisted reproduction technology series no. 11.* Sydney: Australian Institute of Health and Welfare, 2007.
16 Oktay K, Hourvitz A, Sahin G, Oktem O, Safro B, Cil A, et al. Letrozole reduces estrogen and gonadotropin exposure in women with breast cancer undergoing ovarian stimulation before chemotherapy. *J Clin Endocrinol Metab* 2006;91:3885-90.
17 Oktay K, Buyuk E, Libertella N, Akar M, Rosenwaks Z. Fertility preservation in breast cancer patients: a prospective controlled comparison of ovarian stimulation with tamoxifen and letrozole for embryo cryopreservation. *J Clin Oncol* 2005;23:4347-53.
18 Azim AA, Costantini-Ferrando M, Oktay K. Safety of fertility preservation by ovarian stimulation with letrozole and gonadotropins in patients with breast cancer: a prospective controlled study. *J Clin Oncol* 2008;26:2630-5.
19 Reinblatt SL, Buckett W. In vitro maturation for patients with polycystic ovary syndrome. *Semin Reprod Med* 2008;26:121-6.
20 Partridge AH, Ruddy KJ. Fertility and adjuvant treatment in young women with breast cancer. *Breast* 2007;16(suppl 2):S175-81.
21 Ives A, Saunders C, Bulsara M, Semmens J. Pregnancy after breast cancer: population based study. *BMJ* 2007;334:194.
22 Oktay K, Sonmezer M, Oktem O, Fox K, Emons G, Bang H. Absence of conclusive evidence for the safety and efficacy of gonadotropin-releasing hormone analogue treatment in protecting against chemotherapy-induced gonadal injury. *Oncologist* 2007;12:1055-66.
23 Blumenfeld Z, Avivi I, Eckman A, Epelbaum R, Rowe JM, Dann EJ. Gonadotropin-releasing hormone agonist decreases chemotherapy-induced gonadotoxicity and premature ovarian failure in young female patients with Hodgkin lymphoma. *Fertil Steril* 2008;89:166-73.
24 Badawy A, Elnashar A, El-Ashry M, Shahat M. Gonadotropin-releasing hormone agonists for prevention of chemotherapy-induced ovarian

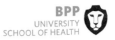

damage: prospective randomized study. *Fertil Steril*2008 Aug 1 Epub ahead of print.

25 Oktay K, Cil AP, Bang H. Efficiency of oocyte cryopreservation: a meta-analysis. *Fertil Steril*2006;86:70-80.

26 Gook DA, Edgar DH. Human oocyte cryopreservation. *Hum Reprod Update*2007;13:591-605.

27 Golombok S, Jadva V, Lycett E, Murray C, Maccallum F. Families created by gamete donation: follow-up at age 2. *Hum Reprod*2005;20:286-93.

28 Hart R, Ruach M, Magos A. Is laparoscopic surgery really worth it? The views of patients, hospital doctors and health care managers. *Gynaecol Endosc*2001;10:289-96.

29 Ahmad G, Duffy JM, Phillips K, Watson A. Laparoscopic entry techniques. *Cochrane Database Syst Rev*2008;(2):CD006583.

30 Newton H, Aubard Y, Rutherford A, Sharma V, Gosden R. Low temperature storage and grafting of human ovarian tissue. *Hum Reprod*1996;11:1487-91.

31 Demeestere I, Simon P, Emiliani S, Delbaere A, Englert Y. Fertility preservation: successful transplantation of cryopreserved ovarian tissue in a young patient previously treated for Hodgkin's disease. *Oncologist*2007;12:1437-42.

32 Donnez J, Dolmans MM, Demylle D, Jadoul P, Pirard C, Squifflet J, et al. Livebirth after orthotopic transplantation of cryopreserved ovarian tissue. *Lancet*2004;364:1405-10.

33 Meirow D, Hardan I, Dor J, Fridman E, Elizur S, Ra'anani H, et al. Searching for evidence of disease and malignant cell contamination in ovarian tissue stored from hematologic cancer patients. *Hum Reprod*2008;23:1007-13.

34 Critchley HO, Wallace WH. Impact of cancer treatment on uterine function. *J Natl Cancer Inst Monogr*2005;34:64-8.

35 Green DM, Fine WE, Li FP. Offspring of patients treated for unilateral Wilms' tumor in childhood. *Cancer*1982;49:2285-8.

36 Holm K, Nysom K, Brocks V, Hertz H, Jacobsen N, Muller J. Ultrasound B-mode changes in the uterus and ovaries and Doppler changes in the uterus after total body irradiation and allogeneic bone marrow transplantation in childhood. *Bone Marrow Transplant*1999;23:259-63.

37 Larsen EC, Schmiegelow K, Rechnitzer C, Loft A, Muller J, Andersen AN. Radiotherapy at a young age reduces uterine volume of childhood cancer survivors. *Acta Obstet Gynecol Scand*2004;83:96-102.

38 Wallace WH, Thomson AB, Saran F, Kelsey TW. Predicting age of ovarian failure after radiation to a field that includes the ovaries. *Int J Radiat Oncol Biol Phys*2005;62:738-44.

39 Hart R, Sawyer E, Magos A. Case report of ovarian transposition and review of literature. *Gynaecol Endosc*1999;8:51-4.

40 Deepinder F, Agarwal A. Technical and ethical challenges of fertility preservation in young cancer patients. *Reprod Biomed Online*2008;16:784-91.

41 Zebrack BJ, Casillas J, Nohr L, Adams H, Zeltzer LK. Fertility issues for young adult survivors of childhood cancer. *Psychooncology*2004;13:689-99.

42 Duffy CM, Allen SM, Clark MA. Discussions regarding reproductive health for young women with breast cancer undergoing chemotherapy. *J Clin Oncol*2005;23:766-73.

BMJ BPP UNIVERSITY SCHOOL OF HEALTH

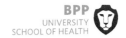

Cancer induced bone pain

Christopher M Kane NIHR academic clinical fellow in palliative medicine[1], Peter Hoskin professor of clinical oncology[2], Michael I Bennett St Gemma's professor of palliative medicine[1]

[1]Academic Unit of Palliative Care, Leeds Institute of Health Sciences, School of Medicine, University of Leeds, Leeds, UK

[2]Mount Vernon Cancer Centre, Northwood, University College London, London, UK

Correspondence to: C M Kane Christopher.Kane@nhs.net

Cite this as: BMJ 2015;350:h315

<DOI> 10.1136/bmj.h315
http://www.bmj.com/content/350/bmj.h315

Bone pain is the most common type of pain from cancer and is present in around one third of patients with bone metastases.[1] [2] Based on postmortem studies of patients with advanced cancer and clinical knowledge of how often bone metastases result in pain, the incidence of cancer induced bone pain is estimated at 30 000 patients in the United Kingdom each year.[3W1] Currently, improvements in cancer treatments mean that many patients are living with metastatic cancer for several years. The prevalence of cancer induced bone pain is therefore likely to be much greater than the annual incidence.[W1] Cancer induced bone pain is considered one of the most difficult pain conditions to treat because of its frequent association with weight bearing and movement. Not surprisingly, it has a major impact on patients' daily functioning and mood and can result in admission to hospital.[W2 W3]

Given the prevalence of cancer induced bone pain, it is likely that clinicians in primary or secondary care will be confronted by patients in pain crises. Recognising and initiating management of this specific pain state, as well as an awareness of the specialist treatments, is important for all clinicians.

What is cancer induced bone pain?

Cancer induced bone pain is a specific pain state with overlapping but distinct features of both inflammatory and neuropathic pain.[4] The most important changes are in bone homeostasis, with corresponding events in the peripheral and central nervous system.[5] In healthy bone, osteoclasts and osteoblasts are highly regulated to maintain balanced resorption and formation of bone respectively, through RANK-ligand (receptor activator of nuclear factor κ). In the presence of a bone metastasis, increased expression of RANK-ligand disrupts this relation leading to increased osteoclast activity and bone destruction. Cancer cells also stimulate local inflammatory mediators and create a highly acidic environment, which sensitises peripheral nerve endings within the bone marrow and bone matrix. When combined with the destruction of nerve endings through cancer invasion, the resulting pain is a mixture of ongoing inflammatory and neuropathic processes, which lead to a hyperexcitability state within the spinal cord. Patients experience this as constant pain, with high sensitivity to movement.[4]

Who gets cancer induced bone pain?

Cancer induced bone pain can occur anywhere that cancer has metastasised to bone. Cancers most often involved are those of the prostate, breast, and lung, as well as myeloma.[3] The most common sites of metastases are vertebrae, pelvis, long bones, and ribs.[3] At postmortem examination, up to 70% of patients who died of cancer will have bone metastases.[3] Bone metastases can be found in a wide range of places (figure). However, not all patients with bone metastases get pain; bone pain was identified in only a third of patients with bone metastases in one

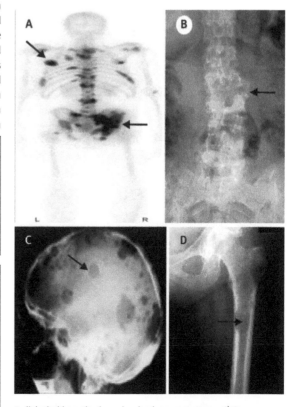

Radiological investigations showing bone metastases. A) Bone scan showing metastatic deposits throughout the skeleton. B) Plain radiography of spine showing lytic vertebral metastasis. C) Plain radiography of a skull showing multiple metastatic deposits. D) Plain radiography showing a lytic lesion of the upper shaft of the left femur

---

SOURCES AND SELECTION CRITERIA

We searched Medline, Clinical Evidence, and the Cochrane Library using the terms "bone metastases", "pain", and "bone pain" and then combined these with the specific treatment terms individually. Where possible we have used systematic reviews but not referenced trials included in these reviews. We limited our search from 1990 to December 2014. We also searched the National Institute for Health and Care Excellence and the Scottish Intercollegiate Guidelines Network. In calculating the numbers needed to treat, we have assumed a conservative placebo response of 25%.

THE BOTTOM LINE

- Cancer induced bone pain is a common problem, which can be extremely debilitating to patients with an already limited life expectancy
- When treating cancer induced bone pain, maintenance of function should be given high priority alongside pain relief
- Early recognition, intervention with functional aids, and behaviour modification, combined with initial titration with analgesia (commonly, strong opioids) are important first steps for non-specialists
- The evidence for early referral for radiotherapy is strong, although bisphosphonates will have an important role for some patients
- Specialist support will be required if pain persists despite initial treatment with behaviour modification, commencement of a non-steroidal anti-inflammatory drug, and initial titration of a strong opioid

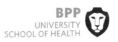

Table 1 Advantages and disadvantages of investigations for bone metastases

Investigation	Advantages	Disadvantages
Plain film radiography	Universal availability; portable films possible, low cost	Low sensitivity: requires >50% cortical destruction to be visible
Computed tomography	More sensitive than plain radiography; best for ribs and pelvic and shoulder girdles; gives information about soft tissue; can be reconstructed in three planes	Access variable outside large hospitals; high cost
Technetium 99m bone scan	Available widely; whole skeleton assessed; intermediate cost	Relatively low sensitivity; reflects osteoblastic activity: non-specific
Magnetic resonance imaging	Optimal images of bone; high sensitivity; detects small metastases before bone damage occurs; optimal for cord compression; gives soft tissue and nerve images; whole body magnetic resonance imaging screens entire skeleton	Access limited; high cost
Fluorodeoxyglucose positron emission tomography	Similar sensitivity to technetium 99m for bone metastases; additional information about other organs	Access limited; high cost; limited specificity: false positives can occur
Fluorine positron emission tomography	Most sensitive detection of bone metastases	Limited experience, evidence, and access; high cost
Choline positron emission tomography	Sensitive for prostate cancer metastases	Access limited but increasing; high cost

large prospective study.[1] It is not yet clear why some bone metastases cause pain and others do not.

What are the clinical features of cancer induced bone pain?

In a cross sectional survey in 2011 patients described their cancer induced bone pain as annoying, gnawing, aching, and nagging.[w4] The pain is commonly a mixture of steady background pain, as well as pain that is exacerbated by weight bearing or movement, called incident or episodic pain.[4] In a recent well conducted European-wide observational study of 1000 patients with cancer, 85.5% reported some form of incident pain episodes.[6] The presence of movement related pain has most impact on function and daily activity.[w4]

Cancer induced bone pain is most commonly experienced in the lower back, pelvis, long bones, and ribs. This can be the presenting feature of the cancer or highlight a recurrence in those previously treated. Therefore in patients with or without active cancer, persistent pain in these areas should alert clinicians to the possibility of bone metastases. Findings on examination are often non-specific with only some tenderness over the site of metastasis or pain specifically related to movement.

A bony metastasis can weaken bone sufficiently such that an innocuous movement, bump, or fall may result in a pathological fracture. Vertebral pain should always alert clinicians to the risk of spinal cord compression, especially in the presence of sensory disturbance, generalised leg weakness, or changes in bladder or bowel function. Even without "red flag" signs, a full neurological examination should be done in these patients, with a low threshold for a spinal magnetic resonance scan.[7] Even if suspicion is low, advice should be sought from the patient's oncologist; retrospective cohort studies have shown that being able to walk at the time of diagnosis of spinal cord compression is correlated with overall survival and the ability to walk after treatment. Early diagnosis and treatment of impending spinal cord compression can drastically improve quality of life for patients.[8][9]

Table 1 outlines the advantages and disadvantages of the various investigations for suspected cancer induced bone pain. Generalists may consider plain film radiography or computed tomography as initial investigations; other investigations are usually undertaken by specialists.

How is cancer induced bone pain initially managed?

The first steps in management are simple measures that can be initiated in non-specialist care, while referral for specialist treatments such as radiotherapy or bisphosphonates is awaited. In the following section we describe the evidence for each treatment that is commonly used for cancer induced bone pain. Consider specialist referral in any patient where pain persists despite these initial steps, those with rapidly increasing pain despite treatment or evidence of toxicity from opioids, and where pathological fracture or spinal cord compression are suspected.

Non-drug interventions

Important aspects of managing cancer induced bone pain are to support patient self management and encourage the use of non-drug measures. An observational study of 1000 European patients with cancer showed that in those who had pain on movement, many of whom had bone metastasis, 43% found consistent pain relief with non-drug measures, often reported as either rest or sleep.[6] Discussing behaviour modifications, such as avoiding strenuous movement, and referring patients for any appropriate movement aids (walking stick, Zimmer frame) or home adaptations (bath rails) can make important contributions to the maintenance of function and quality of life.

World Health Organization pain ladder

For cancer pain in general, the mainstay of treatment has been the World Health Organization's method for the relief of cancer pain, commonly known as the analgesic ladder.[10] Observational studies have shown that about 73% of patients achieved adequate analgesia by following these guidelines, leaving an important minority of patients with inadequately controlled pain despite receiving strong opioids.[11][12]

The first step of the WHO ladder is non-opioid analgesics, such as paracetamol and non-steroidal anti-inflammatory drugs. Although some patients find over the counter analgesics helpful, several systematic reviews that have examined the effectiveness of paracetamol for cancer pain showed that although it was well tolerated there was no significant benefit particularly when added to strong opioids.[13][14] Non-steroidal anti-inflammatory drugs are often perceived to be more efficacious in cancer induced bone pain than in other pain states, and this is a reasonable assumption given the major inflammatory component. However, a well conducted systematic review in 2012 showed

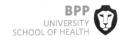
some benefit from adding non-steroidal anti-inflammatory drugs to strong opioids for cancer pain, although this evidence is limited and weak.[13] There are well reported concerns regarding adverse effects of non-steroidal anti-inflammatory drugs; however, this systematic review failed to show any additional harm of adding a non-steroidal anti-inflammatory drug to a strong opioid.[13] The studies did not perform subgroup analysis on cancer induced bone pain. Therefore the assertion that non-steroidal anti-inflammatory drugs are specifically beneficial in cancer induced bone pain cannot be supported.

The next step in the WHO ladder is the use of weak opioids, although a systematic review has only shown marginal benefits of tramadol and codeine in cancer pain, with significant nausea and vomiting associated with tramadol compared with placebo or when added to fentanyl. The authors in these studies did not report the specific proportion of patients with bone metastases.[w5] Therefore it is common to miss this step and start low dose strong opioids if non-opioid analgesia is ineffective.

Strong opioids

Strong opioids are the mainstay of treatment for background pain in patients with cancer induced bone pain. In the United Kingdom, the National Institute for Health and Care Excellence has published extensive guidance on initiating and managing strong opioids in palliative care.[15] This guidance is not specific to cancer induced bone pain, but the principles are directly relevant. Several relatively small randomised controlled trials found no difference between immediate release and sustained release morphine in terms of efficacy or side effects when treatment with opioids was initiated. Therefore this decision should be based on patient and clinician consensus.[16 w6-7]

Several different preparations and types of strong opioid are available. A network meta-analysis showed no important differences in efficacy between morphine and other strong opioids.[17] Based on one well conducted randomised controlled trial, about 75% of patients will achieve good pain control with strong opioids, resulting in a number needed to treat of 2.[18] Within this study, however, there was no subgroup analysis for cancer induced bone pain. Table 2 provides a summary of the numbers needed to treat for various treatments for cancer induced bone pain.

In the United Kingdom, morphine is recommended by NICE as the preferred opioid treatment in patients who can take oral drugs. When morphine was compared with oxycodone no difference was found in pain intensity or adverse effects.[17 18]

Transdermal opioids (fentanyl or buprenophine) are likely to be less constipating than morphine or oxycodone.[17] Specialist advice should be sought if pain control is inadequate after the initial titration of opioid analgesia, or treatment fails.[17]

Management of incident pain is less satisfactory. This is because pain manifests within five minutes, is often movement related, and subsides within 15 minutes in about half of patients with cancer induced bone pain.[w4]

Timing drug treatment to coincide with this pain profile is challenging.

A meta-analysis of fast acting fentanyl preparations found them to be statistically superior over oral morphine in the treatment of incident pain.[19] When compared with oral morphine, however, the numbers needed to treat at 10 and 15 minutes after the drugs have been administered are 18 and 12, respectively.[20] This means that of 12 patients treated with fast acting fentanyl, only one would have gained benefit after 15 minutes of treatment that would not have done so had they been treated with morphine.[20] Given the additional cost of these preparations, current advice is to use immediate release morphine preparations as the preferred treatment and to try a fast acting fentanyl preparation if this treatment fails. Adverse events are difficult to quantify in these studies as patients are already taking regular background opioids. Constipation is a common side effect of opioid treatment and a laxative should be prescribed at the time treatment is started.[17]

WHAT TO DISCUSS WITH PATIENTS WHO ARE STARTING STRONG OPIOIDS

- Address concerns about addiction, tolerance, and side effects, being clear that prescription of strong opioids does not mean patients are in the last stage of life
- Give verbal and written advice on when and how to take opioids for both background and breakthrough pain
- Explain how long the pain relief should last and that patients' ability to drive may be impaired during initiation of treatment or when doses are increased
- Give advice on signs of toxicity, such as drowsiness, twitching, and hallucinations, and who to contact if any occur out of hours
- Provide drugs at the start of treatment, to deal with side effects such as constipation
- Offer regular review

Adapted from NICE clinical guideline 140 (http://guidance.nice.org.uk/CG140)

Other drug interventions

Adjuvant drugs such as antidepressants and anticonvulsants may enhance analgesia from strong opioids and can target neuropathic pain mechanisms. A systematic review in 2011 examined the efficacy of these drugs for the treatment of cancer pain when added to opioids. A modest reduction in pain scores was found in patients with a neuropathic element to their pain, but more adverse effects were reported. Benefit was seen within 4-8 days and did not improve beyond this. These conclusions are limited owing to the quality of the studies included in the review.[21] Although animal studies have suggested that gabapentin can have an important analgesic effect in cancer induced bone pain, there is no evidence confirming the efficacy of this class of drugs in humans.[w8]

Currently there is no evidence to support the use of steroids for cancer induced bone pain; two randomised controlled studies have shown no sustained benefit for cancer pain.[22 23]

Table 2 Numbers needed to treat values for a meaningful clinical response* for various treatments in cancer induced bone pain

Intervention	Numbers needed to treat
Strong opioids for background pain	2
Fast acting fentanyl for incident pain (at 15 mins)	12
Radiotherapy (meaningful response)	2.8
Bisphosphonates (at 12 weeks)	7

*Defined as either 30% or 50% reduction in pain scores or an outcome of partial or complete response.

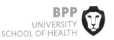

Lidocaine (lignocaine) patches are not absorbed systemically and evidence to support their use for cancer induced bone pain is lacking.[w9][w10]

What further treatment options are available?
Once initial treatment has been started, further treatment options are available to maintain function and quality of life.

Radiotherapy
Radiotherapy has been shown to reduce pain significantly and is the most effective treatment that is specific for cancer induced bone pain. Therefore patients with confirmed cancer induced bone pain should be referred to a clinical oncologist as soon as possible. A well conducted systematic review comparing single dose radiotherapy with multiple doses found no important differences between treatments. Both approaches resulted in a meaningful improvement in pain for about 60% of patients (number needed to treat 2.8).[24][25] Within this group it was reported that approximately 25% would be pain-free. This means that a single dose of radiotherapy can be effective and without major burden for even very frail patients.

In a well conducted randomised trial of 850 patients, where most had had an initial response to radiotherapy but recurrence of pain, 28% experienced a further overall pain response at two months after re-irradiation. This was also associated with improved quality of life.[26][27]

Radioisotopes
Referral to oncology also provides the opportunity to review hormonal treatment and chemotherapy, as well as to consider radioisotope treatment. Some evidence, largely from studies in prostate cancer, indicates that radioisotopes may provide complete reduction in pain over one to six months, with no increase in analgesic use, but severe adverse effects (leucocytopenia and thrombocytopenia) are common.[w11]

Bisphosphonates
Bisphosphonates such as pamidronate and zoledronate are used to reduce both pain and skeletal events in patients with bone metastases. They act by inhibiting osteoclast function. Globally they are used to prevent skeletal related events and reduce pain in breast, prostate, and lung cancer as well as multiple myeloma. In the United Kingdom NICE only recommends early treatment with bisphosphonates for bone pain associated with breast cancer.[28] NICE advise it can be used in lung and prostate cancer once palliative measures and radiotherapy have been given. Several well conducted randomised controlled trials have shown a persistent reduction in pain scores over years with bisphosphonates in patients with breast cancer, and although pain scores increase over time in studies in prostate cancer there is still a significant difference in favour of bisphosphonate compared with placebo.[29] In a large well conducted randomised controlled trial in which patients with bone pain from prostate cancer were randomised to a single infusion of 6 mg of the bisphosphonate ibandronate or a single 8Gy fraction of radiotherapy, overall response rates at four weeks were 49% and 53%, respectively. This non-significant difference was also similar at 12 weeks.[30] This suggests that radiotherapy and bisphosphonates are equally appropriate and effective interventions.

A Cochrane review from 2002 examined the effects of bisphosphonates on cancer induced bone pain and calculated numbers needed to treat of 11 at four weeks after infusion and 7 at 12 weeks after infusion.[31] This review concluded that although evidence supports the use of bisphosphonates they should not be considered as first line management, which is in keeping with the advice from NICE.[31] In patients with cancer induced bone pain from myeloma, a Cochrane review showed benefit from bisphosphonates in pain management.[32]

Denosumab
Denosumab is a novel agent that specifically inhibits RANK-ligand. Clinical trials have shown important benefits in reducing skeletal related events. One randomised controlled trial recruited patients with breast cancer with mild levels of pain. The median time for moderate or severe pain to develop in those receiving denosumab was significantly delayed when compared with bisphosphonate zolendronic acid, although there was no difference in the use of strong analgesics at the end of the study.[33]

Interventional procedures
If patients have ongoing complex cancer induced bone pain despite receiving opioids, radiotherapy, or bisphosphonates, referral to pain services should be considered. There is good evidence from a randomised controlled trial that implantable intrathecal devices lead to a reduction in pain and increased survival in patients taking high dose opiates for refractory pain.[w12]

Surgery
In patients with a good performance status, prophylactic surgery may be considered for relief of cancer induced bone pain. One randomised controlled trial showed that percutaneous stabilisation in the long bones of leg can significantly reduce pain.[w13] Once a pathological fracture has occurred, however, orthopaedic intervention can stabilise the fracture.

Complementary therapies
Complementary therapies may be considered, but as yet they are supported by weak evidence. A Cochrane systematic review of acupuncture acknowledged that there were studies showing benefit in cancer pain, but that evidence was insufficient to recommend this as a treatment.[w14] Evidence was also insufficient to support TENS (transcutaneous electrical nerve stimulation), but one small feasibility randomised controlled trial in patients with cancer induced bone pain suggests that verbal rating scores of pain on movement are reduced with active TENS

> **QUESTIONS FOR FUTURE RESEARCH**
> - Why do some bone metastases cause pain and others do not?
> - What are the disease processes that are responsible for some bone metastases causing pain and others not, and are there any associations with cancer type?
> - Are there specific phenotypes of cancer bone pain that might predict response to analgesia?
> - What is the contribution of spinal hyperexcitability in the experience of bone pain, and how best can this be identified and managed?
> - What non-drug treatments may offer patients benefit in managing movement related pain?

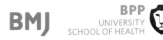

TIPS FOR NON-SPECIALISTS

- The focus of management should be maintenance of function
- Non-steroidal anti-inflammatory drugs may be helpful for some patients but most will require strong opioids
- Early referral for single fraction radiotherapy should be sought, even in relatively frail patients
- Referral for treatment with bisphosphonates can be helpful for some patients
- Consider early referral to specialist services in patients with refractory pain despite initial measures

A PATIENT'S PERSPECTIVE

I was diagnosed with cancer on my wedding anniversary a year ago. I developed back pain, which felt exactly the same as sciatica; however, it wasn't getting any better. One Saturday it became so unbearable that I went to A and E and they diagnosed a water infection and sent me home with antibiotics. I saw my general practitioner and he sent me back to A and E where they did a scan and told me my kidney looked slightly inflamed. They said it would settle down in a few days with antibiotics. They called me back a few days later to tell me they'd found cancer in the bones in my back and my pelvis on the scan I'd had.

Since then the pain has been bad but it's the things that it stops me from doing that I get upset about. I can't swim or walk anymore and it really wears you down. It's affected my marriage so we now sleep in separate beds.

I've really appreciated the doctors' help but they don't understand that I don't just want to lie in bed all day, because the tablets have made me sleepy. I want to be able to do things and this is so important to me. I'd really like doctors to think about trying to make sure I'm able to do things still rather than just giving me tablets.

ADDITIONAL EDUCATIONAL RESOURCES

Resources for healthcare professionals

- National Comprehensive Cancer Network (www.nccn.org)—Provides guidelines for the management of adult cancer pain and treatment of specific cancers (free with registration)
- European Society for Medical oncology (www.esmo.org)—Guidelines for pain management in cancer with access to a smartphone app
- National Institute for Health and Care Excellence (www.nice.org.uk)—Evidence based guidance for specific treatments and an online treatment algorithm for initiating strong opioids and managing side effects

Resources for patients

- Macmillan Cancer Support (www.macmillan.org.uk)—Provides information and help on cancer and the management of symptoms, including bone pain; provides links to local support groups in the United Kingdom
- Cancer Research UK (www.cancerresearchuk.org)—Contains information about cancer and the management of specific symptoms such as pain and includes a forum for patients to discuss their illness
- American Cancer Society (www.cancer.org)—Has general information about bone metastases, and enables patients to search for local support services in the United States

compared with sham TENS.[34][w15] Patients may appreciate non-drug measures that they can manage themselves and so TENS may be of value.

Contributors: CK conceived, drafted, and revised the paper and interviewed a patient to develop the patient's story. PH revised the paper and provided tables and images for inclusion. MIB conceived and revised the paper and calculated the numbers needed to treat. All authors approved the final manuscript. MIB is the guarantor.

Competing interests: We have read and understood the BMJ policy on declaration of interests and declare the following interests: none.

Provenance and peer review: Not commissioned; externally peer reviewed.

1   Grond S, Zech D, Diefenbach C, Radbruch L, Lehmann KA Assessment of cancer pain: a prospective evaluation in 2266 cancer patients referred to a pain service. Pain1996;64:107-14.
2   Caraceni A, Portenoy RK. An international survey of cancer pain characteristics and syndromes. IASP Task Force on Cancer Pain. International Association for the Study of Pain. Pain1999;82:263-74.
3   Coleman RE. Clinical features of metastatic bone disease and risk of skeletal morbidity. Clin Cancer Res2006;12(20 Pt 2):6243s-49s.
4   Falk S, Dickenson AH. Pain and nociception: mechanisms of cancer-induced bone pain. J Clin Oncol2014;32:1647-54.
5   Middlemiss T, Laird BJ, Fallon MT. Mechanisms of cancer-induced bone pain. Clin Oncol2011;23:387-92.
6   Davies A, Buchanan A, Zeppetella G, Porta-Sales J, Likar R, Weismayr W, et al. Breakthrough cancer pain: an observational study of 1000 European oncology patients. J Pain Symptom Manage2013;46:619-28.
7   White BD, Stirling AJ, Paterson E, Asquith-Coe K, Melder A. Diagnosis and management of patients at risk of or with metastatic spinal cord compression: summary of NICE guidance. BMJ2008;337:a2538.
8   Chaichana KL, Woodworth GF, Sciubba DM, McGirt MJ, Witham TJ, Bydon A, et al Predictors of ambulatory function after decompressive surgery for metastatic epidural spinal cord compression. Neurosurgery2008;62:683-92; discussion 83-92.
9   Brown PD, Stafford SL, Schild SE, Martenson JA, Schiff D. Metastatic spinal cord compression in patients with colorectal cancer. J Neuro-oncol1999;44:175-80.
10   World Health Organization. Cancer pain relief. 2nd ed. WHO, 1996. http://whqlibdoc.who.int/publications/9241544821.pdf.
11   Zech DF, Grond S, Lynch J, Hertel D, Lehmann KA. Validation of World Health Organization guidelines for cancer pain relief: a 10-year prospective study. Pain1995;63:65-76.
12   Bennet MI. What evidence do we have that the WHO analgesic ladder is effective in cancer pain? In: McQuay HJ, Moore R, Kalso E, eds. Systematic reviews in pain research; methodology refined. IASP Press, 2008.
13   Nabal M, Librada S, Redondo MJ, Pigni A, Brunelli C, Caraceni A. The role of paracetamol and nonsteroidal anti-inflammatory drugs in addition to WHO Step III opioids in the control of pain in advanced cancer. A systematic review of the literature. Palliat Med2012;26:305-12.
14   McNicol E, Strassels SA, Goudas L, Lau J, Carr DB. NSAIDS or paracetamol, alone or combined with opioids, for cancer pain. Cochrane Database Syst Rev2005;1:CD005180.
15   Bennett MI, Graham J, Schmidt-Hansen M, Prettyjohns M Arnold S. Prescribing strong opioids for pain in adult palliative care: summary of NICE guidance. BMJ2012;344:e2806.
16   Klepstad P, Kaasa S, Jystad A, Hval B, Borchgrevink PC. Immediate- or sustained-release morphine for dose finding during start of morphine to cancer patients: a randomized, double-blind trial. Pain2003;101:193-8.
17   National Institute for Health and Care Excellence. Opioids in palliative care. (Glinical guideline 140.) 2012. www.nice.org.uk/cg140.
18   Riley J, Branford R, Droney J, Gretton S, Sato H, Kennett A, et al. Morphine or oxycodone for cancer-related pain? A randomized, open-label, controlled trial. J Pain Sympt Manage2014; published online 26 Jun. doi: 10.1016/j.jpainsymman.2014.05.021.
19   Jandhyala R, Fullarton JR, Bennett MI. Efficacy of rapid-onset oral fentanyl formulations vs. oral morphine for cancer-related breakthrough pain: a meta-analysis of comparative trials. J Pain Sympt Manage2013;46:573-80.
20   Davis MP. Efficacy of rapid-onset oral fentanyl: what does it mean? J Pain Sympt Manage2014;48:e2-3.
21   Bennett MI. Effectiveness of antiepileptic or antidepressant drugs when added to opioids for cancer pain: systematic review. Palliat Med2011;25:553-9.
22   Yennurajalingam S, Frisbee-Hume S, Palmer JL, Delgado-Guay MO, Bull J, Phan AT, et al. Reduction of cancer-related fatigue with dexamethasone: a double-blind, randomized, placebo-controlled trial in patients with advanced cancer. J Clin Oncol2013;31:3076-82.
23   Paulsen O, Klepstad P, Rosland JH, Aass N, Albert E, Fayers P, et al. Efficacy of methylprednisolone on pain, fatigue, and appetite loss in patients with advanced cancer using opioids: a randomized, placebo-controlled, double-blind trial. J Clin Oncol2014;32:3221-8.
24   Dennis K, Makhani L, Zeng L, Lam H, Chow E. Single fraction conventional external beam radiation therapy for bone metastases: a systematic review of randomised controlled trials. Radiother Oncol2013;106:5-14.
25   Chow E, Zeng L, Salvo N, Dennis K, Tsao M, Lutz S. Update on the systematic review of palliative radiotherapy trials for bone metastases. Clin Oncol2012;24:112-24.
26   Chow E, Meyer RM, Chen BE, van der Linden YM, Roos D, Hartsell WF, et al. Impact of reirradiation of painful osseous metastases on quality of life and function: a secondary analysis of the NCIC CTG SC.20 randomized trial. J Clin Oncol2014; published online 27 Oct.
27   Chow E, van der Linden YM, Roos D, Hartsell WF, Hoskin P, Wu JS et al. Single versus multiple fractions of repeat radiation for painful bone metastases: a randomised, controlled, non-inferiority trial. Lancet Oncol 2014;15:164-71.
28   National Institute for Health and Care Excellence Advancerd breast cancer. (Clinical guideline 81.) 2014. www.nice.org.uk/guidance/cg81.
29   Gralow J, Tripathy D. Managing metastatic bone pain: the role of bisphosphonates. J Pain Sympt Manage2007;33:462-72.
30   Hoskin P, Sundar S, Reczko K, Forsyth S, Mithal N, Sizer B et al. A Multicentre Randomised Trial of Ibandronate Compared to Single Dose Radiotherapy for Localised Metastatic Bone Pain in Prostate Cancer (RIB). Eur J Cancer2011;47:6.
31   Wong R, Wiffen PJ. Bisphosphonates for the relief of pain secondary to bone metastases. Cochrane Database Syst Rev2002;2:CD002068.
32   Mhaskar R, Redzepovic J, Wheatley K, Clark OA, Miladinovic B, Glasmacher A, et al. Bisphosphonates in multiple myeloma: a network meta-analysis. Cochrane Database Syst Rev2012;5:CD003188.
33   Stopeck AT, Lipton A, Body JJ, et al. Denosumab compared with zoledronic acid for the treatment of bone metastases in patients with advanced breast cancer: a randomized, double-blind study. J Clin Oncol2010;28:5132-9.

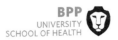

34 Hurlow A, Bennett MI, Robb KA, Johnson MI, Simpson KH, Oxberry SG
    Transcutaneous electric nerve stimulation (TENS) for cancer pain in
    adults. *Cochrane Database Syst Rev*2012;3:CD006276.

Related links

bmj.com/archive
Previous articles in this series
- Managing patients with multimorbidity in primary care (BMJ
  2015;350:h176)
- The prevention and management of rabies (BMJ 2015;350:g7827)
- Heparin induced thrombocytopenia (BMJ 2014;349:g7566)
- The management of chronic breathlessness in patients with
  advanced and terminal illness (BMJ 2015;350:g7617)
- Ebola virus disease (BMJ 2014;349:g7348)

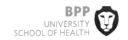

Advances in radiotherapy

Saif S Ahmad specialist registrar in clinical oncology[1], Simon Duke senior house officer in clinical oncology[1], Rajesh Jena consultant clinical oncologist[1], Michael V Williams consultant clinical oncologist[1], Neil G Burnet professor of radiation oncology and honorary consultant clinical oncologist[2]

[1]Clinical Oncology, Cambridge University Hospitals NHS Foundation Trust, Cambridge CB2 0QQ, UK

[2]University of Cambridge, Cambridge

Correspondence to: S S Ahmad saif. ahmad@nhs.net

Cite this as: *BMJ* 2012;345:e7765

‹DOI› 10.1136/bmj.e7765
http://www.bmj.com/content/345/
bmj.e7765

Radiotherapy plays an important role in the care of patients with cancer and forms part of the management of 40% of patients cured of their disease.[1] Advances have been made in the past two decades, as improvements in engineering and computing have enabled technologies such as intensity modulated radiotherapy (IMRT), image guided radiotherapy (IGRT), and stereotactic radiotherapy (SRT) to be used in routine clinical practice.

This article explains newer radiotherapy techniques and aims to enable general practitioners and non-specialist clinicians to advise patients who come to them with questions. It will focus on external beam radiotherapy (EBRT), which is the most common form of treatment, delivered to 125 000 patients a year in England.[2]

How does radiotherapy work?

X rays are a form of electromagnetic radiation that deliver their energy through waves called photons. These photons are produced by accelerating a stream of electrons and colliding them with a metal target. High energy photons produce secondary electrons in human tissue. Electrons cause DNA damage which, if not repaired, proves fatal at cell division. Absorbed radiation doses are measured as joules per kilogram, expressed in the unit gray (Gy).

EBRT is administered using a linear accelerator. These machines are roughly the size of computed tomography (CT) scanners and, for radiation protection purposes, are housed in thick walled bunkers.

EBRT usually uses high energy x rays, which penetrate deep into body tissue while relatively sparing the skin. Electrons can also be used for superficial treatments. These electrons can be derived from most linear accelerators (by removing the metal target) and provide a high dose to a few centimetres depth, with little dose beyond. Electrons are therefore often used to treat skin tumours. Proton beams (discussed later) can also be used for EBRT; the dose builds up to a peak and then falls off steeply with no dose beyond their finite range.

EBRT is normally delivered over multiple sessions (or fractions) to exploit differences in repair and repopulation between tumour cells and normal cells. For example, treatment for prostate and head and neck cancer can extend to 40 fractions over eight weeks. By contrast, in palliative settings, single fraction treatment is common. This is because low doses of radiotherapy can provide tumour control for a short time (range of months) with minimal side effects.

Most EBRT is planned using CT imaging to locate the tumour and provide information on the patient's shape and tissue density. Correlation with diagnostic imaging is essential. The diagnostic imaging modality that provides the best possible information on the position and extent of the tumour is used. For many tumours this will be magnetic resonance imaging (MRI). For some sites such as the brain, computerised image fusion is used alongside the planning CT scan to improve the accuracy of tumour localisation. Positron emission tomography-CT can aid radiotherapy planning for lung cancers and lymphoma by showing which anatomical areas contain tumour. Over the past 20 years, techniques that can align treatment more closely to the tumour have been developed. This approach is known as three dimensional conformal radiotherapy (3D-CRT), and it enables oncologists to spare more healthy tissue and reduce toxicity.[3] IMRT represents a further development of this concept and will be discussed later.

Who needs radiotherapy?

A systematic review of national and international guidelines linked to detailed information on cancer incidence and stage estimated that 52% of patients with cancer should receive radiotherapy at some time during their illness, either for cure or palliation.[4] The authors developed an optimal radiotherapy utilisation tree for each cancer based on indications for radiotherapy taken from evidence based treatment guidelines and correlated this with epidemiological data.

In the curative setting, radical radiotherapy can be offered as the sole treatment. It can also be used with surgery, being given before (neoadjuvant) or after resection (adjuvant) (table).

Palliative radiotherapy plays a vital role in cancer care. A systematic review of 25 randomised controlled trials showed that it can reduce or eliminate pain from bone metastases in 60% of cases.[5] Radiotherapy can also be used to palliate brain metastases, spinal cord compression, compressive symptoms from visceral metastases, and uncontrolled bleeding—for example, haemoptysis or haematuria.

SOURCES AND SELECTION CRITERIA

This article is an evidence based review of clinical radiotherapy. We searched PubMed and the Cochrane databases between 1990 and 2012 using the search terms radiotherapy, intensity modulated radiotherapy, image guided radiotherapy, stereotactic radiotherapy, and proton beam therapy to identify observational studies, randomised trials, meta-analyses, and systematic reviews.

SUMMARY POINTS

- Radiotherapy forms part of the management of 40% of patients who are cured of cancer
- Advances in technology mean that more patients now receive efficacious treatment with less toxicity
- Newer technologies are increasingly available in the UK
- These technologies include intensity modulated radiotherapy, image guided radiotherapy, stereotactic radiotherapy, stereotactic ablative radiotherapy, and proton beam therapy
- Toxicity can develop early or late, and non-specialist clinicians should be aware of the more common side effects, which typically relate to the anatomical site treated

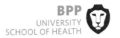

Common indications for radiotherapy

Cancer	Role of radiotherapy	Example of indication	Comments	Outcomes
Breast	Adjuvant treatment	Early stage after wide local excisions	In selected cases may be given intraoperatively (mature data awaited)[w1]	Reduces first recurrence at 10 years (from 35.0% to 19.3%); reduces 15 year absolute risk of death from breast cancer by 3.8% (from 25.2% to 21.4%) compared with no radiotherapy[w2]
		High risk mastectomy patients		Reduces local recurrence at 5 years (from 23% to 6%) and reduces 15 year absolute risk of death from breast cancer by 5.4% (from 60.1% to 54.7%) compared with no radiotherapy[w2]
				After breast radiotherapy the hazard ratio for death from heart disease is 1.27 and lung cancer 1.78 compared with no radiotherapy (overall mortality still reduced)[w3]
Prostate	Primary treatment	Early stage	Radiotherapy alone (brachytherapy in some cases) as a treatment option rather than surveillance or surgery	Similar outcomes to surgery[w4]; 93% prostate specific antigen control with brachytherapy at 7 years in low risk disease[w5]
		Locally advanced	EBRT is often used in combination with androgen deprivation therapy	74.1% and 71.4% prostate specific antigen control and overall survival, respectively, at 10 years for inoperable tumours[w6]
Lung	Primary treatment	Locally advanced tumours or comorbidity	Optimal outcomes using CHART or chemoradiation; radical high dose treatment for small tumours	Concurrent chemoradiation improves 2 year survival by 8% compared with radiotherapy alone[w7]; CHART improves 2 year survival from 20% to 29% compared with conventional radiotherapy[w8]
	Stereotactic ablative radiotherapy	Medically inoperable tumours		Mature outcome data awaited
Head and neck	Primary and adjuvant treatment	Can be used in most cancers to aid organ preservation	Often given with cisplatin	5 year survival: 80-90% in stage 1-2 tumours, 60-70% in stage 3-4 tumours[w9]
Rectum	Neoadjuvant treatment	To downstage bulky tumours at risk of involved resection margins	Given as short course (5 days) or long course (5 weeks) treatment	Cochrane review shows improved overall survival (by 2%) and local recurrence rates (heterogeneous across trials) compared with no radiotherapy[w10]
Gynaecological	Primary and adjuvant treatment	Cervical cancer	Primary chemoradiotherapy is standard of care in all but early stage I cervical cancers	Concurrent cisplatin and radiotherapy improves 5 year survival from 60% to 66%[w11]
		Endometrial cancer		Adjuvant EBRT reduces locoregional recurrence from 8.5% to 2.5% compared with surgery alone but has no effect on survival[w12]
Brain	Primary and adjuvant	After debulking surgery	Concurrent temozolamide improves survival	At doses above 60 Gy improves median survival from 18 to 42 weeks compared with surgery alone[w13]

CHART=continuous hyperfractionated accelerated radiotherapy; EBRT=external beam radiotherapy.

What are the side effects?

With the exception of fatigue, toxicity is associated with the anatomical location of the radiotherapy fields. Common side effects are summarised in web table 1 (see bmj.com).[w1-w13] A detailed discussion of the side effects of treatment is outside the aims of this review.

Toxicity can broadly be divided into early and late. Early toxicity is generally reversible, but it must be managed appropriately to avoid unnecessary gaps in treatment. It begins around two weeks into treatment, but symptoms tend to peak at two to four weeks after completion. Late toxicity occurs at least six months after treatment and may present after many years. Unlike early effects, these late effects are often irreversible. A multinational peer reviewed collection of guidelines has been developed that details these risks and their relation to dose. The guidelines are limited by being based on pooled data from individual studies, but if interpreted appropriately during radiotherapy planning this information can help minimise toxicity.[6]

Fatigue occurs in around 80% of patients receiving radiotherapy and tends to peak in the second week, improving around four weeks after completing treatment.[7] A thorough but non-systematic review reported that fatigue persists in a chronic form in about 30% of cases.[7] Patients are advised to remain as active as possible. Exercise programmes may help, but robust data supporting fatigue prevention strategies are lacking.

Other toxicities are specifically associated with the area of the body treated. The skin is commonly affected during treatment for more superficial tumours. Early skin effects include erythema and desquamation, whereas late effects are characterised by atrophy and telangiectasia.

For example, 23% of women who received adjuvant breast radiotherapy within the phase III trial, START B, at a dose of 40 Gy in 15 fractions (current UK standard of care) reported a change in skin appearance of the treated breast at five years.[8]

Pelvic radiotherapy—for indications such as urological, bowel, and gynaecological cancers—is associated with several early and late effects (see web table 1). The likelihood of certain side effects is largely dictated by the dose fractionation schedule, site treated, and any pre-existing comorbidities. Chronic symptoms such as dyspareunia, urinary incontinence, and faecal incontinence can have a serious impact on quality of life. Their management should be coordinated with the treating oncologist, and in some cases further specialist opinions may be needed.[9]

Does radiotherapy increase the risk of subsequent cancer?

The risk of second cancers after radiotherapy increases over the decades after treatment and depends on the treated volume and dose.[10] The risk is particularly relevant for younger patients with a good prognosis. A cohort study of more than 25 000 patients established that patients with stage I seminoma have a relapse rate of 4% but an excess second cancer risk of 6% at 25 years after radiotherapy.[11] Radiotherapy is now rarely used for these patients. For early treatment of breast cancer, the risks are lower. A cohort study of more than 180 000 patients that used the SEER (surveillance, epidemiology, and end results) database found an excess absolute risk of radiotherapy related second breast cancers and other solid cancers (such as lung cancer and sarcoma) of two and four cases per 10 000 person years, respectively.[12] This slight increase in second cancers is insignificant in most cases when compared with the risk of recurrence and death from the primary lesion. Nevertheless, patients must be fully informed because these data might affect their decisions about radiotherapy when alternative treatment are available.

Breast screening by mammography or MRI is an important consideration for people at higher risk of second cancers. A UK based cohort study in young patients who received supradiaphragmatic radiotherapy for Hodgkin's disease found that the risk of breast cancer was similar to that of women with *BRCA* mutations.[13] This was especially true in women who were treated under the age of 20 years. The maximum absolute excess risk of breast cancer occurred at age 50-59 years (87.9 cases/10 000). In the United Kingdom, women given radiotherapy for Hodgkin's lymphoma under the age of 35 years are advised to have annual breast screening starting eight years after treatment. At the age of 50 years, they then join the national breast screening programme (mammography every three years) but, because this is the time of the maximum excess risk, it has been argued that more intensive screening may be needed.[13]

Increased risks of cardiovascular events and stroke are also important, and the evidence has recently been reviewed.[10] A key retrospective study of survivors of Hodgkin's disease showed a relative risk of 3.5 for death from myocardial infarction in patients receiving high dose radiotherapy.[14] The risk varies greatly according to dose and tumour site.[10] However, these findings are largely based on treatments using older techniques and may be overestimates. Smoking cessation and other lifestyle advice should be as standard. Moreover, the additional risk should be considered when using tools for estimating the risk of cardiovascular disease. Similarly, hypothyroidism occurs in almost 50% of patients after radiotherapy for head and neck cancer, necessitating regular thyroid function checks, at least annually, for 10 years or more.[15]

How safe is radiotherapy?

The potentially devastating effects of maladministration reinforce the need to avoid complacency.[16] The risk of death directly caused by radiotherapy errors is estimated at two per million courses in the UK and 15 per million courses in an international systematic review. For comparison, the risk of a crash on a commercial air flight is four per million departures.[17] Within the UK, detailed national checks and procedures are in place to ensure that the right patient receives the right treatment. In developed countries robust error reporting systems are an important learning tool.

Patients often ask if they will be "radioactive," but once the beam is turned off there is no radiation exposure. This makes the treatment environment safe for relatives and staff, although they must vacate the room while the beam is on.

How is radiotherapy initiated?

Once a patient has consented to treatment they will attend a "planning CT scan." Using these images, the precise arrangement of radiotherapy beams for treatment is planned, usually by an oncologist in conjunction with a radiographer and medical physicist. Simpler plans, such as single fraction palliative treatments, can be completed within an hour. More complex ones, such as those using IMRT, may take up to a week to allow for checking and verification of the plan. Each treatment session, or fraction,

takes around 10-20 minutes, including time spent ensuring the patient is correctly positioned on the treatment couch. Patients receiving multiple fractions are usually reviewed, at least weekly, by a doctor to help manage treatment related side effects.

Newly introduced techniques in radiotherapy

IMRT, IGRT, and SRT are newer techniques that should be routinely available for all patients within the appropriate clinical context.

Intensity modulated radiotherapy (IMRT)

IMRT can create concave treatment shapes and steep dose gradients. This maximises the sparing of normal tissues, particularly if the tumour is wrapped around normal structures such as the spinal cord. Conventional radiotherapy typically uses a small number of beams, each with uniform intensity across the field. In contrast, IMRT uses multiple beams with a highly non-uniform dose across the field. This is achieved by dividing the beam into multiple "beamlets," so that doses of varying intensity can be delivered to different parts of the field (figure).

IMRT is particularly useful for head and neck cancers because of the high number of important normal tissue structures within close proximity to the tumour. A phase III study randomised patients with squamous cell cancers of the oropharynx to conventional 3D-CRT or parotid sparing IMRT. It found a significant reduction in dry mouth at two years (29% v 83%; P<0.0001) with IMRT compared with 3D-CRT.[18] A systematic review published in 2010 of the benefits of IMRT identified 61 studies that compared it with conventional radiotherapy.[19] It found similar benefits at many other treatment sites, including reduced rectal toxicity in patients with prostate cancer.

In breast cancer, improved dose distributions in patients with larger breasts decrease the risk of breast pain and improve long term cosmesis. Findings on local control and overall survival were generally inconclusive. However, consequent sparing of normal tissue means that higher and potentially more effective doses could be used without the risk of increased toxicity; this is being investigated in current trials.

IMRT does have disadvantages. A consequence of using multiple beams to deliver radiation is that despite normal tissue being spared higher doses, a greater volume of tissue receives a lower dose. As a result, it has been suggested that IMRT may increase the risk of a second cancer from 1% for conventional radiotherapy to 1.75% at 10 years.[20] It has been counter-argued that these figures are an overestimate and that risks from 3D-CRT and IMRT are similar.[21] Considerable uncertainty surrounds these estimates because they are generated from models of risk that are based on long term data obtained mainly from the follow-up of atomic bomb survivors. These people were exposed to a single whole body dose rather than fractionated high doses to specific parts of the body as used in radiotherapy.[21]

Provision of IMRT is variable worldwide, although availability is generally increasing. For example, a survey of all cancer centres in Canada showed that the proportion of centres offering IMRT rose from 37% to 87% between 2006 and 2010.[22] In the UK, it increased from 46% to 81% between 2007 and 2012.[23] [24] The key indicator for patients is access to this treatment when needed: it has been estimated that about 33% of radically treated patients should receive IMRT.[25] In the United States, 50% of patients receive IMRT,

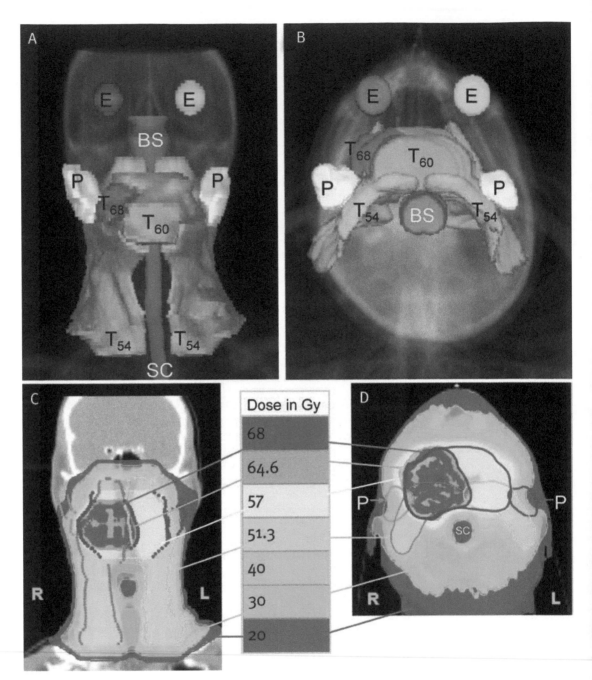

Example of an intensity modulated radiotherapy plan for head and neck cancer. Panels A and B: Target and normal tissue structures are outlined before preparation of the dose plan. The complex three dimensional shapes and anatomical associations can be seen. The tumour target is delineated into three parts, representing different levels of tumour burden. The primary gross tumour itself (T68 red) will receive 68 Gy, the surrounding area with high risk of direct tumour involvement (T60 light brown) will receive 60 Gy, and the nodal areas at risk of microscopic disease (T54 pink) will receive 54 Gy. Some of the important normal structures—the eyes, parotid salivary glands, brain stem, and spinal cord—are also shown. Other structures have been omitted for clarity. Panels C and D: Intensity modulated radiotherapy dose plan. Use of advanced computing techniques allows different doses to be "painted" on to different target areas, while minimising the dose to important structures. The high dose is delivered to the complex target, which is concave posteriorly, avoiding the spinal cord

whereas in the UK this figure is currently 19%.[23] Access in the UK is increasing rapidly and the 33% figure is expected to be reached by 2014.[23]

Despite its importance, there are few cost effectiveness data for IMRT and other newer radiotherapy techniques. A UK study reviewed 13 non-randomised studies in prostate cancer.[26] The authors estimated the additional staff costs of providing IMRT at £1100 (€1370; $1750) per case. Using models of clinical outcome, the authors concluded that if the higher doses possible with IMRT (up to 81 Gy) improve overall survival, then IMRT would be cost effective. At the lower dose of 74 Gy currently recommended by the National Institute for Health and Clinical Excellence, conformal radiotherapy is safe and the cost benefit depends on the size of the reduction in gastrointestinal toxicity that can be achieved by using IMRT rather than conformal treatment. The authors concluded that the size of the benefit and its cost are unclear, which makes cost effectiveness uncertain. Further studies investigating cost effectiveness are needed.

Image guided radiotherapy (IGRT)
All radiotherapy is delivered with imaging at the beginning and intermittently throughout treatment to ensure accuracy. IGRT uses imaging (often on a daily basis) just before radiotherapy is delivered to allow positional correction if necessary so that the dose is correctly delivered to

the target.[27] This can be achieved with CT imaging or by implanting radio-opaque seeds, which allows the target to be identified using treatment x rays. This assures accurate treatment of the tumour and potentially allows smaller safety margins to be used, thereby sparing healthy tissue. The prostate, for example, is subject to a daily positional change of 15 mm or more in relation to bony landmarks; a recent review summarises evidence from the pre-IGRT era showing that this movement contributes to underdosage and reduced control of biochemical disease.[28]

Image guidance is crucial to the use of IMRT because steep dose gradients carry a risk of the target being given too low a dose and normal tissue being overdosed. Most machines that deliver IMRT also have IGRT capabilities, allowing imaging and treatment in a single session.

Lung cancers move with respiration and if this variation is great, four dimensional CT can be used to obtain a series of CT scans at different phases of the respiratory cycle.[28] The information can help define the motion of the tumour, which can then be targeted with respiratory gating. This involves tracking the patient's respiratory cycle, commonly using surface markers, and delivering treatment at specific phases of the cycle.

The provision of IGRT is increasing in the UK, but reliable national data on its availability are not yet available. There is an associated additional cost, but no robust cost effectiveness studies have yet been published.

Stereotactic radiotherapy (SRT)

SRT involves highly targeted treatment. It has been used for many years to treat a variety of brain lesions, using traditional fractionations such as 60 Gy in 30 fractions. More recently it has been used to treat small discrete lesions in a limited number (one to five) of higher dose fractions.[29] SRT is often administered using a frame to fully immobilise the patient, although frameless techniques are also available. Stereotactic radiosurgery refers to SRT delivered in just one session. SRT can be delivered using several different machines. These include specifically adapted standard linear accelerators, which use multiple beams from different angles centred on the tumour, and the Gamma Knife, which is designed exclusively to treat intracranial lesions.

Stereotactic ablative radiotherapy (SABR), also known as stereotactic body radiotherapy, refers to precise irradiation of extracranial lesions. As a result of improvements in image guidance, it is now increasingly offered for sites including the lung, prostate, liver, and pancreas.[30] It can be delivered using a standard linear accelerator, equipped for image guided IMRT. For mobile lesions tracking or gating technology can be used. The CyberKnife is a frameless robotic system consisting of a linear accelerator mounted on a robotic arm. It can deliver treatment with high accuracy and uses real time image guidance to track the tumour. To allow this, most tumours require implantation of metal markers. This can lead to complications, including pneumothorax in lung cancers, but newer software can track some peripheral tumours without markers.[30]

Clinical outcomes for SABR within early phase trials are promising, particularly in the radical treatment of inoperable lung cancers. Trials have shown excellent local control but less of an impact on overall survival.[31] Similar results have been seen for other tumours. Accurate delineation of the tumour is essential, so lesions with unclear or infiltrative margins should be avoided. Because the volume of normal tissue within the periphery of the target is proportional

to the cube of the target's radius, this treatment is most suitable for smaller lesions.

SABR has challenged our approach towards small volume metastatic disease. Selected patients can now be treated with high doses of SABR with the aim of achieving a long disease-free interval.[30] Small phase I-II studies of this technique have reported encouraging short term outcomes. Mature phase III comparisons with surgery, or other modalities, are needed to establish its place within clinical practice.[30]

At present within the UK, SRT and SABR are mainly available only at specialist cancer centres. Consequently, referral pathways are in place that allow patients from peripheral hospitals to be treated centrally. Robust cost effectiveness data are not available.

What is the role of proton beam therapy?

Proton beam therapy is an established technology that uses protons rather than photons to deliver the radiation dose. The physical properties of protons enable the dose to be deposited up to, but not beyond, a specific depth within tissue. When compared with photons, this limited range allows improved target volume coverage, with reduced doses to the normal tissue beyond.[32] [33] This is expected to reduce the risks of late effects, including second cancers and cardiovascular risk, which are particularly relevant when treating children and young adults.[34]

A recent systematic review that summarised the current evidence base for proton beam therapy noted a lack of evidence from randomised phase III trials.[34] Current indications in adults include spinal and base of the skull tumours, although this is based on single institution cohort studies.[35] In the US this treatment is widely used for prostate cancer. Although excellent results can be obtained, the only clinical trials compared different doses given with protons, and there is no evidence from randomised trials that protons improve outcomes compared with photons when given at the same dose.[33]

In the UK, patients suitable for proton beam therapy can now be referred abroad under the NHS Proton Overseas Programme. The government has committed to fund two proton therapy units for children and adults with specific indications. It is intended that clinical provision will be combined with high quality research to help expand the evidence base for this treatment.[36]

What is the future of radiotherapy?

The evolution of radiotherapy will continue, fuelled by improvements in imaging, computing, and engineering, combined with a greater understanding of tumour biology. Radiotherapy trials currently recruiting within the UK are shown in web table 2 (see bmj.com). Ensuring the availability of newly established techniques to patients who would benefit from them poses an important challenge, particularly in the face of economic constraints. It is hoped that more precise delivery of radiotherapy coupled with strategies to enhance tumour cell killing, such as chemoradiation, will enable more cancers to be cured with fewer side effects. As these strategies are developed, it is vital that their implementation is supported by evidence from intelligently designed phase III trials.[37]

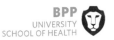

TIPS FOR NON-SPECIALISTS

- The term radiotherapy encompasses a wide range of different techniques. Establish precisely which has been used when discussing treatment and complications with patients
- Newer techniques, such as intensity modulated radiotherapy and image guided radiotherapy, generally reduce toxicity
- Because interruptions in treatment can lead to poorer outcomes in patients receiving curative radiotherapy, manage early toxicity promptly, coordinating with the treating oncologist
- Late toxicity can sometimes occur years after radiotherapy, so determine the details of anticancer treatments in patients with a history of cancer
- Long term effects include an increased risk of second cancer and cardiovascular disease

ADDITIONAL EDUCATIONAL RESOURCES

Resources for healthcare professionals

- Begg AC, Stewart FA, Vens C. Strategies to improve radiotherapy with targeted drugs. *Nat Rev Cancer* 2011;11:239-53. Review of biological basis for combining targeted drugs with radiotherapy
- Bortfeld T, Jeraj R. The physical basis and future of radiation therapy. *Br J Radiol* 2011;84:485-98. Summarises the importance of medical physics within radiotherapy
- Towards safer radiotherapy (https://www.rcr.ac.uk/docs/oncology/pdf/Towards_saferRT_final.pdf)—Report detailing strategies to optimise radiotherapy safety
- The Clinical and Translational Radiotherapy Research Working Group (www.ncri.org.uk/ctrad/)—National programme of collaborative radiotherapy research activity

Resources for patients

- Cancer Research UK (www.cancerresearchuk.org)—Overview of current news stories in cancer and information on active research studies
- Macmillan Cancer Support (www.macmillan.org.uk)—Information on cancer treatments and support networks
- Patient.co.uk (www.patient.co.uk)—Lifestyle and cancer related discussion forums

Thanks to Kate Burton (consultant radiographer at Addenbrooke's Hospital, Cambridge) for help in revising this article.

Contributors: SSA did the literature review, wrote the initial draft, and collated subsequent revisions; SD helped design the figures and tables; RJ developed the IMRT image figure and provided the first review of the text; MVW oversaw all subsequent reviews and contributed to all sections of the text; NB conducted all subsequent reviews, contributed to all sections of the text, and contributed the IMRT image figure. NGB is guarantor

Funding: NGB is supported by the NIHR Cambridge Biomedical Research Centre.

Competing interests: All authors have completed the ICMJE uniform disclosure form at www.icmje.org/coi_disclosure.pdf (available on request from the corresponding author) and declare: no support from any organisation for the submitted work; no financial relationships with any organisations that might have an interest in the submitted work in the previous three years; no other relationships or activities that could appear to have influenced the submitted work.

Provenance and peer review: Not commissioned; externally peer reviewed.

1   Tubiana M. The role of local treatment in the cure of cancer. *Eur J Cancer* 1992;28A:2061-9.
2   Department of Health. Radiotherapy dataset annual report 2009/2010. 2011. www.dh.gov.uk/en/Publicationsandstatistics/Publications/PublicationsPolicyAndGuidance/DH_128357.
3   Dearnaley DP, Khoo VS, Norman AR, Meyer L, Nahum A, Tait D, et al. Comparison of radiation side-effects of conformal and conventional radiotherapy in prostate cancer: a randomised trial. *Lancet* 1999;353:267-72.
4   Delaney G, Jacob S, Featherstone C, Barton M. The role of radiotherapy in cancer treatment: estimating optimal utilization from a review of evidence-based clinical guidelines. *Cancer* 2005;104:1129-37.
5   Chow E, Zeng L, Salvo N, Dennis K, Tsao M, Lutz S. Update on the systematic review of palliative radiotherapy trials for bone metastases. *Clin Oncol (R Coll Radiol)* 2012;24:112-24.
6   Marks LB, Yorke ED, Jackson A, Ten Haken RK, Constine LS, Eisbruch A, et al. Use of normal tissue complication probability models in the clinic. *Int J Radiat Oncol Biol Phys* 2010;76(3 suppl):S10-9.
7   Jereczek-Fossa BA, Marsiglia HR, Orecchia R. Radiotherapy-related fatigue. *Crit Rev Oncol Hematol* 2002;41:317-25.
8   Hopwood P, Haviland JS, Sumo G, Mills J, Bliss JM, Yarnold JR. Comparison of patient-reported breast, arm, and shoulder symptoms and body image after radiotherapy for early breast cancer: 5-year follow-up in the randomised Standardisation of Breast Radiotherapy (START) trials. *Lancet Oncol* 2010;11:231-40.
9   Andreyev J. Gastrointestinal symptoms after pelvic radiotherapy: a new understanding to improve management of symptomatic patients. *Lancet Oncol* 2007;8:1007-17.
10   Travis LB, Ng AK, Allan JM, Pui CH, Kennedy AR, Xu XG, et al. Second malignant neoplasms and cardiovascular disease following radiotherapy. *J Natl Cancer Inst* 2012;104:357-70.
11   Travis LB, Curtis RE, Storm H, Hall P, Holowaty E, Van Leeuwen FE, et al. Risk of second malignant neoplasms among long-term survivors of testicular cancer. *J Natl Cancer Inst* 1997;89:1429-39.
12   Berrington de Gonzalez A, Curtis RE, Gilbert E, Berg CD, Smith SA, Stovall M, et al. Second solid cancers after radiotherapy for breast cancer in SEER cancer registries. *Br J Cancer* 2010;102:220-6.
13   Swerdlow AJ, Cooke R, Bates A, Cunningham D, Falk SJ, Gilson D, et al. Breast cancer risk after supradiaphragmatic radiotherapy for Hodgkin's lymphoma in England and Wales: a national cohort study. *J Clin Oncol* 2012;30:2745-52.
14   Hancock SL, Tucker MA, Hoppe RT. Factors affecting late mortality from heart disease after treatment of Hodgkin's disease. *JAMA* 1993;270:1949-55.
15   Miller MC, Agrawal A. Hypothyroidism in postradiation head and neck cancer patients: incidence, complications, and management. *Curr Opin Otolaryngol Head Neck Surg* 2009;17:111-5.
16   Marks LB, Rose CM, Hayman JA, Williams TR. The need for physician leadership in creating a culture of safety. *Int J Radiat Oncol Biol Phys* 2011;79:1287-9.
17   Williams MV, Frew TL. How dangerous is radiotherapy? *Int J Radiat Oncol Biol Phys* 2011;79:1601.
18   Nutting CM, Morden JP, Harrington KJ, Urbano TG, Bhide SA, Clark C, et al. Parotid-sparing intensity modulated versus conventional radiotherapy in head and neck cancer (PARSPORT): a phase 3 multicentre randomised controlled trial. *Lancet Oncol* 2011;12:127-36.
19   Staffurth J. A review of the clinical evidence for intensity-modulated radiotherapy. *Clin Oncol (R Coll Radiol)* 2010;22:643-57.
20   Hall EJ, Wuu CS. Radiation-induced second cancers: the impact of 3D-CRT and IMRT. *Int J Radiat Oncol Biol Phys* 2003;56:83-8.
21   Ruben JD, Davis S, Evans C, Jones P, Gagliardi F, Haynes M, et al. The effect of intensity-modulated radiotherapy on radiation-induced second malignancies. *Int J Radiat Oncol Biol Phys* 2008;70:1530-6.
22   AlDuhaiby EZ, Breen S, Bissonnette JP, Sharpe M, Mayhew L, Tyldesley S, et al. A national survey of the availability of intensity-modulated radiation therapy and stereotactic radiosurgery in Canada. *Radiat Oncol* 2012;7:18.
23   Mayles WP, Cooper T, Mackay R, Staffurth J, Williams M. Progress with intensity-modulated radiotherapy implementation in the UK. *Clin Oncol (R Coll Radiol)* 2012;24:543-4.
24   Jefferies S, Taylor A, Reznek R. Results of a national survey of radiotherapy planning and delivery in the UK in 2007. *Clin Oncol (R Coll Radiol)* 2009;21:204-17.
25   Williams MV, Cooper T, Mackay R, Staffurth J, Routsis D, Burnet N. The implementation of intensity-modulated radiotherapy in the UK. *Clin Oncol (R Coll Radiol)* 2010;22:623-8.
26   Hummel S, Simpson EL, Hemingway P, Stevenson MD, Rees A. Intensity-modulated radiotherapy for the treatment of prostate cancer: a systematic review and economic evaluation. *Health Technol Assess* 2010;14:1-108, iii-iv.
27   Verellen D, De Ridder M, Linthout N, Tournel K, Soete G, Storme G. Innovations in image-guided radiotherapy. *Nat Rev Cancer* 2007;7:949-60.
28   Button MR, Staffurth JN. Clinical application of image-guided radiotherapy in bladder and prostate cancer. *Clin Oncol (R Coll Radiol)* 2010;22:698-706.
29   Short S, Tobias J. Radiosurgery for brain tumours. *BMJ* 2010;340:c3247.
30   Martin A, Gaya A. Stereotactic body radiotherapy: a review. *Clin Oncol (R Coll Radiol)* 2010;22:157-72.
31   Chi A, Liao Z, Nguyen NP, Xu J, Stea B, Komaki R. Systematic review of the patterns of failure following stereotactic body radiation therapy in early-stage non-small-cell lung cancer: clinical implications. *Radiother Oncol* 2010;94:1-11.
32   Schulz-Ertner D, Tsujii H. Particle radiation therapy using proton and heavier ion beams. *J Clin Oncol* 2007;25:953-64.
33   Allen AM, Pawlicki T, Dong L, Fourkal E, Buyyounouski M, Cengel K, et al. An evidence based review of proton beam therapy: the report of ASTRO's emerging technology committee. *Radiother Oncol* 2012;103:8-11.
34   Brodin NP, Vogelius IR, Maraldo MV, Munck Af Rosenschold P, Aznar MC, Kiil-Berthelsen A, et al. Life years lost-comparing potentially fatal

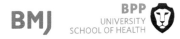

late complications after radiotherapy for pediatric medulloblastoma on a common scale. *Cancer*2012;118:5432-40.

35 DeLaney TF. Proton therapy in the clinic. *Front Radiat Ther Oncol*2011;43:465-85.

36 Maughan TS, Illidge TM, Hoskin P, McKenna WG, Brunner TB, Stratford IJ, et al. Radiotherapy research priorities for the UK. *Clin Oncol (R Coll Radiol)*2010;22:707-9.

37 Burnet NG, Billingham LJ, Chan CS, Hall E, Macdougall J, Mackay RI, et al; on behalf of the National Cancer Research Institute Clinical and Translational Radiotherapy Research Working Group Executive Group. Methodological considerations in the evaluation of radiotherapy technologies. *Clin Oncol (R Coll Radiol)*2012; published online 12 July.

Related links

bmj.com/archive
Previous articles in this series

- Generalized anxiety disorder: diagnosis and treatment (2012;345:e7500)
- Resistant hypertension (2012;345:e7473)
- Childhood constipation (2012;345:e7309)
- Preparing young travellers for low resource destinations (2012;345:e7179)
- Management of chronic rhinosinusitis (2012;345:e7054)

More titles in
The BMJ Clinical
Review Series

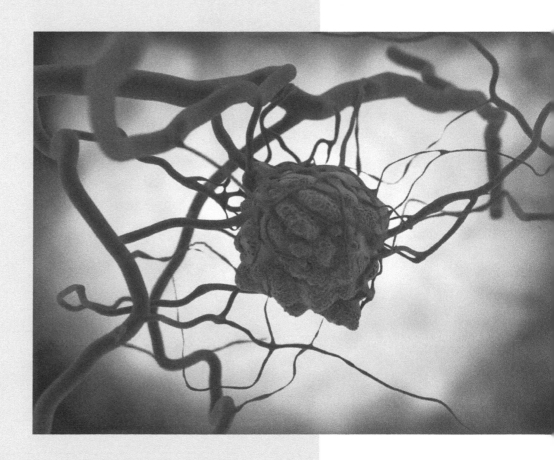

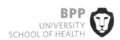
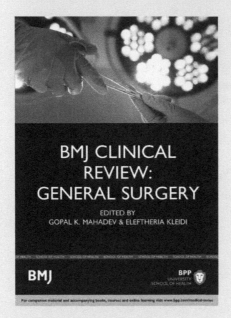
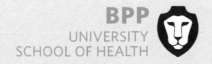

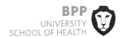

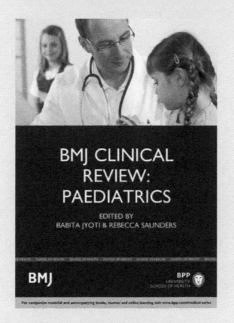
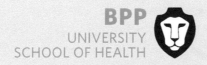

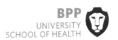

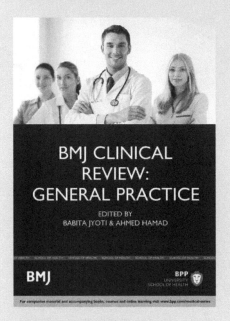
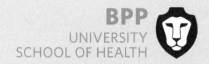

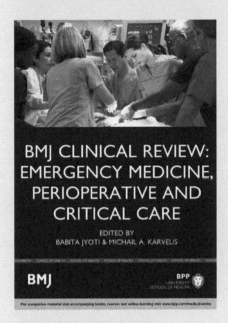
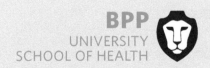

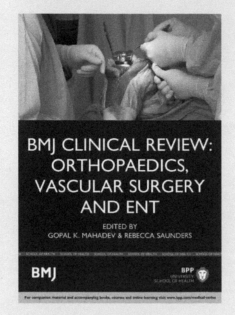
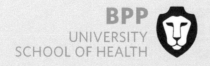

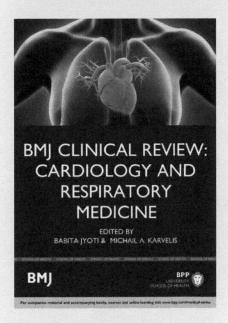
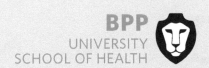

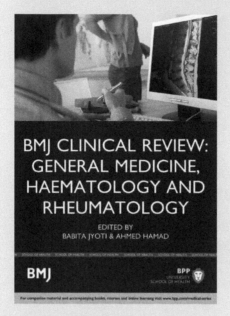
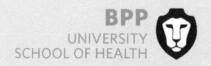

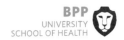
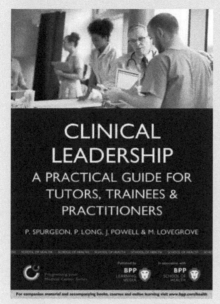
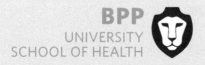

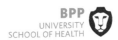
More titles in The Progressing your Medical Career Series

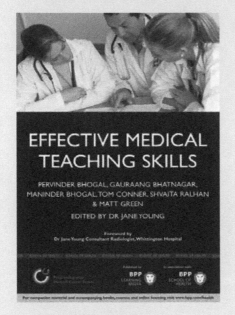

EFFECTIVE MEDICAL TEACHING SKILLS

PERVINDER BHOGAL, GAURAANG BHATNAGAR,
MANINDER BHOGAL, TOM CONNER, SHVAITA RALHAN
& MATT GREEN

EDITED BY DR JANE YOUNG

Foreword by
Dr Jane Young Consultant Radiologist, Whittington Hospital

£19.99

September 2011

Paperback

978-1-445379-56-2

We can all remember a teacher that inspired us, encouraged us and helped us to excel. But what is it that makes a good teacher and are these skills that can be learned and improved?

As doctors and healthcare professionals we are all expected to teach, to a greater or lesser degree, and this carries a great deal of responsibility. We are helping to develop the next generation and it is essential to pass on the knowledge that we have gained during our experience to date.

This book aims to cover the fundamentals of medical education. It has been designed to be a guide for the budding teacher with practical advice, hints, tips and essential points of reflection designed to encourage the reader to think about what they are doing at each step.

By taking the time to read through this book and completing the exercises contained within it you should:

- Understand the needs of the learner

- Understand the skills required to be an effective teacher

- Understanding the various different teaching scenarios, from lectures to problem based teaching, and how to use them effectively

- Understand the importance and sources of feedback

- Be aware of assessment techniques, appraisal and revalidation

This book aims to provide you with a foundation in medical education upon which you can build the skills and attributes to become a competent and skilled teacher.

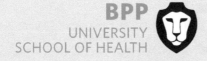

BPP
UNIVERSITY
SCHOOL OF HEALTH

www.bpp.com/medical-series

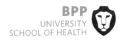

More titles in The Progressing your Medical Career Series

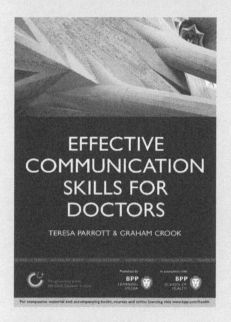

£19.99

September 2011

Paperback

978-1-445379-56-2

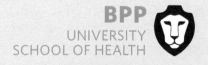

Would you like to know how to improve your communication skills? Are you looking for a clearly written book which explores all aspects of effective medical communication?

There is an urgent need to improve doctors' communication skills. Research has shown that poor communication can contribute to patient dissatisfaction, lack of compliance and increased medico-legal problems. Improved communication skills will impact positively on all of these areas.

The last fifteen years have seen unprecedented changes in medicine and the role of doctors. Effective communication skills are vital to these new roles. But communication is not just related to personality. Skills can be learned which can make your communication more effective, and help you to improve your relationships with patients, their families and fellow doctors.

This book shows how to learn those skills and outlines why we all need to communicate more effectively. Healthcare is increasingly a partnership. Change is happening at all levels, from government directives to patient expectations. Communication is a bridge between the wisdom of the past and the vision of the future.

Readers of this book can also gain free access to an online module which upon successful completion can download a certificate for their portfolio of learning/Revalidation/CPD records.

This easy-to-read guide will help medical students and doctors at all stages of their careers improve their communication within a hospital environment.

www.bpp.com/medical-series

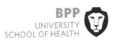

More titles in The Progressing your Medical Career Series

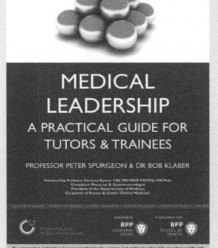

MEDICAL LEADERSHIP
A PRACTICAL GUIDE FOR TUTORS & TRAINEES

PROFESSOR PETER SPURGEON & DR BOB KLABER

£19.99
November 2011
Paperback
978-1-445379-57-9

Are you a doctor or medical student who wishes to acquire and develop your leadership and management skills? Do you recognise the role and influence of strong leadership and management in modern medicine?

Clinical leadership is something in which all doctors should have an important role in terms of driving forward high quality care for their patients. In this up-to-date guide Peter Spurgeon and Robert Klaber take you through the latest leadership and management thinking, and how this links in with the Medical Leadership Competency Framework. As well as influencing undergraduate curricula and some of the concepts underpinning revalidation, this framework forms the basis of the leadership component of the curricula for all medical specialties, so a practical knowledge of it is essential for all doctors in training.

Using case studies and practical exercises to provide a strong work-based emphasis, this practical guide will enable you to build on your existing experiences to develop your leadership and management skills, and to develop strategies and approaches to improving care for your patients.

This book addresses:

- Why strong leadership and management are crucial to delivering high quality care

- The theory and evidence behind the Medical Leadership Competency Framework

- The practical aspects of leadership learning in a wide range of clinical environments (eg handover, EM, ward etc)

- How Consultants and trainers can best facilitate leadership learning for their trainees and students within the clinical work-place

Whether you are a medical student just starting out on your career, or an established doctor wishing to develop yourself as a clinical leader, this practical, easy-to-use guide will give you the techniques and knowledge you require to excel.

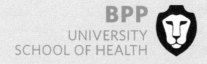

www.bpp.com/medical-series

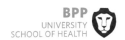

More titles in The MediPass Series

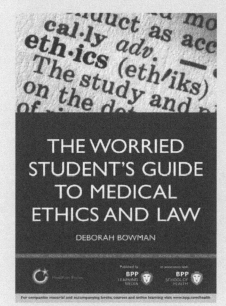

Are you confused about medical ethics and law? Are you looking for a definitive book that will explain clearly medical ethics and law?

This book offers a unique guide to medical ethics and law for applicants to medical school, current medical students at all stages of their training, those attending postgraduate ethics courses and clinicians involved in teaching. It will also prove a useful guide for any healthcare professional with an interest in medical ethics and law. This book provides comprehensive coverage of the core curriculum (as recently revised) and clear demonstration of how to pass examinations, both written and practical. The title also considers the ethical dilemmas that students can encounter during their training.

This easy to use guide sets out to provide:

- Comprehensive coverage of the recently revised core curriculum

- Consideration of the realities of medical student experiences and dilemmas with reference to recently published and new GMC guidance for medical students

- Practical guidance on applying ethics in the clinical years, how to approach all types of examinations and improve confidence regarding the moral aspects of medicine

- A single, portable volume that covers all stages of the medical student experience

In addition to the core curriculum, this book uniquely explains the special priveleges and responsibilities of being a healthcare professional and explores how professional behaviour guidance from the General Medical Council applies to students and medical professionals. The book is a single, accessible volume that will be invaluable to all those who want to thrive, not merely survive, studying and applying medical ethics day to day, whatever their stage of training.

£19.99

October 2011

Paperback

978-1-445379-49-4

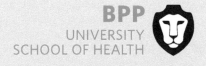

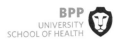
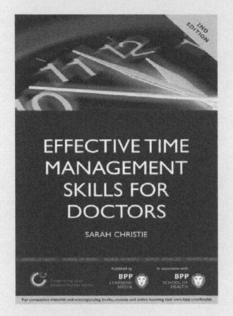
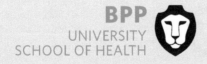

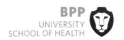
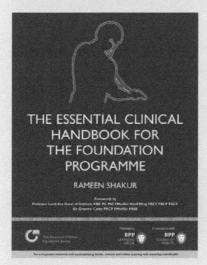
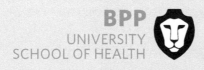

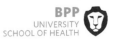

More titles in The Essential Clinical Handbook Series

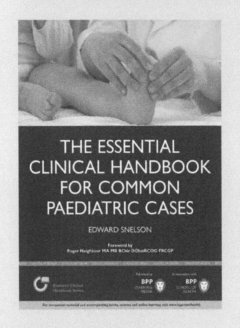

THE ESSENTIAL CLINICAL HANDBOOK FOR COMMON PAEDIATRIC CASES

EDWARD SNELSON

Foreword by
Roger Neighbour MA MB BChir DObstRCOG FRCGP

September 2011

Paperback

978-1-445379-60-9

Not sure what to do when faced with a crying baby and demanding parent on the ward? Would you like a definitive guide on how to manage commonly encountered paediatric cases?

This clear and concise clinical handbook has been written to help healthcare professionals approach the initial assessment and management of paediatric cases commonly encountered by Junior Doctors, GPs, GP Specialty Trainee's and allied healthcare professionals. The children who make paediatrics so fun, can also make it more than a little daunting for even the most confident person. This insightful guide has been written based on the author's extensive experience within both a General Practice and hospital setting.

Intended as a practical guide to common paediatric problems it will increase confidence and satisfaction in managing these conditions. Each chapter provides a clear structure for investigating potential paediatric illnesses including clinical and non-clinical advice covering: background, how to assess, pitfalls to avoid, FAQs and what to tell parents. This helpful guide provides :

- A problem/symptom based approach to common paediatric conditions

- As essential guide for any doctor assessing children on the front line

- Provides easy-to-follow and step-by-step guidance on how to approach different paediatric conditions

- Useful both as a textbook and a quick reference guide when needed on the ward

This engaging and easy to use guide will provide you with the knowledge, skills and confidence required to effectively diagnose and manage commonly encountered paediatric cases both within a primary and secondary care setting.

BPP
UNIVERSITY
SCHOOL OF HEALTH